Interstitial Lung Disease

Editors

JOSHUA J. SOLOMON
KEVIN K. BROWN

IMMUNOLOGY AND ALLERGY CLINICS OF NORTH AMERICA

https://www.immunology.theclinics.com/

May 2023 • Volume 43 • Number 2

ELSEVIER

1600 John F. Kennedy Boulevard • Suite 1800 • Philadelphia, Pennsylvania, 19103-2899

http://www.theclinics.com

IMMUNOLOGY AND ALLERGY CLINICS OF NORTH AMERICA Volume 43, Number 2

May 2023 ISSN 0889-8561, ISBN-13: 978-0-443-18181-8

Editor: Taylor Hayes

Developmental Editor: Jessica Cañaberal

Immunology and Allergy Clinics of North America (ISSN 0889–8561) is published quarterly by Elsevier Inc., 360 Park Avenue South, New York, NY 10010-1710. Months of issue are February, May, August, and November. Periodicals postage paid at New York, NY and additional mailing offices. Subscription prices are $365.00 per year for US individuals, $704.00 per year for US institutions, $100.00 per year for US students and residents, $445.00 per year for Canadian individuals, $100.00 per year for Canadian students, $895.00 per year for Canadian institutions, $470.00 per year for international individuals, $895.00 per year for international institutions, $220.00 per year for international students. To receive student/resident rate, orders must be accompanied by name of affiliated institution, date of term, and the *signature* of program/residency coordinator on institution letterhead. Orders will be billed at individual rate until proof of status is received. Foreign air speed delivery is included in all *Clinics* subscription prices. All prices are subject to change without notice. **POSTMASTER:** Send address changes to *Immunology and Allergy Clinics of North America,* Elsevier Health Sciences Division, Subscription Customer Service, 3251 Riverport Lane, Maryland Heights, MO 63043. **Customer Service: 1-800-654-2452 (U.S. and Canada); 314-447-8871 (outside U.S. and Canada). Fax: 314-447-8029. E-mail: journalscustomerservice-usa@elsevier.com (for print support); journalsonlinesupport-usa@elsevier.com (for online support).**

Reprints. For copies of 100 or more, of articles in this publication, please contact the Commercial Reprints Department, Elsevier Inc., 360 Park Avenue South, New York, New York 10010-1710. Tel. 212-633-3874, Fax: 212-633-3820, E-mail: reprints@elsevier.com.

Immunology and Allergy Clinics of North America is covered in MEDLINE/PubMed (Index Medicus), Current Contents/Life Sciences, Science Citation Index, ISI/BIOMED, Chemical Abstracts, and EMBASE/Excerpta Medica.

Contributors

EDITORS

JOSHUA J. SOLOMON, MD
Associate Professor of Medicine, National Jewish Health and University of Colorado School of Medicine, Director, Interstitial Lung Disease Program, Department of Medicine, National Jewish Health, Denver, Colorado, USA

KEVIN K. BROWN, MD
Chair, Department of Medicine, Professor of Medicine, National Jewish Health and University of Colorado School of Medicine, Denver, Colorado, USA

AUTHORS

AYODEJI ADEGUNSOYE, MD, MS
Assistant Professor of Medicine, Scientific Director, Interstitial Lung Disease Program, Section of Pulmonary/Critical Care, University of Chicago, Chicago, Illinois, USA

AMARILYS ALARCON-CALDERON, MD
Division of Pulmonary and Critical Care Medicine, Mayo Clinic College of Medicine and Science, Rochester, Minnesota, USA

HAYLEY BARNES, PhD, MPH, MBBS
Department of Respiratory Medicine, Alfred Hospital, Monash Centre for Occupational and Environmental Health, Monash University, Central Clinical School, Monash University, Melbourne, Australia

NICOL BERNARDINELLO, MD
Respiratory Disease Unit, Department of Cardiac, Thoracic, Vascular Sciences and Public Health, University of Padova, Padova, Italy

PHILIPPE CAMUS, MD
Professor Emeritus, Pulmonary and Intensive Care at Université de Bourgogne, Dijon, France

NAZIA CHAUDHURI, MD, PhD
University of Ulster Magee Campus, Londonderry, Northern Ireland, United Kingdom

CARLYNE D. COOL, MD
Clinical Professor, Department of Pathology, University of Colorado School of Medicine Anschutz Medical Campus, Aurora, Colorado, USA; Division of Pathology, Department of Medicine, National Jewish Health, Denver, Colorado, USA

VINCENT COTTIN, MD, PhD
Service de pneumologie, Hospices Civils de Lyon, Hôpital Louis Pradel, Centre de référence coordonnateur des maladies pulmonaires rares (OrphaLung), Université Lyon 1, INRAE, UMR754, Lyon, France

M. KRISTEN DEMORUELLE, MD, PhD
Associate Professor of Medicine, Division of Rheumatology, University of Colorado
School of Medicine, Aurora, Colorado, USA

GREGORY P. DOWNEY, MD, FRCPC
Professor, Departments of Medicine, Pediatrics and Immunology and Genomic Medicine,
National Jewish Health, Denver, Colorado, USA; Associate Dean and Professor,
Departments of Medicine and Immunology and Microbiology, University of Colorado
School of Medicine, Aurora, Colorado, USA

DAFFOLYN RACHAEL FELS ELLIOTT, MD, PhD, FRCPC
University of Kansas Medical Center, Kansas City, Kansas, USA

MICHAEL A. GIBBONS, PhD, FRCP
Professor, Academic Department of Respiratory Medicine, Royal Devon University
Healthcare NHS Foundation Trust, Department of Clinical and Biomedical Sciences,
University of Exeter Medical School, Exeter, United Kingdom

IAN GLASPOLE, PhD, MBBS
Department of Respiratory Medicine, Alfred Hospital, Central Clinical School, Monash
University, Melbourne, Australia

STEVE D. GROSHONG, MD
Chief of Pathology, Professor, Department of Medicine, National Jewish Health, Denver,
Colorado, USA

MARK J. HAMBLIN, MD, FCCP
University of Kansas Medical Center, Kansas City, Kansas, USA

KERRI-MARIE HEENAN, MB Bch, BAO
Department of Respiratory Medicine, Antrim Area Hospital, Northern Health and Social
Care Trust, Antrim, Northern Ireland, United Kingdom

ELLA A. KAZEROONI, MD, MS
Professor, Division of Pulmonary and Critical Care Medicine, Department of Internal
Medicine, Division of Cardiothoracic Radiology, Department of Radiology, University of
Michigan, Ann Arbor, Michigan, USA

NAMRATA KEWALRAMANI, MD
Department for BioMedical Research DBMR, Department of Pulmonary Medicine,
Inselspital, Bern University Hospital, University of Bern, Switzerland

DINESH KHANNA, MD, MS
Professor, Scleroderma Program, Division of Rheumatology, Department of Internal
Medicine, University of Michigan, Ann Arbor, Michigan, USA

MATTHEW KOSLOW, MD
Assistant Professor of Medicine, Division of Pulmonary, Critical Care, and Sleep
Medicine, Department of Medicine, Associate Co-Director of LAM and Rare Lung Disease
Clinic, National Jewish Health, Denver, Colorado, USA

DAVID A. LYNCH, MB
Professor, Department of Radiology, National Jewish Health, Denver, Colorado,
USA

SCOTT M. MATSON, MD
Assistant Professor of Medicine, Division of Pulmonary, Critical Care and Sleep Medicine, University of Kansas School of Medicine, Kansas City, Kansas, USA

DENISE MCKEEGAN, MB Bch, BAO, MSc
Department of Respiratory Medicine, Antrim Area Hospital, Northern Health and Social Care Trust, Antrim, Northern Ireland, United Kingdom

AYE MYAT NOE KHIN, MBBS
Academic Department of Respiratory Medicine, Royal Devon University Healthcare NHS Foundation Trust, Exeter, United Kingdom

NICOLE NG, MD, PharmD
Division of Pulmonary, Critical Care, and Sleep Medicine, Icahn School of Medicine at Mount Sinai Hospital, New York, New York, USA

JUSTIN OLDHAM, MD, MS
Associate Professor, Division of Pulmonary and Critical Care Medicine, Department of Internal Medicine, Department of Epidemiology, University of Michigan, Ann Arbor, Michigan, USA

MARIA L. PADILLA, MD
Professor of Medicine, Division of Pulmonary, Critical Care, and Sleep Medicine, Icahn School of Medicine at Mount Sinai Hospital, New York, New York, USA

AARTI P. PANDYA, MD
Children's Mercy Hospital, Kansas City, Missouri, USA

SAHIL M. PANDYA, MD, FCCP
University of Kansas Medical Center, Kansas City, Kansas, USA

JANELLE VU PUGASHETTI, MD, MS
Clinical Instructor, Division of Pulmonary and Critical Care Medicine, Department of Internal Medicine, University of Michigan, Ann Arbor, Michigan, USA

JAY H. RYU, MD
Dr. David E. and Bette H. Dines Professor of Pulmonary Medicine, Division of Pulmonary and Critical Care Medicine, Mayo Clinic College of Medicine and Science, Rochester, Minnesota, USA

PAOLO SPAGNOLO, MD, PhD
Respiratory Disease Unit, Department of Cardiac, Thoracic, Vascular Sciences and Public Health, University of Padova, Padova, Italy

MATTHEW STEWARD, BMBS, MRCP
Academic Department of Respiratory Medicine, Royal Devon University Healthcare NHS Foundation Trust, Department of Clinical and Biomedical Sciences, University of Exeter Medical School, Exeter, United Kingdom

RACHEL STRYKOWSKI, MD
Fellow, Section of Pulmonary/Critical Care, University of Chicago, Chicago, Illinois, USA

HANNAH THOULD, BA, BMBCh, MRCP
Academic Department of Respiratory Medicine, Royal Devon University Healthcare NHS
Foundation Trust, Exeter, United Kingdom

ROBERT VASSALLO, MD
Professor of Medicine, Division of Pulmonary and Critical Care Medicine, Mayo Clinic
College of Medicine and Science, Rochester, Minnesota, USA

EUNHEE S. YI, MD
Professor of Pathology, Department of Laboratory Medicine and Pathology, Mayo Clinic
College of Medicine and Science, Rochester, Minnesota, USA

Contents

Idiopathic pulmonary fibrosis (IPF), a common interstitial lung disease (ILD), is a chronic, progressive fibrosing interstitial pneumonia, with an unknown cause. IPF has been linked to several genetic and environmental risk factors. Disease progression is common and associated with worse outcomes. Management often encompasses pharmacotherapy, supportive interventions, addressing comorbidities when present, and treating hypoxia with ambulatory O2. Consideration for antifibrotic therapy and lung transplantation evaluation should occur early. Patients with ILD other than IPF, and who have radiological evidence of pulmonary fibrosis, may have progressive pulmonary fibrosis.

Connective tissue disease associated interstitial lung disease (CTD-ILD) is a heterogenous collection of conditions with a diverse spectrum of interstitial lung disease (ILD) manifestations. Currently, clinical practice of lung-directed immunosuppression in CTD-ILD is supported by several randomized, placebo-controlled trials (RCTs) in patients with scleroderma and several observational, retrospective studies in other autoimmune conditions. However, given the harm of immunosuppression in idiopathic pulmonary fibrosis, there is an urgent need for RCTs of immunosuppression and antifibrotic agents in fibrotic CTD-ILD populations as well as the study of intervention in patients with subclinical CTD-ILD.

Hypersensitivity pneumonitis (HP) is a heterogenous disease entity characterized by an aberrant immune response to inhalational antigens. Disease modification hinges on early antigen remediation with a goal to attenuate immune dysregulation. Disease severity and progression are mediated by an interface between degree, type and chronicity of exposure, genetic predisposition, and biochemical properties of the inducing agent. Guidelines have provided a standardized approach; however, decision-making remains with many clinical dilemmas. The delineation of fibrotic and nonfibrotic HP is crucial to identify the differences in clinical trajectories, and further clinical trials are needed to understand optimal therapeutic strategies.

Sarcoidosis is a disease of unknown cause characterized by granulomatous inflammation. Although the lung is almost universally involved, any organ can be affected. Complex pathogenesis and protean clinical manifestations are additional features of the disease. The diagnosis is one of exclusion, although the presence of noncaseating granulomas at disease sites is a prerequisite in most cases. The management of sarcoidosis requires a multidisciplinary approach, particularly when the heart, the brain, or the eyes are involved. The paucity of effective therapies and the lack of reliable predictors of disease behavior greatly contribute to making sarcoidosis a challenging disease to manage.

Smoking-related interstitial lung diseases (ILDs) are a group of heterogeneous, diffuse pulmonary parenchymal disease processes associated with tobacco exposure. These disorders include pulmonary Langerhans cell histiocytosis, respiratory bronchiolitis-associated ILD, desquamative interstitial pneumonia, acute eosinophilic pneumonia, and combined pulmonary fibrosis and emphysema. This review summarizes the current evidence of pathogenesis, clinical manifestations, diagnostic approach, prognosis, and treatment modalities for these diseases. We also discuss the interstitial lung abnormalities incidentally detected in radiologic studies and smoking-related fibrosis identified on lung biopsies.

The eosinophilic lung diseases may manifest as chronic eosinophilic pneumonia, acute eosinophilic pneumonia, or as the Löffler syndrome. The diagnosis is made when both characteristic clinical-imaging features and alveolar eosinophilia are present. Peripheral blood eosinophils are generally markedly elevated. Lung biopsy is not indicated. The inquiry to possible causes (medications, toxic drugs, exposures, and infections especially parasitic) must be meticulous. Extrathoracic manifestations raise the suspicion of a systemic disease especially eosinophilic granulomatosis with polyangiitis. Airflow obstruction is frequent. Corticosteroids are the cornerstone of therapy, but relapses are common. Therapies targeting the interleukin 5 pathway are increasingly used.

Occupational exposures are directly causal or partially contributory to the development of interstitial lung diseases. A detailed occupational history, relevant high-resolution computed tomography findings, and where relevant additional histopathology, are required to make a diagnosis. Treatment options are limited, and further exposure avoidance is likely to reduce disease progression.

> Drug-induced interstitial lung disease (DI-ILD) is an increasingly common cause of morbidity and mortality as the list of culprit drugs continues to grow. Unfortunately, DI-ILD is difficult to study, diagnose, prove, and manage. This article attempts to raise awareness of the challenges in DI-ILD and discusses the current clinical landscape.

> Cysts and cavities in the lung are commonly encountered on chest imaging. It is necessary to distinguish thin-walled lung cysts ($\leq$2 mm) from cavities and characterize their distribution as focal or multifocal versus diffuse. Focal cavitary lesions are often caused by inflammatory, infectious, or neoplastic processes in contrast to diffuse cystic lung diseases. An algorithmic approach to diffuse cystic lung disease can help narrow the differential diagnosis, and additional testing such as skin biopsy, serum biomarkers, and genetic testing can be confirmatory. An accurate diagnosis is essential for the management and disease surveillance of extrapulmonary complications.

> Interstitial lung disease is a common complication of anti-neutrophil cytoplasmic antibody-associated vasculitis (AAV). It is seen most commonly in microscopic polyangiitis owing to the pathogenic effect of myeloperoxidase in the lung. Oxidative stress, neutrophil elastase release, and expression of inflammatory proteins by neutrophil extracellular traps result in fibroblast proliferation and differentiation and therefore fibrosis. Usual interstitial pneumonia pattern fibrosis. Treatment for patients with AAV and interstitial lung disease lacks evidence, and those with vasculitis are treated with immunosuppression, whereas those with progressive fibrosis may well benefit from antifibrotic therapy.

> The proportion of symptomatic patients with post-coronavirus 2019 (COVID-19) condition (long COVID) represents a significant burden on the individual as well as on the health care systems. A greater understanding of the natural evolution of symptoms over a longer period and the impacts of interventions will improve our understanding of the long-term impacts of the COVID-19 disease. This review will discuss the emerging evidence for the development of post-COVID interstitial lung disease focusing on the pathophysiological mechanisms, incidence, diagnosis, and impact of this potentially new and emerging respiratory disease.

Interstitial lung disease (ILD) complicates connective tissue disease (CTD) with variable incidence and is a leading cause of death in these patients. To improve CTD-ILD outcomes, early recognition and management of ILD is critical. Blood-based and radiologic biomarkers that assist in the diagnosis CTD-ILD have long been studied. Recent studies, including -omic investigations, have also begun to identify biomarkers that may help prognosticate such patients. This review provides an overview of clinically relevant biomarkers in patients with CTD-ILD, highlighting recent advances to assist in the diagnosis and prognostication of CTD-ILD.

IMMUNOLOGY AND ALLERGY CLINICS OF NORTH AMERICA

SERIES OF RELATED INTEREST

Medical Clinics
https://www.medical.theclinics.com/

THE CLINICS ARE AVAILABLE ONLINE!
Access your subscription at:
www.theclinics.com

Preface

Interstitial Lung Disease: 150 Years of Progress

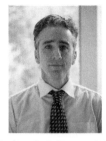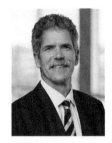

Joshua J. Solomon, MD   Kevin K. Brown, MD
Editors

In 1873, von Buhl published one of the earliest histologic descriptions of interstitial lung disease (ILD) in *Tuberkulose und Schwindsucht*.[1] He described a disorder pathologically characterized by "degeneration and desquamation of alveolar and bronchiolar epithelium" likely caused by tuberculosis or syphilis and coined the term "chronic interstitial pneumonia." The first histologic description of what today we call idiopathic pulmonary fibrosis (IPF) was published in 1897 by Rindfleisch, calling the new entity "Cirrhosis Cystica Pulmonum.[2]" In 1912, von Hansemann described cases of organizing pneumonia secondary to tuberculosis and suggested the term "Lymphangitis Reticularis Pulmonum.[3]" In the early 1930s, Hamman and Rich described a rapidly progressive ILD that they called "Acute Diffuse Interstitial Fibrosis of the Lungs," later colloquially termed "Hamman-Rich Syndrome.[4]" This description was an early step toward the recognition of IPF as a distinct clinical entity with a high mortality. Dr Averill Liebow was the first to recognize the distinct pathologic pattern of fibrosis in IPF, using the term "Usual Interstitial Pneumonia" to reflect that this was the most common pattern of fibrosis seen in his practice. In the mid-1960s, Liebow and Carrington extended these findings by describing and naming five common histopathologic patterns of ILD and argued that the pattern suggested cause.[5] These observations set the stage for the first international consensus on ILD, summarized by the 2000 American Thoracic Society and European Respiratory Society statement on the diagnosis and treatment of IPF.

These humble beginnings have prepared us for our current era of understanding, ushered in by advances in omics (genomics, epigenomics, transcriptomics, proteomics, and metabolomics), and a rapidly expanding era of drug development. The first effective medications for IPF were approved in 2014, and we now have over 20 promising drugs in phase 2 or 3 trials.

As we have made progress, in this issue of *Immunology and Allergy Clinics of North America* on "Interstitial Lung Disease," we summarize our current understanding of

Immunol Allergy Clin N Am 43 (2023) xiii–xv
https://doi.org/10.1016/j.iac.2023.03.001
0889-8561/23/© 2023 Published by Elsevier Inc.

immunology.theclinics.com

both the common and the uncommon disorders. Drs Strykowski and Adegunsoye update us on the most common and lethal of the ILDs, IPF. In addition, they review progressive pulmonary fibrosis, a new concept that groups together ILDs based on shared pathologic features, longitudinal behavior, and a poor prognosis. Drs Matson and Demoruelle help us navigate the ever-growing field of connective tissue disease–associated ILD (CTD-ILD) with a review of both the clinical features and the potential pathogenic pathways. Dr Pandya and her colleagues skillfully outline the complexities of the diagnosis and management of hypersensitivity pneumonitis (HP), a heterogenous disease that can mimic others and one where management involves more than just pharmacotherapy. In the words of Drs Spagnolo and Nicol Bernardinello, sarcoidosis remains a diagnostic challenge by virtue of its "complex multidimensional nature…coupled with its wide range of clinical manifestations," and their review helps us navigate the diagnosis and management of the multiorgan system involvement. The spectrum of smoking-related ILDs is nicely reviewed by Dr Alarcon-Calderon and colleagues, and Dr Cottin provides us with a thorough review of the wide range of pulmonary diseases associated with eosinophils. Drs Glaspole and Barnes' review on occupational lung disease reminds us that occupational exposures can cause primary disease as well as contribute to the development of more common forms of ILD, such as HP and CTD-ILD. Dr Ng and colleagues ask us to consider drug-induced lung disease in our differential diagnoses and that this diagnosis is fraught with challenges. The next two articles cover less-common ILDs; Dr Koslow and colleagues cover the range of rare cystic lung diseases and provide us with an algorithmic approach to their diagnosis. ILD associated with anti-neutrophil cytoplasm antibody (ANCA) vasculitis is a challenge both diagnostically and therapeutically; Dr Stewards and colleagues review our current understanding of this rare but serious ILD. The recent pandemic has provided us with a potentially new disorder to add to our list—COVID-induced ILD. Dr Kewalrammani and colleagues take us through this developing body of literature. In our final article, Dr Pugashetti and colleagues provide us with a thorough review of the ever-growing list of biomarkers in the world of CTD-ILD.

We recognize the outstanding combined efforts of these authors and trust that this issue of *Immunology and Allergy Clinics of North America* will give you an appreciation of the breadth and complexity of ILD; insight into their clinical presentations, diagnostic pathways, and management; as well as a glimpse into the future.

Joshua J. Solomon, MD
Department of Medicine
National Jewish Health
University of Colorado School of Medicine
1400 Jackson Street
Denver, CO 80206, USA

Kevin K. Brown, MD
Department of Medicine
National Jewish Health
University of Colorado School of Medicine
1400 Jackson Street
Denver, CO 80206, USA

E-mail addresses:
solomonj@njhealth.org (J.J. Solomon)
brownk@njhealth.org (K.K. Brown)

REFERENCES

1. Buhl L. Lungenentzündung, Tuberkulose und Schwindsucht: zwö lf Briefe an einen Freund. Oldenbourg: Bayrische Staatsbibliothek München; 1873.
2. Rindfleisch G. Ueber cirrhosis cystica pulmonum. Zentralbl Pathol 1897;8:864–5.
3. Von Hansemann D. Die Lymphangitis reticularis der Lungen als selbstandige Erkrankung. Vilrhows Arch [Pathol Anaq 1912;220:311–21.
4. Hamman L, Rich AR. Fulminating diffuse interstitial fibrosis of the lungs. Trans Am Clin Climatol Assoc 1935;51:154–63.
5. Liebow AA, Carrington CB. The interstitial pneumonias, frontiers of pulmonary radiology. New York: Grune and Stratton; 1969.

Idiopathic Pulmonary Fibrosis and Progressive Pulmonary Fibrosis

Rachel Strykowski, MD[a], Ayodeji Adegunsoye, MD, MS[b],*

KEYWORDS

- Idiopathic pulmonary fibrosis • Progressive pulmonary fibrosis
- Interstitial lung disease • Diffuse parenchymal lung disease

KEY POINTS

- When diagnosing idiopathic pulmonary fibrosis (IPF), it is important to consider the demographic features of the patient, the physical examination, computed tomography (CT) chest results, and laboratory data.
- If a patient has a high pretest probability for IPF, chest CT is usually sufficient for the diagnosis without the need for a bronchoscopy or surgical biopsy.
- Disease progression should be tracked by clinical symptoms and pulmonary function testing, particularly forced vital capacity and diffusing capacity of the lungs for carbon monoxide values, and can guide when to start antifibrotic therapy.
- There is a formal definition of non-IPF progressive pulmonary fibrosis that incorporates symptoms, lung function data, and imaging changes.
- Treatment of IPF and progressive pulmonary fibrosis may involve nintedanib or pirfenidone and should follow a shared and informed decision-making process with the patient.

IDIOPATHIC PULMONARY FIBROSIS
Introduction

Interstitial lung diseases (ILDs) are a heterogeneous group of disorders that are classified together because of similar clinical, physiologic, radiographic, and pathologic manifestations.[1] ILDs are characterized by cellular proliferation, interstitial inflammation, and fibrosis within the wall of the alveolus, with findings not attributed to cancer or infection.[2] There are more than 200 types of known ILDs,[3] with interstitial fibrosis often predominating as a frequent phenotype. Among these, a large majority will receive a diagnosis of fibrotic hypersensitivity pneumonitis (sometimes attributable to an identified exposure), pulmonary sarcoidosis (granulomas as cause of fibrosis),

[a] Section of Pulmonary and Critical Care, Department at University of Chicago, 5841 South Maryland Avenue, MC 6076, Chicago, IL 60637, USA; [b] Interstitial Lung Disease Program, Section of Pulmonary/Critical Care, University of Chicago, Chicago, IL, USA
* Corresponding author.
E-mail address: deji@uchicago.edu

Immunol Allergy Clin N Am 43 (2023) 209–228
https://doi.org/10.1016/j.iac.2023.01.010
0889-8561/23/© 2023 Elsevier Inc. All rights reserved.

connective tissue disease [CTD-ILD] related interstitial lung disease (autoimmune related), or idiopathic interstitial pneumonia (IIP, cause unknown).[2] Idiopathic pulmonary fibrosis (IPF) is the most common subtype among the different IIPs.[4] IPF is a specific form of chronic, progressive fibrosing interstitial pneumonia, with an unknown cause, and is limited to the lungs.[5] This book chapter explores the clinical manifestations, pathogenesis, treatment, and outcomes in IPF.

Clinical Manifestations and Diagnosis of Idiopathic Pulmonary Fibrosis

Epidemiology

The exact prevalence and incidence of IPF vary and depend on methodology as well as demographics of the geographic population from which the data are being collected. Both prevalence and incidence increase with age, and it is known that IPF most commonly occurs in the sixth and seventh decades of life. It is rare in patients younger than 50 years. Further, both the prevalence and incidence are higher in men compared with women.[5,6] Thus, the pretest probability of the disease can increase by using basic data such as age greater than 60 years and male sex.[7,8] In a recent systematic review,[9] the prevalence of IPF was 0.5 to 27.9/100,000 and the incidence ranged from 0.22 to 8.8/100,000.[10] US population estimates of IPF incidence ranged between 7 and 16/100,000. Comparatively, the Medicare population between 2000-2011 had an IPF yearly incidence of 93.7 cases per 100,000 person years.[11] In Europe, IPF prevalence ranges from 1.25 to 23.4 cases per 100,000 in the population and incidence of 0.22 to 7.9 cases per 100,000 population.[12] In a worldwide systematic review, the overall incidence of IPF is increasing, with conservative estimates revealing an incidence range from 3 to 9 per 100,000 per year for Europe and North America.[13]

The role that race/ethnicity plays in IPF diagnosis is less clear given variation in the pretest probabilities across demographic groups and geographic locations. One large study[14] evaluating IPF diagnoses among decedents in a national database found that Black patients are significantly less likely than White and Hispanic patients to be diagnosed with IPF at time of death, but among those Black patients diagnosed with IPF, death occurs at a younger age. Further Hispanic patients are more likely than White patients to have IPF present at time of death.[14] A more recent multicenter cohort study demonstrated that ILD diagnoses and death occurred at a much younger age among Black patients with diverse forms of fibrotic ILD.[15]

Pathogenesis and genetic predisposition

The pathogenesis of IPF is complex and likely related to cycles of epithelial cell injury and, subsequent, dysregulation in repair.[8] One prevailing theory proposes that IPF results from abnormal fibroblasts and epithelial cell function, along with abnormal epithelial-mesenchymal interactions with little to no inflammatory component.[16] This notion has been supported histologically with findings of fibroblastic foci directly beneath areas of damaged epithelium without the presence of inflammatory cells.[17] Initiation and progression of this fibrosis may depend on genetic factors, environmental triggers, an imbalance between oxidants and antioxidants, and an imbalance of certain cytokines.[18,19]

Although most cases of IPF are thought to be sporadic, familial cases have been described. Familial pulmonary fibrosis, Hermansky-Pudlak syndrome (HPS), and short telomere syndromes typically present at a younger age than IPF. Further, although a large number of genetic polymorphisms have been reported, few are well established.[5,20] Familial pulmonary fibrosis (FPF) is diagnosed when at least 2 relatives within the same family develop pulmonary fibrosis and seems to follow an autosomal dominant pattern.[21] A number of genetic factors have been attributed to FPF; some notable genes include surfactant-associated proteins A (*SFTPA2*),[22] surfactant protein C (*SFTPC*),[23] and mucin 5B (*MUC5B*).[24] HPS is an autosomal recessive disorder characterized by oculocutaneous albinism and platelet abnormalities, which is a rare cause of usual interstitial pneumonia (UIP) often presenting at an earlier age.[25] Lastly, short telomere syndromes are caused by mutations in genes responsible for maintaining telomere length (eg, *TERT, TERC, PARN, DK1, TINF2, RTEL1*).[26] The disorder is characterized by severely short telomeres (often less than the first percentile for age and frequently less than the tenth percentile) along with dysfunction of one or more target organs. Short telomeres have been identified in about 25% of sporadic IPF and about 15% of families with FPF.[27]

Risk factors

Cigarette smoking has been identified as a potential risk factor for development of IPF with an odds ratio (OR) ranging from 1.6 to 2.9 for developing IPF in ever-smokers.[28,29] This relationship seems to be dose dependent, in that the odds of developing IPF increase with the number of pack-years smoked.[29] Further, chronic aspiration due to gastroesophageal reflux has been implicated in the development of pulmonary fibrosis; however, the direct relationship and degree to which chronic aspiration drives the pathogenesis of IPF remains unclear.[30] Environmental and occupational exposures to stone, metal, wood, and organic dusts has also been suggested as a risk factor.[31,32] Many viruses have been linked to the pathogenesis of IPF, but there is no clear evidence for a viral cause of the disease.[33] Hereditary factors may also contribute to IPF.

Clinical characteristics and diagnosis

History and physical examination. A common clinical presentation for IPF is dyspnea, which is usually progressive, debilitating, and persistent for greater than 6 months in an older adult. Dry cough, unrelieved with antitussives is also common. On physical examination crackles are detected on chest auscultation in more than 80% of patients.[5,8,34] These are often "dry," occur at end-inspiration, and have a "velcro" quality. Rales can also be heard, particularly with disease progression. Clubbing is present in up to half of all patients. Evidence of right-sided heart failure including an accentuated second pulmonic sound, right ventricular heave, and peripheral edema may be seen in the late stage of the disease and associated with cor pulmonale.

Laboratory and serologic tests. There are no laboratory tests to make the diagnosis of IPF, so the role of laboratory testing in patients with newly discovered ILD is to identify or exclude a cause for the disease.[5] These laboratory tests are usually looking for subclinical rheumatologic disease or hypersensitivity pneumonitis. They should, however, be interpreted cautiously, as an antinuclear antibody greater than or equal to 1:40 is present in 17% to 25% of patients with IPF and a positive rheumatoid factor is present in up to 18% of patients with IPF.[35]

Chest imaging. Most patients with IPF have an abnormal chest radiograph at the time of presentation.[36] Peripheral reticular opacities, most profuse at the lung bases, are typical findings on chest radiograph. The opacities are usually bilateral, often asymmetric, and associated with volume loss.[37]

High-resolution computed tomography scanning (HRCT) is the imaging modality of choice for diagnosing IPF and has changed the diagnostic evaluation by allowing for earlier diagnosis of IPF.[37–39] In a trained reviewer, the accuracy of a confident diagnosis of UIP made on HRCT is about 90%.[8,40] The common radiologic findings of IPF on HRCT are patchy, predominantly peripheral, subpleural, and bibasilar reticular abnormalities.[5] There may be a variable, although usually limited, extent of ground-glass opacities (GGOs), and findings of extensive GGOs should prompt alternative diagnoses.[8] In areas of severe involvement there can be traction bronchiectasis and/or subpleural honeycombing.[5]

Pulmonary function testing. Complete pulmonary function testing (PFT with spirometry, lung volumes, diffusing capacity for carbon monoxide [DLCO]) is performed on all patients with suspected IPF.[41] PFTs often occur in conjunction with resting and ambulatory oxygen saturations as well and are done at baseline and at regular intervals to assess the degree of lung involvement and track disease progression. Commonly, IPF presents with a restrictive pattern on PFTs (often a reduced total lung capacity, reduced forced vital capacity [FVC]), a reduced DLCO, and oxygen desaturation or a decrease in 6-minunte walk distance with time and as the disease progresses.[41]

Flexible bronchoscopy. Although invaluable in many other pulmonary diseases, a bronchoalveolar lavage (BAL) has a limited role in evaluating a patient with an HRCT that is suggestive of UIP and is not guideline recommended[34]; this is because there are broad and overlapping range of cell counts that can be seen, none of which are sensitive or specific for IPF. However, when the clinical impression is consistent with IPF but the HRCT pattern is probable UIP or indeterminate then a cellular analysis may be helpful to exclude alternative diagnoses.

Transbronchial lung biopsy and transbronchial cryobiopsy. Transbronchial lung biopsy (TBLB) is a procedure that uses forceps to obtain transbronchial samples that are a few millimeters in size and can be helpful in some ILD diagnoses but often obtains a sample that is too small to definitively diagnose IPF.[41,42] Approximately one-third of TBLB done for new ILD of unknown cause will provide a clear diagnosis, with two-thirds requiring a subsequent lung biopsy.[43] Transbronchial cryobiopsy (TCBC) is a promising technique that is less invasive than a surgical lung biopsy (SLB) and can obtain biopsy samples that are better in size and quality compared with TBLB. Although some evidence suggests that the utility and safety of TBCB for diagnosing ILD in the context of a multidisciplinary discussion (MDD) is similar to that of an SLB, the role it plays in the diagnostic algorithm of ILD remains unestablished.[44,45]

Surgical lung biopsy. SLB remains the gold standard for obtaining histopathologic confirmation of a patient suspected of having IPF. The decision to perform an SLB requires assessing the benefits of making a definitive diagnosis relative to the surgical risks and should be done in the context of an MDD, ideally involving a pulmonologist, radiologist, pathologist, and rheumatologist with expertise in ILD. Per ATS/ERS/JRS/ALAT guidelines an SLB should be considered in a patient with newly detected ILD of uncertain cause and an HRCT pattern of probable UIP, indeterminate UIP, or an alternate diagnosis where the benefits of surgical lung biopsy outweigh the risk, unless the patient has significant hypoxia or medical comorbidities. However, in patients with newly detected ILD without a known cause, but with an HRCT pattern consistent with UIP, a lung biopsy will be unlikely to change management or diagnosis and is not worth the risk. SLB, whether done via a video-assisted thoracoscopic approach or a thoracotomy, leads to a definitive diagnosis (in conjunction with clinical assessment and HRCT) in 89% of patients.[34]

Diagnosis. The diagnosis of IPF is based on an algorithm that is highly reliant on HRCT scans and pathology data, if available, after exclusion of other known causes of ILD (eg, domestic and occupational exposures, CTD, and drug toxicity).[41] The features on HRCT (**Table 1**) and histology patterns from lung biopsies (**Table 2**) can help diagnose IPF based on how similar the findings are to UIP. An algorithmic approach using these 2 diagnostic modalities (**Table 3**) can help determine how likely the diagnosis of IPF is.[8,41] Performance of an MDD is increasingly recommended for diagnosis ascertainment and crafting an optimal plan of management.[41]

Treatment

Nonpharmacotherapeutic and supportive care. The most important aspects of supportive care in IPF includes supplemental oxygen, education (including smoking cessation), pulmonary rehabilitation, management of comorbidities, and vaccinations. A large fraction of patients with IPF will require supplemental oxygen for symptoms and to prevent or delay the onset of secondary pulmonary hypertension due to hypoxemia. Improved education about the disease regarding diagnosis and management is an important component to patient's experience, and often this will include end-of-life discussions, particularly the avoidance of mechanical ventilation.[46] Pulmonary rehabilitation in ILD has resulted in a significant reduction in dyspnea and improvement in 6-minute walk distance.[47,48] Avoidance of pulmonary infections, and vaccinations against respiratory infections including *Streptococcus pneumoniae*, Influenza, *Bordetella pertussis*, and COVID-19, are also an important piece of care.[49,50] Lastly, prompt treatment of respiratory infections, including treatment of COVID-19 and preexposure prophylaxis for COVID-19 are also invaluable.[51]

Pharmacotherapy

Treatment available and target population There are 2 antifibrotic medications available to slow disease progression and reduce the frequency of exacerbations: nintedanib and pirfenidone.[5,52–54] In addition to slowing disease progression, these medications have also been shown to decrease the risk of all-cause mortality (pooled risk ratio [RR] 0.55, 95% confidence interval [CI] 0.45–0.66) and decrease risk of acute exacerbations of IPF (RR 0.63, 95% 0.53–0.76).[55] Between the 2 medications there is no clear agent of choice, but patient preference regarding side-effect profiles should be discussed (see further side-effect profiles in the following section).

In patients with mild-to-moderate disease with IPF without underlying liver disease the recommendation is to treat.[5] Further, in patients with more advanced IPF (FVC < 50% predicted and/or DLCO < 25% predicted) the recommendation is also to treat. Although those with advanced disease were not included in most major trials, studies suggest that both agents slow disease progression even at advanced stages.[56,57]

Nintedanib Nintedanib is a receptor antagonist for multiple tyrosine kinases that mediate the elaboration of fibrogenic growth factors and slows the rate of progression in IPF.[58,59] Based on clinical trials the efficacy of nintedanib is mostly due to a reduction in the rate of decline in lung function (particularly FVC) and a longer time to the first exacerbation of IPF.[56,59,60] The typical dose of nintedanib is 150 mg administered orally twice daily. Liver function testing (LFTs) should be assessed before initiation, and the medication should be avoided in patients with moderate or severe hepatic impairment (Child-Pugh B or C). After starting nintedanib, LFTs should be repeated monthly for 3 months and every 3 months thereafter. A pregnancy test should also be done and conception avoided until at least 3 months after last dose.

Most frequent adverse effects associated with nintedanib include diarrhea (62%), nausea (24%), vomiting (12%), and transaminitis (14%).[60] Diarrhea should be treated with hydration and antidiarrheal medications along with a potential dose reduction to 100 mg twice daily. Although clinical trials revealed that diarrhea leads to a dose reduction in 11% of patients and to discontinuation in 5%, observational/real world

Table 1
High-resolution computed tomography patterns in idiopathic pulmonary fibrosis

		HRCT Pattern		
	UIP Pattern	**Probable UIP Pattern**	**Indeterminate for UIP**	**CT Findings Suggestive of an Alternative Diagnosis**
Level of confidence for UIP histology	Confident (>90%)	Provisional high confidence (70%–89%)	Provisional low confidence (51%–69%)	Low to very low confidence (<50%)
Distribution	• Subpleural and basal predominant • Often heterogeneous (areas of normal lung interspersed with fibrosis) • May be asymmetric	• Subpleural and basal predominant • Often heterogeneous (areas of normal lung interspersed with reticulation and traction bronchiectasis/ bronchiolectasis)	• Diffuse distribution without subpleural predominance	• Peribronchovascular predominant with subpleural sparing (consider NSIP) • Perilymphatic distribution (consider sarcoidosis) • Upper or mid lung (consider fibrotic HP,CTD-LID, and sarcoidosis) • Subpleural sparing (consider NSIP or smoking related IP)

CT features	• Honeycombing with or without traction bronchiectasis/ bronchiolectasis
	• Presence of irregular thickening of interlobular septa
	• Usually superimposed with a reticular pattern, mild GGO
	• May have pulmonary ossification
		• Reticular pattern with traction bronchiectasis/ bronchiolectasis
		• May have mild GGO
		• Absence of subpleural sparing
			• CT features of lung fibrosis that do not suggest any specific etiology	• Lung findings
				  ○ Cysts (consider LAM,PLCH,LIP andDIP)
				  ○ Mosaic attenuation or three-density sign (consider HP)
				  ○ Predominant GGO (consider HP, smoking related disease, drug toxicity, and acute exacerbation of fibrosis)
				  ○ Profuse centrilobular micronodules (consider HP or smoking-related disease)

- Nodules (consider sarcoidosis)
- Consolidation (consider organizing pneumonia, etc.)
- Mediastinal findings
  - Pleural plaques (consider) asbestosis
  - Dilated esophagus (consider CTD)

The previous term, "early UIP pattern," has been eliminated to avoid confusion with "interstitial lung abnormalities" described in the text. The term "indeterminate for UIP" has been retained for situations in which the HRCT features do not meet UIP or probable UIP criteria and do not explicitly suggest an alternative diagnosis.

Abbreviations: CT, computed tomography; CTD, connective tissue disease; DIP, desquamative interstitial pneumonia; GGO, ground-glass opacity; HP, hypersensitivity pneumonitis; HRCT, high-resolution computed tomography; ILD, interstitial lung disease; IP, interstitial pneumonia; LAM, lymphangioleiomyomatosis; LIP, lymphoid interstitial pneumonia; NSIP, nonspecific interstitial pneumonia; PLCH, pulmonary Langerhans cell histiocytosis; UIP, usual interstitial pneumonia.

Table 2
Histopathology patterns and features

UIP	Probable UIP	Indeterminate for UIP	Alternative Diagnosis
• Dense fibrosis with architectural distortion (ie, destructive scarring and/or honeycombing) • Predominant subpleural and/or paraseptal distribution of fibrosis • Patchy involvement of lung parenchyma by fibrosis • Fibroblast foci • Absence of features to suggest an alternate diagnosis	• Some histologic features from column 1 are present but to an extent that precludes a definite diagnosis of UIP/PIF *And* • Absence of features to suggest an alternative diagnosis *Or* • Honeycombing	• Fibrosis with or without architectural distortion, with features favoring either a pattern other than UIP or features favoring UIP secondary to another cause[a] • Some histologic features from column 1, but with other features suggesting an alternative diagnosis[b]	• Features of other histologic patterns of IPS (eg, absence of fibroblast foci or loose fibrosis) in all biopsies • Histologic findings indicative of other diseases (eg, hypersensitivity pneumonitis, Langerhans cell histiocytosis, sarcoidosis, LAM)

Abbreviations: IIP, idiopathic interstitial pneumonia; IPF, idiopathic pulmonary fibrosis; LAM, lymphangioleiomyomatosis; UIP, usual interstitial pneumonia.

[a] Granulomas, hyaline membranes (other than when associated with acute exacerbation of IPF, which may be the presenting manifestation in some patients), prominent airway-centered changes, areas of interstitial inflammation lacking associated fibrosis, marked chronic fibrous pleuritis, organizing pneumonia. Such features may not be overt or easily seen to the untrained eye and often need to be specifically sought.

[b] Features that should raise concerns about the likelihood of an alternative diagnosis include a cellular inflammatory infiltrate away from areas of honeycombing, prominent lymphoid hyperplasia including secondary germinal centers, and a distinctly bronchiolocentric distribution that could include extensive peribronchiolar metaplasia.

Table 3
Idiopathic pulmonary fibrosis diagnosis based on high-resolution computed tomography and biopsy patterns, developed using consensus by discussion

		Histopathology Pattern[b]			
	IPF Suspected[a]	UIP	Probable UIP	Indeterminate for UIP or Biopsy not Performed	Alternative Diagnosis
HRCT pattern	UIP	IPF	IPF	IPF	Non-IPF dx
	Portable UIP	IPF	IPF	IPF (Likely)[c]	Non-IPF dx
	Indeterminate	IPF	IPF (Likely)[c]	Indeterminate[d]	Non-IPF dx
	Alternative diagnosis	IPF (Likely)[c]	Indeterminate[d]	Non-IPF dx	Non-IPF dx

Abbreviations: dx, diagnosis; UIP, usual interstitial pneumonia.

[a] "Clinically suspected of having IPF" is defined as unexplained patterns of bilateral pulmonary fibrosis on chest radiography or chest computed tomography, bibasilar inspiratory crackles, and age >60 y. Middle-aged adults (age >40 and < 60 years) can rarely present with otherwise similar clinical features, especially in patients with features suggesting familial pulmonary fibrosis.

[b] Diagnostic confidence may need to be downgraded if histopathological assessment is based on transbronchial lung cryobiopsy given the smaller biopsy size and greater potential for sampling error compared with surgical lung biopsy.

[c] IPF is the likely diagnosis when any of the following features are present: (1) moderate-to-severe traction bronchiectasis and/or bronchiolectasis (defined as mild traction bronchiectasis and/or bronchiolectasis in 4 or more lobes, including the lingula as a lobe, or moderate-to-severe traction bronchiectasis in 2 or more lobes) in a man >50 years old or in a woman >60 years old; (2) extensive (>30%) reticulation on HRCT and age > 70 years; (3) increased neutrophils and/or absence of lymphocytosis in BAL fluid; and (4) multidisciplinary discussion produces a confident diagnosis of IPF.

[d] Indeterminate for IPF (1) without an adequate biopsy remains indeterminate and (2) with an adequate biopsy may be reclassified to a more specific diagnosis after multidisciplinary discussion and/or additional consultation.

studies suggest a much higher rate of dose reduction (20%–30%) or discontinuation (5%–25%) due to gastrointestinal (GI) side effects.[61,62]

Pirfenidone Pirfenidone is an antifibrotic that inhibits transforming growth factor beta–stimulated collagen synthesis, decreases the extracellular matrix, and blocks fibroblast proliferation in vitro (PMID: 31967851). The dose can be as high as 40 mg/kg/d with a maximum dose of 2403 mg/d, is taken in 3 divided doses, and always with food. It is initiated gradually with 1 capsule (267 mg) 3 times per day for 1 week, then 2 capsules, and then 3 capsules in a stepwise manner. Similar to nintedanib, LFTs should be monitored regularly with the medication, as drug-induced liver disease can range from mild to fatal. The efficacy of pirfenidone is in slowing the progression of IPF in patients with mild-to-moderate disease and a possible mortality benefit in pooled analysis.[63,64]

Most frequent adverse effects associated with pirfenidone include rash (30%), photosensitivity (9%), nausea (36%), diarrhea (26%), abdominal discomfort (24%), dyspepsia (19%), anorexia (13%), and fatigue (26%). Dose reduction or interruption for GI events was required in 18% of patients in the high-dose group, and 2% discontinued the medication. However, some of the GI adverse reactions can be mitigated by taking the medication with food.[65]

Prognosis and monitoring

Assessing disease severity and prognosis. The severity of IPF is assessed based on symptoms, HRCT findings, and PFTs. Although the typical progression is from mild → moderate → severe respiratory disease, the rate of the progression can vary. The median survival of IPF ranges from 2 to 5 years.[66,67] However, this estimate reflects the range of average life expectancies observed in cohorts of patients with IPF before effective therapies, rather than the limits of an individual patient's life expectancy. This is important, as the actual range of survival in IPF is broad, with up to 20% to 25% of patients living beyond 10 years.[66] Further, the role that antifibrotic agents have on potentially extending life expectancies remains unclear.

The Gender-Age-Physiology (GAP) model can be helpful in estimating the prognosis for patients.[67] This widely validated, clinical prediction model incorporates age, gender, FVC, and DLCO into a point system that is predictive of 1-, 2-, and 3-year mortality. When taken together, in conjunction with the patient's overall clinical picture, the GAP scores can help guide patient's prognosis.

Acute exacerbations. Acute exacerbations of IPF (AE-IPF) are defined as "an acute, clinically significant respiratory deterioration characterized by evidence of new widespread alveolar abnormality." They occur in 5% to 10% of patients with IPF annually, carry a poor prognosis with a median survival of only 3 to 4 months after an exacerbation, and have a high in-hospital mortality when presenting in respiratory failure (50% overall and 90% for those requiring mechanical ventilation).[68,69] The following diagnostic criteria for an AE-IPF, from the 2016 guidelines are as follows:[68]

- A known diagnosis of IPF (diagnosis may be made at the time of acute respiratory deterioration)
- Acute worsening, "typically less than 1-month duration"
- HRCT with new bilateral ground-glass opacification and/or consolidation superimposed on a background of findings consistent with UIP
- Heart failure or volume overload does not fully explain the worsening

Broadly speaking, multiple studies[63,64] have shown that worsening respiratory symptoms, regardless of whether or not they meet strict criteria for an acute exacerbation, confer a high risk for subsequent mortality and thus should prompt a discussion of prognosis and goals of care. Treatment often consists of high-dose corticosteroids although data on their efficacy in exacerbations of IPF are lacking with a weak recommendation for their use in guidelines.[5]

Monitoring of disease. The primary reason to monitor the disease progression in patients with IPF is to assess for potential disease progression that may prompt a change in therapy including medication changes, referral to lung transplantation, and goals of care discussions. There is no clear guideline for frequency of monitoring although typically patients are seen every 3 to 6 months, with frequency dependent on clinical status. One of the key components to monitoring in IPF is following PFTs. Both declines in DLCO and FVC are strong predictors of mortality in IPF and may prompt referral to transplant. A decline in FVC or DLCO of at least 10% over 6 to 12 months predicts an increased risk of mortality, although changes as small as 5% over this same period also portend a worse prognosis.[70–73] In addition to PFTs, a decrease in 6-minute walk distance of 30 m is a clinically important change in IPF over 6 months and can predict mortality.[72,73] Further, worsening hypoxemia and increasing oxygen requirements are common indicators of disease progression and increase the risk of mortality.

Lung transplantation. IPF is the most common ILD referred for lung transplantation and is currently the most common disease process for which lung transplant is performed in the United States,[74] with a median survival following lung transplantation of 5.2 years.[75]

Guidelines for placing a referral for transplantation, in a patient with IPF, include the following:[76,77]

- DLCO less than 40% predicted
- FVC less than 80% predicted
- Any dyspnea or functional limitation due to disease
- A decrease in pulse oximetry of less than 89%, even if only on exertion

Criteria for placing a patient with IPF on the transplant list include the following:[76,77]

- Decline in FVC greater than or equal to 10% during 6 months of follow-up
- Decline in DLCO greater than or equal to 15% during 6 months of follow-up
- On 6-minute walk: oxygen desaturation to less than 88% or distance walked less than 250 m or greater than 50 m decline in distance walked over 6 months
- Pulmonary hypertension
- Hospitalization for respiratory decline, pneumothorax, or acute exacerbation

OTHER INTERSTITIAL LUNG DISEASES—PROGRESSIVE PULMONARY FIBROSIS
Introduction

Patients with a spectrum of lung disorders, including IPF, have a progressive fibrosing clinical phenotype that is characterized by an increasing extent of fibrosis on HRCT, decline in lung function, worsening symptoms, and early death.[41,78] These other ILDs include CTD-associated ILD (CTD-ILD), fibrotic hypersensitivity pneumonitis (HP), unclassifiable ILD, idiopathic nonspecific interstitial pneumonia (NSIP), and rarely sarcoidosis, organizing pneumonia, and ILD associated with occupational exposures.[79] (**Fig. 1**)

Based on clinical and pathophysiological similarities, it has been hypothesized that disorders with this progressive phenotype have a common mechanism, regardless of cause, and thus have a similar response to treatment.[78,80] This section aims to outline

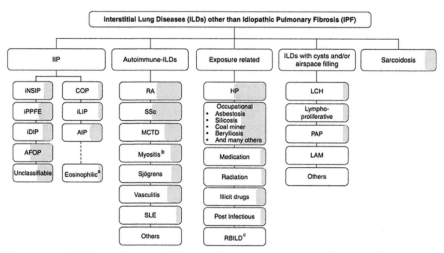

Fig. 1. Interstitial lung diseases (ILDs) manifesting progressive pulmonary fibrosis (PPF), developed using consensus by discussion. The shaded area represents the estimated proportion of patients with various types of ILD who manifest PPF. Note that idiopathic pulmonary fibrosis (IPF) is not included in the figure, because it is excluded from the definition of PPF. Although virtually all patients with IPF will manifest disease progression similar to PPF, the proportion of patients with ILDs other than IPF who manifest PPF is based on the consensus of opinions and the perception of the international committee. There are no data to provide the exact or estimated proportion of patients manifesting PPF in ILDs, other than IPF. [a]The committee acknowledges that eosinophilic pneumonia of unknown cause was not included in the IIP classification. [b]Myositis includes PM/DM/antisynthetase syndrome, which may be amyopathic. [c]Although respiratory bronchiolitis interstitial lung disease (RBILD) is acknowledged to be a consequence of exposure to cigarette smoke in virtually all patients with RBILD, RBILD and desquamative interstitial pneumonia (DIP) often coexist. Although DIP is also related to exposure to cigarette smoke in most of the patients, DIP is also seen in some patients with connective tissue disease, without exposure to cigarette smoke, and without a known cause. Antifibrotic treatment is indicated for patients diagnosed with IPF (3). Antifibrotic treatment of the other types of ILD upon manifesting PPF is as suggested/recommended in this guideline. AFOP, acute fibrinous and organizing pneumonia; AIP, acute interstitial pneumonia; COP, cryptogenic organizing pneumonia; DM, dermatomyositis; HP, hypersensitivity pneumonitis; iDIP, idiopathic DIP; IIP, idiopathic interstitial pneumonia; iLIP, idiopathic lymphoid interstitial pneumonia; iNSIP, idiopathic nonspecific interstitial pneumonia; iPPFE, idiopathic pleuroparenchymal fibroelastosis; LAM, lymphangioleiomyomatosis; LCH, Langerhans cell histiocytosis; MCTD, mixed connective tissue disease; PAP, pulmonary alveolar proteinosis; PM, polymyositis; RA, rheumatoid arthritis; SLE, systemic lupus erythematosus; SSc, systemic sclerosis. Reprinted with permission of the American Thoracic Society. Copyright © 2022 American Thoracic Society. All rights reserved. Raghu G, Remy-Jardin M, Richeldi L, et al. Idiopathic Pulmonary Fibrosis (an Update) and Progressive Pulmonary Fibrosis in Adults: An Official ATS/ERS/JRS/ALAT Clinical Practice Guideline. *Am J Respir Crit Care Med.* 2022;205(9):e18-e47. The American Journal of Respiratory and Critical Care Medicine is an official journal of the American Thoracic Society.

the diagnosis and treatment of progressive pulmonary fibrosis (PPF) in fibrotic ILD, other than IPF.

Although guidelines on PPF were being developed, there was a clinical trial (INBUILD trial, described in more detail in the later section[16]) reporting the beneficial effect of antifibrotic medication in ILDs other than IPF, which manifests with this

PPF phenotype. Given the significance of these findings, and the shift in treatment patterns toward a broader application of antifibrotics, a guideline committee was formed to define the diagnosis of PPF and decide on formal treatment recommendations. The guidelines,[41] established in 2022, for the diagnosis and treatment of PPF are a collaboration between ATS (American Thoracic Society), ERS (European Respiratory Society), JRS (Japanese Respiratory Society), and ALAT (Asociacion Latinoamericana de Torax) and are summarized below.

Definition of Progressive Pulmonary Fibrosis

In patients with ILD other than IPF, and who have radiological evidence of pulmonary fibrosis, PPF is defined as at least 2 of the following 3 criteria occurring within the past year with no alternative explanation.[70]

1. Worsening respiratory symptoms
2. Physiologic evidence of disease progression (either of the following; of note, much of these data have been extrapolated from data on IPF[81,82]):
   a. Absolute decline in FVC $\geq$ 5% predicted within 1 year of follow-up
   b. Absolute decline in DLCO (corrected for hemoglobin) $\geq$ 10% predicted within 1 year of follow-up
3. Radiological evidence of disease progression[83,84] (one or more of the following):
   a. Increased extent or severity of traction bronchiectasis and bronchiolectasis
   b. New GGO with traction bronchiectasis
   c. New fine reticulation
   d. Increased extent or increased coarseness of reticular abnormality
   e. New or increased honeycombing
   f. Increased lobar volume loss

As part of the diagnosis, it is important to exclude alternative explanations of worsening features with suspected progression; this is particularly true in those with worsened respiratory symptoms and/or a decline in DLCO, given the lower specificity of these features of PPF compared with FVC and chest CT.

It is important to highlight that PPF is defined separate from IPF (see **table 3**). Further PPF is not a diagnosis, and the definition is independent of the underlying condition. PPF has been associated only with prognosis, and it remains unclear if it also identifies patients best suited for antifibrotic therapy.[41]

Treatment of Progressive Pulmonary Fibrosis, Other than Idiopathic Pulmonary Fibrosis

Nintedanib
Available evidence for efficacy in progressive pulmonary fibrosis. As previously discussed, nintedanib has been shown to slow disease progression in IPF; as such, the guidelines looked to explore, based on evidence available, if it is a beneficial treatment of non-IPF PPF.[41] To guide this decision, investigators assessed data from a randomized clinical trial (RCT) (INBUILD)[78] that assigned 663 patients with progressive fibrosing ILD (PF-ILD) to nintedanib or placebo for 52 weeks, with a post hoc analysis that further broke down this relationship based on type of ILD. It should be noted that subtle differences in diagnostic criteria exist between the PF-ILD applied in the INBUILD study, and current PPF criteria.[41,78] Among all patients with PPF, FVC declined in both the treatment (nintedanib) and control (placebo) arms of the INBUILD trial, but the mean annual decline was significantly less (107 mL) in the nintedanib arm. The difference in the annual decline in FVC between nintedanib and placebo arms was 128 mL/y among patients who had a radiological UIP pattern, whereas it was 75.3 mL/

y in patients with a radiologic non-UIP pattern. More recent efforts assessing the PPF criteria identify the FVC decline of 10% points or greater as being integral to determination of outcomes among patients with PPF.[85,86] The trial further found that the adverse effect of "progression of ILD" was 2.4 times less likely in the nintedanib compared with the placebo arm. The INBUILD trial showed no significant difference in all-cause mortality or fatal acute exacerbations among all patients with PPF. Similarly, there was no difference in all-cause mortality among patients with PPF who had a radiological UIP pattern. Side effects from the medications were most commonly GI in nature, or transaminitis, as previously outlined in the section on IPF.

Guideline recommendations. Based on the earlier discussion, there is a conditional recommendation for nintedanib in patients with PPF based on 2 major factors:[41]

- There was a statistically significant reduction in disease progression, measured as the annual decline of FVC.
- The side effects are reversible with discontinuation of the medication.

Pirfenidone

Available evidence for efficacy in progressive pulmonary fibrosis. Pirfenidone, similarly, has been shown to slow disease progression in IPF; thus the committee looked to explore, based on evidence available, if it is a beneficial treatment of PPF. To guide this decision, the investigators primarily looked at 2 RCT that enrolled patients with PPF and evaluated the effects of pirfenidone or placebo.[87,88] One of the trials,[78] looking at patients with unclassifiable fibrotic ILD, randomly assigned 253 patients to receive pirfenidone or placebo with a 24-week follow-up period. The second trial,[77] randomly assigned 127 patients with PPF (chronic HP, CTD-ILD, NSIP, and asbestosis-induced lung disease) to receive pirfenidone or placebo with a 48-week follow-up period. Of note, the second trial was terminated early because of futility due to slow recruitment but imputations were made for the missing data.[41]

When the 2 RCTs were combined into a meta-analysis, pirfenidone was found to decrease FVC by 100 mL or by 2.3% over 24 weeks.[87,88] Pirfenidone reduced by 1.6 times the likelihood that percentage predicted of FVC would decline by greater than 5% and reduce by 1.9 times the likelihood that percentage predicted FVC would decline greater than 10%. Neither trial showed a statistically significant difference in progression-free survival, nor was there a difference in mortality.

Guideline recommendations. Based on the earlier discussion, and the fact that one-third of the committee abstained from voting for or against the use of pirfenidone, the committee made the following recommendation[41]:

- The recommendation is for further research into the efficacy, effectiveness, and safety of pirfenidone in both non-IPF PPF in general and specific types of non-IPF PPF.

CLINICS CARE POINTS

- IPF is defined by an UIP pattern after excluding other known causes of ILD.
- Indices of disease progression in IPF include lung function decline, worsening dyspnea, and greater extent of HRCT fibrosis. The GAP model can be helpful in prognosticating outcomes.
- Approach to management of IPF includes pharmacotherapy, nonpharmacotherapeutic interventions, and supportive care. Comorbidities should be addressed when present, and hypoxia treated with ambulatory O2.

- Consideration for antifibrotic therapy and lung transplantation evaluation should occur early.
- Patients with ILD other than IPF, and who have radiological evidence of pulmonary fibrosis, may have PPF with disease behavior similar to IPF.
- PPF is defined by the presence of 2 out of 3 criteria including worsening respiratory symptoms, physiologic evidence of disease progression, or radiological evidence of disease progression.

FUNDING

NIH, United States K23HL146942. Final approval of the submitted manuscript and accountability for all aspects: R. Strykowski, A. Adegunsoye.

CONFLICT OF INTEREST DISCLOSURES

A. Adegunsoye is supported by a career development award from the National Heart, Lung, and Blood Institute, United States (K23HL146942) and has received speaking and advisory board fees from Boehringer Ingelheim and Roche and grant funding for interstitial lung disease research from the Pulmonary Fibrosis Foundation. R. Strykowki has no relevant disclosures.

REFERENCES

1. Meyer KC. Diagnosis and management of interstitial lung disease. Transl Respir Med 2014;2:4.
2. Lederer DJ, Martinez FJ. Idiopathic Pulmonary Fibrosis. N Engl J Med 2018; 378(19):1811–23.
3. Cottin V, Hirani NA, Hotchkin DL, et al. Presentation, diagnosis and clinical course of the spectrum of progressive-fibrosing interstitial lung diseases. Eur Respir Rev 2018;27(150).
4. Oliveira DS, Araujo Filho JA, Paiva AFL, et al. Idiopathic interstitial pneumonias: review of the latest American Thoracic Society/European Respiratory Society classification. Radiol Bras 2018;51(5):321–7.
5. Raghu G, Collard HR, Egan JJ, et al. An official ATS/ERS/JRS/ALAT statement: idiopathic pulmonary fibrosis: evidence-based guidelines for diagnosis and management. Am J Respir Crit Care Med 2011;183(6):788–824.
6. American Thoracic Society. Idiopathic pulmonary fibrosis: diagnosis and treatment. International consensus statement. American Thoracic Society (ATS), and the European Respiratory Society (ERS). Am J Respir Crit Care Med 2000; 161(2 Pt 1):646–64.
7. Fell CD, Martinez FJ, Liu LX, et al. Clinical predictors of a diagnosis of idiopathic pulmonary fibrosis. Am J Respir Crit Care Med 2010;181(8):832–7.
8. Marinescu DC, Raghu G, Remy-Jardin M, et al. Integration and Application of Clinical Practice Guidelines for the Diagnosis of Idiopathic Pulmonary Fibrosis and Fibrotic Hypersensitivity Pneumonitis. Chest 2022;162(3):614–29.
9. Kaunisto J, Salomaa ER, Hodgson U, et al. Idiopathic pulmonary fibrosis–a systematic review on methodology for the collection of epidemiological data. BMC Pulm Med 2013;13:53.
10. Raghu G, Weycker D, Edelsberg J, et al. Incidence and prevalence of idiopathic pulmonary fibrosis. Am J Respir Crit Care Med 2006;174(7):810–6.

11. Raghu G, Chen SY, Yeh WS, et al. Idiopathic pulmonary fibrosis in US Medicare beneficiaries aged 65 years and older: incidence, prevalence, and survival, 2001-11. Lancet Respir Med 2014;2(7):566–72.

12. Nalysnyk L, Cid-Ruzafa J, Rotella P, et al. Incidence and prevalence of idiopathic pulmonary fibrosis: review of the literature. Eur Respir Rev 2012;21(126):355–61.

13. Hutchinson J, Fogarty A, Hubbard R, et al. Global incidence and mortality of idiopathic pulmonary fibrosis: a systematic review. Eur Respir J 2015;46(3):795–806.

14. Swigris JJ, Olson AL, Huie TJ, et al. Ethnic and racial differences in the presence of idiopathic pulmonary fibrosis at death. Respir Med 2012;106(4):588–93.

15. Adegunsoye A, Oldham JM, Bellam SK, et al. African-American race and mortality in interstitial lung disease: a multicentre propensity-matched analysis. Eur Respir J 2018;51(6).

16. Selman M, King TE, Pardo A. American Thoracic S, European Respiratory S, American College of Chest P. Idiopathic pulmonary fibrosis: prevailing and evolving hypotheses about its pathogenesis and implications for therapy. Ann Intern Med 2001;134(2):136–51.

17. Hecker L, Thannickal VJ. Nonresolving fibrotic disorders: idiopathic pulmonary fibrosis as a paradigm of impaired tissue regeneration. Am J Med Sci 2011; 341(6):431–4.

18. Hunninghake GW. Antioxidant therapy for idiopathic pulmonary fibrosis. N Engl J Med 2005;353(21):2285–7.

19. Fries KM, Blieden T, Looney RJ, et al. Evidence of fibroblast heterogeneity and the role of fibroblast subpopulations in fibrosis. Clin Immunol Immunopathol 1994;72(3):283–92.

20. Adegunsoye A, Vij R, Noth I. Integrating Genomics Into Management of Fibrotic Interstitial Lung Disease. Chest 2019;155(5):1026–40.

21. Zhang D, Newton CA. Familial Pulmonary Fibrosis: Genetic Features and Clinical Implications. Chest 2021;160(5):1764–73.

22. Wang Y, Kuan PJ, Xing C, et al. Genetic defects in surfactant protein A2 are associated with pulmonary fibrosis and lung cancer. Am J Hum Genet 2009; 84(1):52–9.

23. van Moorsel CH, van Oosterhout MF, Barlo NP, et al. Surfactant protein C mutations are the basis of a significant portion of adult familial pulmonary fibrosis in a dutch cohort. Am J Respir Crit Care Med 2010;182(11):1419–25.

24. Seibold MA, Wise AL, Speer MC, et al. A common MUC5B promoter polymorphism and pulmonary fibrosis. N Engl J Med 2011;364(16):1503–12.

25. Vicary GW, Vergne Y, Santiago-Cornier A, et al. Pulmonary Fibrosis in Hermansky-Pudlak Syndrome. Ann Am Thorac Soc 2016;13(10):1839–46.

26. Snetselaar R, van Moorsel CHM, Kazemier KM, et al. Telomere length in interstitial lung diseases. Chest 2015;148(4):1011–8.

27. Armanios MY, Chen JJ, Cogan JD, et al. Telomerase mutations in families with idiopathic pulmonary fibrosis. N Engl J Med 2007;356(13):1317–26.

28. Iwai K, Mori T, Yamada N, et al. Idiopathic pulmonary fibrosis. Epidemiologic approaches to occupational exposure. Am J Respir Crit Care Med 1994; 150(3):670–5.

29. Baumgartner KB, Samet JM, Stidley CA, et al. Cigarette smoking: a risk factor for idiopathic pulmonary fibrosis. Am J Respir Crit Care Med 1997;155(1):242–8.

30. Lee JS. The Role of Gastroesophageal Reflux and Microaspiration in Idiopathic Pulmonary Fibrosis. Clin Pulm Med 2014;21(2):81–5.

31. Baumgartner KB, Samet JM, Coultas DB, et al. Occupational and environmental risk factors for idiopathic pulmonary fibrosis: a multicenter case-control study. Collaborating Centers. Am J Epidemiol 2000;152(4):307–15.

32. Taskar VS, Coultas DB. Is idiopathic pulmonary fibrosis an environmental disease? Proc Am Thorac Soc 2006;3(4):293–8.

33. Sheng G, Chen P, Wei Y, et al. Viral Infection Increases the Risk of Idiopathic Pulmonary Fibrosis: A Meta-Analysis. Chest 2020;157(5):1175–87.

34. Raghu G, Remy-Jardin M, Myers JL, et al. Diagnosis of Idiopathic Pulmonary Fibrosis. An Official ATS/ERS/JRS/ALAT Clinical Practice Guideline. Am J Respir Crit Care Med 2018;198(5):e44–68.

35. Moua T, Maldonado F, Decker PA, et al. Frequency and implication of autoimmune serologies in idiopathic pulmonary fibrosis. Mayo Clin Proc 2014;89(3): 319–26.

36. Johnston ID, Prescott RJ, Chalmers JC, et al. British Thoracic Society study of cryptogenic fibrosing alveolitis: current presentation and initial management. Fibrosing Alveolitis Subcommittee of the Research Committee of the British Thoracic Society. Thorax 1997;52(1):38–44.

37. Muller NL, Guerry-Force ML, Staples CA, et al. Differential diagnosis of bronchiolitis obliterans with organizing pneumonia and usual interstitial pneumonia: clinical, functional, and radiologic findings. Radiology 1987;162(1 Pt 1):151–6.

38. Souza CA, Muller NL, Flint J, et al. Idiopathic pulmonary fibrosis: spectrum of high-resolution CT findings. AJR Am J Roentgenol 2005;185(6):1531–9.

39. Orens JB, Kazerooni EA, Martinez FJ, et al. The sensitivity of high-resolution CT in detecting idiopathic pulmonary fibrosis proved by open lung biopsy. A prospective study. Chest 1995;108(1):109–15.

40. Lynch DA, Newell JD, Logan PM, et al. Can CT distinguish hypersensitivity pneumonitis from idiopathic pulmonary fibrosis? AJR Am J Roentgenol 1995;165(4): 807–11.

41. Raghu G, Remy-Jardin M, Richeldi L, et al. Idiopathic Pulmonary Fibrosis (an Update) and Progressive Pulmonary Fibrosis in Adults: An Official ATS/ERS/JRS/ ALAT Clinical Practice Guideline. Am J Respir Crit Care Med 2022;205(9): e18–47.

42. Tomassetti S, Ravaglia C, Wells AU, et al. Prognostic value of transbronchial lung cryobiopsy for the multidisciplinary diagnosis of idiopathic pulmonary fibrosis: a retrospective validation study. Lancet Respir Med 2020;8(8):786–94.

43. Wells AU, Hirani N. Interstitial lung disease guideline. Thorax 2008;63(Suppl 5): v1–58.

44. Hetzel J, Wells AU, Costabel U, et al. Transbronchial cryobiopsy increases diagnostic confidence in interstitial lung disease: a prospective multicentre trial. Eur Respir J 2020;56(6).

45. Maldonado F, Danoff SK, Wells AU, et al. Transbronchial Cryobiopsy for the Diagnosis of Interstitial Lung Diseases: CHEST Guideline and Expert Panel Report. Chest 2020;157(4):1030–42.

46. Collard HR, Tino G, Noble PW, et al. Patient experiences with pulmonary fibrosis. Respir Med 2007;101(6):1350–4.

47. Ferreira A, Garvey C, Connors GL, et al. Pulmonary rehabilitation in interstitial lung disease: benefits and predictors of response. Chest 2009;135(2):442–7.

48. Al-Ghimlas F, Todd DC. Predictors of success in pulmonary rehabilitation for patients with interstitial lung disease. Chest 2009;136(4):1183–4.

49. Zhao J, Metra B, George G, et al. Mortality among Patients with COVID-19 and Different Interstitial Lung Disease Subtypes: A Multicenter Cohort Study. Ann Am Thorac Soc 2022;19(8):1435–7.

50. Marcon A, Schievano E, Fedeli U. Mortality Associated with Idiopathic Pulmonary Fibrosis in Northeastern Italy, 2008-2020: A Multiple Cause of Death Analysis. Int J Environ Res Public Health 2021;18(14).

51. Levin MJ, Ustianowski A, De Wit S, et al. Intramuscular AZD7442 (Tixagevimab-Cilgavimab) for Prevention of Covid-19. N Engl J Med 2022;386(23):2188–200.

52. Raghu G, Rochwerg B, Zhang Y, et al. An Official ATS/ERS/JRS/ALAT Clinical Practice Guideline: Treatment of Idiopathic Pulmonary Fibrosis. An Update of the 2011 Clinical Practice Guideline. Am J Respir Crit Care Med 2015;192(2): e3–19.

53. Carlos WG, Strek ME, Wang TS, et al. Treatment of Idiopathic Pulmonary Fibrosis. Ann Am Thorac Soc 2016;13(1):115–7.

54. Adegunsoye A, Strek ME. Therapeutic Approach to Adult Fibrotic Lung Diseases. Chest 2016;150(6):1371–86.

55. Petnak T, Lertjitbanjong P, Thongprayoon C, et al. Impact of Antifibrotic Therapy on Mortality and Acute Exacerbation in Idiopathic Pulmonary Fibrosis: A Systematic Review and Meta-Analysis. Chest 2021;160(5):1751–63.

56. Wuyts WA, Kolb M, Stowasser S, et al. First Data on Efficacy and Safety of Nintedanib in Patients with Idiopathic Pulmonary Fibrosis and Forced Vital Capacity of </=50 % of Predicted Value. Lung 2016;194(5):739–43.

57. Harari S, Caminati A, Poletti V, et al. A Real-Life Multicenter National Study on Nintedanib in Severe Idiopathic Pulmonary Fibrosis. Respiration 2018;95(6):433–40.

58. Wollin L, Wex E, Pautsch A, et al. Mode of action of nintedanib in the treatment of idiopathic pulmonary fibrosis. Eur Respir J 2015;45(5):1434–45.

59. Richeldi L, du Bois RM, Raghu G, et al. Efficacy and safety of nintedanib in idiopathic pulmonary fibrosis. N Engl J Med 2014;370(22):2071–82.

60. Richeldi L, Cottin V, du Bois RM, et al. Nintedanib in patients with idiopathic pulmonary fibrosis: Combined evidence from the TOMORROW and INPULSIS((R)) trials. Respir Med 2016;113:74–9.

61. Galli JA, Pandya A, Vega-Olivo M, et al. Pirfenidone and nintedanib for pulmonary fibrosis in clinical practice: Tolerability and adverse drug reactions. Respirology 2017;22(6):1171–8.

62. Harari S, Pesci A, Albera C, et al. Nintedanib in IPF: Post hoc Analysis of the Italian FIBRONET Observational Study. Respiration 2022;101(6):577–84.

63. Raghu G, Johnson WC, Lockhart D, et al. Treatment of idiopathic pulmonary fibrosis with a new antifibrotic agent, pirfenidone: results of a prospective, open-label Phase II study. Am J Respir Crit Care Med 1999;159(4 Pt 1):1061–9.

64. Noble PW, Albera C, Bradford WZ, et al. Pirfenidone for idiopathic pulmonary fibrosis: analysis of pooled data from three multinational phase 3 trials. Eur Respir J 2016;47(1):243–53.

65. Valeyre D, Albera C, Bradford WZ, et al. Comprehensive assessment of the long-term safety of pirfenidone in patients with idiopathic pulmonary fibrosis. Respirology 2014;19(5):740–7.

66. Nathan SD, Shlobin OA, Weir N, et al. Long-term course and prognosis of idiopathic pulmonary fibrosis in the new millennium. Chest 2011;140(1):221–9.

67. Ley B, Ryerson CJ, Vittinghoff E, et al. A multidimensional index and staging system for idiopathic pulmonary fibrosis. Ann Intern Med 2012;156(10):684–91.

68. Collard HR, Ryerson CJ, Corte TJ, et al. Acute Exacerbation of Idiopathic Pulmonary Fibrosis. An International Working Group Report. Am J Respir Crit Care Med 2016;194(3):265–75.

69. Ryerson CJ, Cottin V, Brown KK, et al. Acute exacerbation of idiopathic pulmonary fibrosis: shifting the paradigm. Eur Respir J 2015;46(2):512–20.

70. Durheim MT, Collard HR, Roberts RS, et al. Association of hospital admission and forced vital capacity endpoints with survival in patients with idiopathic pulmonary fibrosis: analysis of a pooled cohort from three clinical trials. Lancet Respir Med 2015;3(5):388–96.

71. Paterniti MO, Bi Y, Rekic D, et al. Acute Exacerbation and Decline in Forced Vital Capacity Are Associated with Increased Mortality in Idiopathic Pulmonary Fibrosis. Ann Am Thorac Soc 2017;14(9):1395–402.

72. Singh SJ, Puhan MA, Andrianopoulos V, et al. An official systematic review of the European Respiratory Society/American Thoracic Society: measurement properties of field walking tests in chronic respiratory disease. Eur Respir J 2014;44(6): 1447–78.

73. Holland AE, Spruit MA, Troosters T, et al. An official European Respiratory Society/American Thoracic Society technical standard: field walking tests in chronic respiratory disease. Eur Respir J 2014;44(6):1428–46.

74. Chambers DC, Perch M, Zuckermann A, et al. The International Thoracic Organ Transplant Registry of the International Society for Heart and Lung Transplantation: Thirty-eighth adult lung transplantation report - 2021; Focus on recipient characteristics. J Heart Lung Transplant 2021;40(10):1060–72.

75. Chambers DC, Cherikh WS, Harhay MO, et al. The International Thoracic Organ Transplant Registry of the International Society for Heart and Lung Transplantation: Thirty-sixth adult lung and heart-lung transplantation Report-2019; Focus theme: Donor and recipient size match. J Heart Lung Transplant 2019;38(10): 1042–55.

76. Weill D, Benden C, Corris PA, et al. A consensus document for the selection of lung transplant candidates: 2014–an update from the Pulmonary Transplantation Council of the International Society for Heart and Lung Transplantation. J Heart Lung Transplant 2015;34(1):1–15.

77. Kapnadak SG, Raghu G. Lung transplantation for interstitial lung disease. Eur Respir Rev 2021;30(161).

78. Flaherty KR, Wells AU, Cottin V, et al. Nintedanib in Progressive Fibrosing Interstitial Lung Diseases. N Engl J Med 2019;381(18):1718–27.

79. Wong AW, Ryerson CJ, Guler SA. Progression of fibrosing interstitial lung disease. Respir Res 2020;21(1):32.

80. Wells AU, Brown KK, Flaherty KR, et al. What's in a name? That which we call IPF, by any other name would act the same. Eur Respir J 2018;51(5).

81. Brown KK, Martinez FJ, Walsh SLF, et al. The natural history of progressive fibrosing interstitial lung diseases. Eur Respir J 2020;55(6).

82. Karimi-Shah BA, Chowdhury BA. Forced vital capacity in idiopathic pulmonary fibrosis–FDA review of pirfenidone and nintedanib. N Engl J Med 2015;372(13): 1189–91.

83. Akira M, Inoue Y, Arai T, et al. Long-term follow-up high-resolution CT findings in non-specific interstitial pneumonia. Thorax 2011;66(1):61–5.

84. Silva CI, Muller NL, Hansell DM, et al. Nonspecific interstitial pneumonia and idiopathic pulmonary fibrosis: changes in pattern and distribution of disease over time. Radiology 2008;247(1):251–9.

85. Pugashetti JV, Adegunsoye A, Wu Z, et al. Validation of Proposed Criteria for Progressive Pulmonary Fibrosis. Am J Respir Crit Care Med 2023;207(1):69–76.
86. Khor YH, Farooqi M, Hambly N, et al. Patient Characteristics and Survival for Progressive Pulmonary Fibrosis Using Different Definitions. Am J Respir Crit Care Med 2023;207(1):102–5.
87. Behr J, Prasse A, Kreuter M, et al. Pirfenidone in patients with progressive fibrotic interstitial lung diseases other than idiopathic pulmonary fibrosis (RELIEF): a double-blind, randomised, placebo-controlled, phase 2b trial. Lancet Respir Med 2021;9(5):476–86.
88. Maher TM, Corte TJ, Fischer A, et al. Pirfenidone in patients with unclassifiable progressive fibrosing interstitial lung disease: a double-blind, randomised, placebo-controlled, phase 2 trial. Lancet Respir Med 2020;8(2):147–57.

Connective Tissue Disease Associated Interstitial Lung Disease

Scott M. Matson, MD[a], M. Kristen Demoruelle, MD, PhD[b],*

KEYWORDS

- Autoimmunity • Interstitial lung disease • Connective tissue disease
- Immunosuppression • Subclinical interstitial lung disease • Antifibrotic

KEY POINTS

- Connective tissue disease associated interstitial lung disease (CTD-ILD) is a heterogenous collection of autoimmune and CTDs with myriad manifestations of interstitial lung disease (ILD) including cellular, inflammatory lung disease and progressive, fibrotic manifestations.
- Subclinical CTD-ILD may offer an important treatment window; however, with the lack of clinical data to guide clinicians, there are currently only expert consensus guidelines within SSc to guide screening for ILD in CTD populations, and it remains unclear how early intervention will impact these conditions.
- Immunosuppression in CTD-ILD is supported by several randomized, placebo-controlled trials (RCTs) in patients with scleroderma and several observational, retrospective studies in other autoimmune conditions.
- There is increasing data and clinical interest in the addition of antifibrotic therapy for patients with CTD-ILD.
- There are urgent needs for RCTs, which test the efficacy of immunosuppression and antifibrotic agents, including in combination and the sequence of use, in fibrotic CTD-ILD populations as well as study of intervention in subclinical CTD-ILD populations.

INTRODUCTION

Interstitial lung disease (ILD) occurs in a portion of patients with underlying connective tissue disease (CTD), most commonly effecting patients with rheumatoid arthritis (RA), systemic sclerosis (SSc), and idiopathic inflammatory myositis (IIM). The field of connective tissue disease associated interstitial lung disease (CTD-ILD) has seen major

[a] Division of Pulmonary, Critical Care and Sleep Medicine, University of Kansas School of Medicine, 3901 Rainbow boulevard, Mailstop 3007, Kansas City, KS 66160, USA; [b] Division of Rheumatology, University of Colorado School of Medicine, 1775 Aurora Court, Mail Stop B-115, Aurora, CO 80045, USA
* Corresponding author.
E-mail address: kristen.demoruelle@cuanschutz.edu

Immunol Allergy Clin N Am 43 (2023) 229–244
https://doi.org/10.1016/j.iac.2023.01.005
immunology.theclinics.com

advances in the past several years. However, there remain many unanswered questions for which further study is critically needed. In this review, we will discuss recent advances in treatment options that have had a major influence on the clinical approach to patients with CTD-ILD. We will also review what is known about pathogenic pathways in different CTD-ILDs and the entity of subclinical CTD-ILD, both areas in which further research is likely to change the current paradigm of CTD-ILD management.

EPIDEMIOLOGY AND CLINICAL OUTCOMES

ILD is one of the more severe forms of pulmonary involvement in patients with CTD. It involves varying degrees of inflammation and fibrosis in the interstitial compartment of the lung. For effected patients, it is a common cause of poor quality of life and early mortality. ILD can affect any patient with any CTD but the prevalence is higher in certain types of CTD and in patients with certain risk factors. Clinically diagnosed CTD-ILD is most common in patients with RA, SSc, and IIM, ranging from 5% to 10% in RA to 20% to 60% in SSc and 20% to 80% in IIM.[1–3] It is of note, that despite the lower rates of ILD in patients with RA, the number of patients affected by RA-ILD is similar or higher compared with the number of patients affected by SSc-ILD and IIM-ILD, given the overall higher prevalence of RA in the population. Moreover, it is notable that studies report a wide range of CTD-ILD prevalence, often differing based on the population studied, mode of detection, retrospective versus prospective data collection, clinical cohort versus claims-based cohort, and whether subclinical ILD was included along with clinically diagnosed ILD.

It is well established that different CTD-ILDs have different patterns of lung involvement. For example, SSc and IIM commonly display a pattern of nonspecific interstitial pneumonia (NSIP) with or without organizing pneumonia, whereas patients with RA are more likely to have a pattern of usual interstitial pneumonia (UIP). Overall, patients with CTD-ILD have a more favorable outcome compared with those with idiopathic disease,[4] although patients with RA with a UIP pattern are a notable exception and can progress at rates similar to those seen in idiopathic pulmonary fibrosis (IPF).[5] Different predictors of prognosis have been reported in the different CTD-ILDs but significant impairment in physiology at baseline or worsening in physiology over time as measured by percent predicted forced vital capacity (FVC) is associated with a poor prognosis across CTD-ILDs.[6–8]

More clarity is needed to understand the exact prevalence of CTD-ILDs, and a major gap in the field continues to be a lack of standardized screening guidelines, which can lead to delays in diagnosis or diagnosis at late-stage disease when treatment options are less effective. As therapeutic options for CTD-ILD increase (discussed further below), prompt identification of CTD-ILD will become increasing necessary for optimal patient care, and consensus guidelines on who and how to screen as well as what constitutes clinically significant disease will be critical. Of note, consensus statements for SSc-ILD have been published[9] and support screening with high-resolution computed tomography (HRCT), pulmonary function tests (PFTs), and chest auscultation in all patients with SSc. However, given the much higher prevalence of RA, HRCT, and PFT, screening of all patients with RA presents logistical and financial challenges. As such, the use of HRCT or PFTs for ILD screening in patients with RA is often reserved for patients with respiratory symptoms, although screening may also be appropriate in asymptomatic patients with RA with multiple ILD risk factors (eg, male sex, older age, smoking history). In addition to a lack of screening guidelines, there are also no standardized guidelines for monitoring ILD progression once CTD-ILD has been identified, a gap in the field made more critical with the approval of treatments for patients with

CTD-ILD with progressive pulmonary fibrosis (PPF).[10] A common clinical approach is to repeat PFTs every 3 months and HRCT annually but evidence-based guidelines are needed. Given the uncertainties highlighted, a multidisciplinary approach between pulmonologists, rheumatologists, radiologists, pathologists, and other health-care providers can be beneficial in the clinical management of patients with CTD-ILD.[10]

THERAPEUTIC OPTIONS AND ADVANCES

Clinicians approaching treatment options for CTD-ILD face several important decision points and currently many of these questions lack high-quality data to answer. It is important to highlight that nearly all randomized, controlled trials for CTD-ILD are derived from scleroderma ILD (SSc-ILD) and subsequently extrapolated to other autoimmune lung diseases. However, many questions remain about the applicability of SSc-ILD broadly across all types of CTD-ILDs and patterns, that is, do more fibrotic ILDs represent the same conditions as more cellular, inflammatory ILD patterns commonly encountered in SSc-ILD? There is increasingly more interest in the expanded use of antifibrotic therapy to non-IPF conditions including CTD-ILD, and many questions remain regarding sequencing of therapies in these patients.

This field is dynamic and evolving but for the purposes of this review, the authors have chosen to highlight 3 important stages of CTD-ILD treatment considerations: (1) considerations of medication-induced lung injury in the baseline autoimmune regimen, (2) role of added "ILD-specific" immunosuppression, and (3) the role of antifibrotic therapy in CTD-ILD.

Considerations of Medication-Induced Lung Injury in Baseline Autoimmune Regimens

Retrospective, observational data in CTD-ILD led to a persistent and common vagary that has driven many of the considerations in this field for decades. For instance, methotrexate is a first-line disease modifying anti-rheumatic drug (DMARD) for patients with RA.[11] It is typically continued for many years, either as monotherapy or as a foundation to which other conventional or biologic DMARDs are added. As such, methotrexate is broadly applied to the most severe patients with the condition during times of most significant disease progression. Therefore, it was difficult to differentiate this temporal relationship in historical records, that is, did these patients with RA who developed RA-ILD do so because of the risk from methotrexate or because those patients with RA on methotrexate represented a progressive phenotype of patients with RA and thus the most likely to develop ILD as an extra-articular manifestation.[12] For decades, the clinical management of patients with CTD-ILD was influenced by this observation and clinicians were faced with a difficult decision, that is, do you remove an effective DMARD when patients develop ILD given this concern for its role in ILD risk. However, recent evidence has absolved methotrexate from its previous putative role in causing or contributing to progressive fibrotic ILDs in patients with RA, indicating that the relationship was correlative and not causative.[13]

This pursuit of high-quality evidence in CTD-ILD has led to a paradigm shift in newly diagnosed fibrotic ILDs where there is no longer concern for continuing methotrexate. Subsequently, clinicians can safely continue methotrexate as an effective DMARD in patients with ILD who were achieving adequate articular disease control.[14] However, important caveats remain, including the rare potential for methotrexate to cause a cellular, acute hypersensitivity pneumonitis, which is clinically distinct from fibrotic ILDs and can typically be differentiated based on cellular analysis of bronchoalveolar lavage if indicated for diagnostic uncertainty.[15]

Methotrexate is illustrative in CTD-ILD treatment where it is often difficult to separate the temporal relationship between DMARD use and the underlying autoimmune disease progression. For instance, a similar controversy still surrounds the use of biologic anti-tumor necrosis factor (TNF) therapy in patients with CTD-ILD given observational associations with ILD exacerbations and potential harm in a meta-analysis of retrospective studies[16–18] despite several initial reports of improved ILD-specific outcomes with these agents.[19]

Table 1 highlights several known toxicities of medications used in the baseline treatment of autoimmune diseases, which may complicate ILD diagnosis and treatment in CTD-ILD.

Finally, there is an important observed association between autoimmune disease activity and ILD prognosis, which is important to consider for baseline autoimmune therapy in patients with ILD. For instance, RA disease activity is associated with both incidence of ILD and severity/prognosis of ILD in 2 recent studies.[20,21] This evidence supports the role of optimizing typical DMARD therapy in patients with ILD aside from ILD-specific immunosuppression given the association with disease activity and ILD outcomes. As mentioned above, for these complex clinical decisions, the authors of this review strongly endorse the use of multidisciplinary discussions to place the patient's baseline therapy in context, which requires the balance of autoimmune disease activity with the potential impact of current therapies on ILD exacerbation such as the use of anti-TNF therapy in patients with previous difficult-to-control autoimmune disease.

Interstitial Lung Disease-Specific Immunosuppression

There are 3 randomized, placebo-controlled trials (RCTs) that address the important question of the impact of immunosuppression in CTD-ILD (**Fig. 1**).[22–24] As mentioned

Table 1
Baseline autoimmune therapies with potential for lung toxicity

Drug	Toxicity
Methotrexate	Most commonly presents with acute hypersensitivity pneumonitis, up to 50% will have peripheral eosinophilia and associated with broncho-alveolar lymphocytosis[15]
Leflunomide	Associated with low risk of alveolar pneumonitis, especially in those patients with underlying ILD or history of methotrexate-induced lung toxicity[69]
Biologic agents	Direct inflammatory pneumonitis resulting from treatment with biologic agents in RA is reported. However, a direct pathogenic link between the agent and the pneumonitis has not been shown. Given the clinical efficacy of these agents in treating the synovial manifestations of RA, their use in patients with autoimmune-ILD remains controversial[16,19,70]
Gold	Although no longer commonly used, a typical but rare pulmonary toxicity was known to be associated with gold administration. Patients with gold-induced pulmonary toxicity have a fever and develop an NSIP pattern with lymphocytes in the lung[71]
Sulfasalazine and non-steroidal anti-inflammatory drugs (NSAIDs)	Associated with an eosinophilic alveolar infiltrate with fever which is steroid-responsive[72,73]

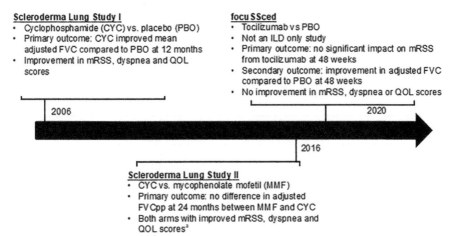

Scleroderma Lung Study I
- Cyclophosphamide (CYC) vs. placebo (PBO)
- Primary outcome: CYC improved mean adjusted FVC compared to PBO at 12 months
- Improvement in mRSS, dyspnea and QOL scores

focuSSced
- Tocilizumab vs PBO
- Not an ILD only study
- Primary outcome: no significant impact on mRSS from tocilizumab at 48 weeks
- Secondary outcome: improvement in adjusted FVC compared to PBO at 48 weeks
- No improvement in mRSS, dyspnea or QOL scores

2006

2020

2016

Scleroderma Lung Study II
- CYC vs. mycophenolate mofetil (MMF)
- Primary outcome: no difference in adjusted FVCpp at 24 months between MMF and CYC
- Both arms with improved mRSS, dyspnea and QOL scores[a]

Fig. 1. *Timeline of randomized, controlled trials for immunosuppression in SSc-ILD* with primary efficacy results highlighted in each study. [a]Quality of life evaluation from SLSII was published in a second article, separate from the main article.[80] CYC, cyclophosphamide; FVC, forced vital capacity; FVCpp, forced vital capacity percent predicted; ILD, Interstitial lung disease; MMF, mycophenolate mofetil; mRSS, modified Rodnan skin score; PBO, placebo; QOL, quality of life.

previously, all 3 of these seminal RCTs were performed in patients with SSc-ILD. However, there are important lessons learned from these data and each study can inform current clinical practice in CTD-ILD.

The first RCT in CTD-ILD was the initial Scleroderma Lung Study (SLS), which compared cyclophosphamide with placebo. SLS found that cyclophosphamide preserved decline in FVC compared with placebo and had important improvements in skin thickening scores and health-related quality of life metrics.[23] Given the toxicity profile of cyclophosphamide, investigators performed SLS II where mycophenolate mofetil (MMF) was compared with cyclophosphamide. SLS II demonstrated an improvement in FVC during the intervention period from both therapies.[24] More recently, tocilizumab was studied in SSc-ILD in the focuSSced trial (which included patients with SSc with ILD and was enriched for a progressive phenotype including patients with elevated interleukin-6).[22] In this 48-week, placebo-controlled, randomized, double-blind study, the primary endpoint (change in modified Rodnan skin fibrosis score [mRSS]) was not significant between groups.[22] However, the investigators report a prespecified secondary endpoint which showed preservation in FVC % predicted with tocilizumab compared with placebo at 48 weeks (-0.4 vs -4.6 change in % predicted FVC).[22]

These 3 studies and their therapies make up the primary backbone of immunosuppression used in clinical practice in CTD-ILD given their data, which confirms efficacy when compared with placebo. All other clinical agents used in CTD-ILD lack confirmatory efficacy trials. However, various levels of evidence exist in CTD-ILD from prospective studies of therapy without control arms to multisite observational studies to single-site retrospective study design (**Table 2**). Further specific discussion of individual choice of immunosuppressive agent for each specific CTD-ILD is beyond the scope of this review; however, it is worth addressing one important question that remains in CTD-ILD treatment: the impact of immunosuppression on outcomes for patients with CTD-ILD with the UIP pattern ILD.

Table 2
Immunosuppression therapy in autoimmune interstitial lung diseases and level of evidence

Therapy	Highest Level of Evidence	Outcome	Study
Glucocorticoids	Observational in multiple autoimmune ILDs	Lung function stability	Cassone et al,[74] 2020
Cyclophosphamide	Randomized, placebo-controlled	Improves lung function, QOL	Tashkin et al,[23] 2006
Mycophenolate	Randomized, noninferiority to CYC	Improves lung function, QOL	Tashkin et al,[24] 2016
Azathioprine	Multisite observational (fibrotic autoimmune ILD)	Lung function stability	Oldham et al,[75] 2016
Rituximab	Observational	Lung function stability	Md Yusof et al,[76] 2017
Anti-TNF biologics	Observational	Mixed outcomes	16–18
Abatacept	Prospective, observational (RA)	Lung function stability, steroid-sparing effect	Mena-Vázquez et al,[77] 2022
Tocilizumab	Randomized, placebo controlled (SSc)	Lung function with less decline compared with placebo	Khanna et al,[22] 2020
IVIG	Observational (Myositis)	Lung function stability	Huapaya et al,[78] 2019
Tacrolimus	Observational	Lung function improvement	Witt et al,[79] 2016

Abbreviations: CYC, cyclophosphamide; ILD, interstitial lung disease; IVIG, intravenous immuno-globulin; QOL, quality of life; RA, rheumatoid arthritis; SSc, systemic scleroderma; TNF, tumor necrosis factor.

In 2012, investigators revealed the results of Prednisone, Azathioprine, and *N*-Acetylcysteine: A Study That Evaluates Response in Idiopathic Pulmonary Fibrosis (PANTHER-IPF), an RCT comparing the effect of combined azathioprine, prednisone, and N-acetylcysteine to placebo for patients with IPF. In this study, there was harm associated with the treatment arm with worse survival from the immunosuppression-based strategy.[25] Although IPF is not thought to be an autoimmune disease, there was significant observational data before the PANTHER study to support an anti-inflammatory strategy, and these results highlight the limitations of retrospective treatment data. However, there are potentially important implications of the PANTHER outcomes considering the clinical, genetic, and radiographic overlaps between IPF and several autoimmune conditions, most notably RA-ILD.[26]

The observed similarities between CTD-ILDs with the UIP pattern and IPF lead to an important clinical quandary in CTD-ILD: how do clinicians safely approach immunosuppression in patients with CTD-ILD in UIP patterns? The current state of the literature offers only expert opinion as guidance for now, with observational level evidence to guide these decisions. It is the opinion of the authors of this review that UIP represents a pathologic, end-stage fibrotic pattern, which is corollary to "cirrhosis" in hepatic disease, and that treatment should be directed at the underlying cause of the pattern and not the pattern itself including, when appropriate, immunosuppression to improve autoimmune disease activity.[27] However, we continue to stress the need for prospective, randomized data to address this important question.

Antifibrotics in Autoimmune Interstitial Lung Disease

Antifibrotics are a broad "class" of therapies that include 2 Federal Drug Administration (FDA)-approved therapies (nintedanib and pirfenidone) that have been shown to reduce the decline of FVC in patients with IPF in 3 RCTs published in 2014.[28,29] Given the overlaps of CTD-ILD and IPF as mentioned previously, there has been interest in expanding the use of these novel therapies beyond only IPF.

In the SENSCIS trial, nintedanib was found to slow the decline in FVC over time compared with placebo in a study that allowed for the background immunosuppression in SSc-ILD.[30] Additionally, in 2022, the results of the Safety, tolerability, and efficacy of pirfenidone in patients with rheumatoid arthritis-associated interstitial lung disease: a randomised, double-blind, placebo-controlled, phase 2 study (TRAIL-1) were published, the first-ever RCT in RA-ILD, which found no statistically significant difference between pirfenidone and placebo in their primary endpoint (proportion of RA-ILD subjects with more than 10% or more FVC decline from baseline or death).[31] It is important to point out that FVC decline as a secondary endpoint in TRAIL-1 was similar to the trends seen in all other RCTs of antifibrotic therapy and reached statistical significance but the study was underpowered and underrecruited for multiple reasons including the coronavirus disease 2019 pandemic. It is also important to point out that patients with autoimmune ILD made-up 24.7% of the treatment arm of an RCT of nintedanib versus placebo that explored the role of nintedanib in a subset of patients with PPF, which met its primary end-point.[32]

Considered in totality, these studies highlight primarily one major takeaway: for patients with CTD-ILD with fibrotic features who have progressive loss of lung function, the addition of an antifibrotic agent is associated with slower lung function decline compared with placebo. However, these data fail to address the impact of these therapies on survival or quality of life; they also are unable to properly guide clinicians on choice or sequence of therapy when several other immunosuppressive agents would be available to a clinician when a patient with CTD-ILD experiences progression.

There is a reasonably renewed interest and excitement regarding this era of treatment afforded by this novel modality of treatment in CTD-ILD. However, we currently lack data regarding many of the important questions that these therapies raise in CTD-ILD. For instance, are there particular features of CTD-ILD that should guide treatment approaches such as earlier antifibrotic use for those patients with the UIP featured ILD?

Multidisciplinary discussion between rheumatologists and pulmonologists with experience treating these conditions and familiarity with these therapies remains the gold-standard for clinical decision-making in the absence of the level of data required to fully guide these complex decisions. However, there is hope that adaptive randomized trial platforms and global collaborative initiatives will fill these large clinical gaps in knowledge for patients with CTD-ILD in the coming decade.

PATHOGENIC PATHWAYS IN CONNECTIVE TISSUE DISEASE ASSOCIATED INTERSTITIAL LUNG DISEASE

As discussed above, CTD-ILD can be challenging to treat. The treatment approach may differ based on the ILD subtype (ie, UIP vs NSIP) but the treatment approach is not often specific for the underlying CTD despite marked differences in the clinical phenotypes associated with each CTD. These differences raise the question of whether the pathogenesis of ILD is also markedly different among different CTDs, in such a way that should be considered when investigating new treatment targets. Understanding more about the overlapping and distinct pathogenic pathways across CTD-ILDs could lead to improved screening and potentially more effective treatment approaches in CTD-ILD.

The pathogenesis of all CTD-ILDs includes interactions among genetic, environmental, and immunologic risk factors. In general, ILDs develop following repetitive alveolar epithelial and endothelial damage and activation of lung fibroblasts that transform into profibrotic myofibroblasts.[33,34] However, the initiating and propagating factors that ultimately lead to ILD in a patient with CTD likely have both shared and distinct features based on the underlying CTD. For the purposes of this review, we will highlight 4 areas that are of interest in considering whether CTD-ILDs develop through distinct pathways based on the underlying CTD: (1) genetics, (2) environmental risk factors, (3) autoantibodies, and (4) neutrophil extracellular traps (NETs).

Genetic Risk Alleles in Autoimmune Interstitial Lung Disease

As with autoimmune diseases, in general, genetics clearly play a role in CTD-ILD development. One of the strongest genetic links in CTD-ILD has been demonstrated between the gain-of-function polymorphism in the promoter of the mucin 5b (*MUC5B*) gene and RA-ILD, particularly the UIP pattern of RA-ILD.[35,36] The same polymorphism has also been strongly linked to risk of IPF,[37] suggesting shared pathways of disease development between RA-ILD and IPF. However, in SSc-ILD and IIM-ILD, other genetic variants have been identified, and the MUC5B genetic risk variant has not been associated with these forms of ILD (reviewed in ref[38]). Overall suggesting the likelihood that distinct pathogenic pathways contribute to the development of RA-ILD compared with other NSIP-predominant CTD-ILDs such as SSc-ILD and IIM-ILD.

Environmental Risk Factors and Autoimmune Interstitial Lung Disease

A number of environmental factors have been identified that are associated with increased CTD-ILD risk. However, they often vary depending on the underlying CTD. For example, cigarette smoking is consistently associated with increased RA-ILD risk but not with risk of ILD in SSc or IIM.[39–42] Longer disease duration is often associated with ILD risk in RA, whereas shorter disease duration is associated with ILD risk in SSc. These differences are likely informative regarding distinct pathways of ILD development across CTD-ILDs. However, there are also risk factors shared across CTD-ILDs, such as older age,[39,41] and shared risk factors likely inform overlapping pathways of ILD development. A deeper understanding of the mechanisms by which each risk factor leads to ILD development, including immunologic responses in the lung associated with each risk factor, will likely be informative to an improved understanding of the distinct and shared pathways in CTD-ILDs.

Autoantibodies and Autoimmune Interstitial Lung Disease

Autoantibodies play a critical role in the clinical diagnosis of most CTDs because they are often distinguishing between different CTDs. When considering how autoantibodies may be informative of CTD-ILD pathogenesis, it is of interest that there are typically a small subset of autoantibodies within a larger group of CTD-specific autoantibodies that are associated with ILD. For example, there are 3 common SSc-associated autoantibodies but antitopoisomerase I is consistently associated with SSc-ILD.[43,44] Similarly, there are multiple myositis-associated and myositis-specific autoantibodies but antisynthetase antibodies and antimelanoma differentiation-associated gene 5 carry the strongest association with IIM-ILD.[45] In RA-ILD, rheumatoid factor, anticyclic citrullinated peptide, and antipeptidylarginine deiminase-4 antibodies have been associated with RA-ILD.[39,40,46] The strong association of specific autoantibodies with CTD-ILD suggest a potential role in pathogenesis but more research is needed to understand whether these autoantibodies are directly pathogenic or an epiphenomenon arising from a separate pathogenic process. It is of note that each CTD-ILD has its own ILD-associated autoantibodies, perhaps suggesting distinct pathways by which ILD develops but it may also be that different autoantibodies trigger similar pathways that culminate in a similar downstream pathway of ILD development.

Neutrophil Extracellular Traps and Autoimmune Interstitial Lung Disease

NET formation (termed NETosis) is an innate immune response to infection or inflammation that is distinct from neutrophil apoptosis or necrosis.[47] During NETosis, neutrophils decondense and expel their DNA in complex with intracellular proteins. Proteins contained within NET remnants have antimicrobial properties but can also induce inflammation, damage surrounding tissues, and enhanced NETosis has been associated with multiple autoimmune diseases, including RA, SSc, and IIM.[48–50] Relevant to this review, NETs have also been associated with several forms of chronic lung disease, including ILD.[51,52] Several key pathways implicated in ILD pathogenesis can be influenced by NETs including that several NET-bound proteins are cytotoxic to alveolar epithelial cells,[51] NETs can activate human lung fibroblasts to differentiate into myofibroblasts,[52,53] and NETs can be a source of matrix-metalloproteinase-9 (MMP-9).[54] Moreover, in animal models, NET inhibition has been associated with a reduction in lung fibrosis.[55]

NETs in the lung have not been well studied in CTD-ILD. Our group has reported that neutrophils isolated from the sputum of patients with RA demonstrate enhanced NET formation[56] but it is unknown if this phenomenon is further exaggerated in patients with RA with ILD. It is notable that lung neutrophilia has been associated with increased mortality in IPF,[57] and based on unpublished data from our group, we suspect that this association is mediated through increased NET formation in the lung. Given these data in aggregate, it will be highly informative to better understand the function of neutrophils in the lung in different CTD-ILDs, particularly lung neutrophil predilection for NET formation. It is of note that distinct protein cargo is expressed in the NETs generated in patients with RA compared with osteoarthritis controls.[49] It will therefore be of particular interest to identify the protein content of NETs generated in the lung in different CTDs because differences could potentially inform distinct pathways of CTD-ILD development, whereas similarities could potentially identify common pathways of CTD-ILD pathogenesis.

SUBCLINICAL DISEASE

Disease modification in autoimmune conditions such as RA highlights the positive impact that translational biomedical research can have on human disease. For instance, the identification of highly sensitive biomarkers in RA and research-based screening in the first-degree family members has led to identification of a "preclinical" state in which an individual does not meet classification for RA but has demonstrated features that strongly increase that individual's risk for developing RA in the future. In RA, the identification of this preclinical state has provided valuable lessons regarding pathogenesis and has also led to several clinical trials aimed at an early intervention with the goal of prevention.[58,59] In the preclinical state of RA, joint disease has not yet developed but similar concepts can be applied to a "subclinical" state of ILD during which lung fibrosis is present on imaging but pulmonary function testing and symptoms do not indicate a clinically significant level of ILD.

There are 2 primary principles of fibrotic ILD that make the identification of a subclinical fibrotic ILD state important: (1) pulmonary fibrosis is devastating and irreversible for patients and (2) treatment exists but often patients present in late stages of disease severity when therapy only offers to reduce the rate of progression. The long-range goal of pulmonary fibrosis research is the development of reliable clinical or molecular-based prediction systems to facilitate reliable, early identification of subclinical ILD states. Autoimmune conditions at risk for ILD could allow for novel insights into subclinical ILD states, including the identification of factors associated with the progression to clinically meaningful disease and, in time, could facilitate early intervention trials to alter the natural history of ILD.

Rates of Subclinical Interstitial Lung Disease in Autoimmune Disease States

Recently, 2 large RA cohorts were screened, prospectively, for the presence of sub-clinical ILD via high-resolution cross-sectional chest imaging.[60,61] These 2 studies identified subclinical ILD in 21% and 18% of the screened patients with RA, respectively. Both studies found associations between subclinical ILD and the previously discussed *MUC5B* promoter polymorphism that is a primary genetic risk factor for IPF and clinical RA-ILD.[37,62] Estimates of lifetime risk for the development of clinical ILD within RA cohorts vary but typically they are thought to be between 5% and 10%.[1,63]

SSc cohorts without known lung disease have also undergone prospective evaluation for subclinical ILD via high-resolution cross-sectional computed tomography (CT) chest imaging.[64–66] Although the methods differ in these 3 studies, the primary takeaway is that SSc cohorts have high rates of subclinical ILD when screened (as high as 197/305 with 1 to >20% fibrosis on CT chest from Hoffman-Vold and colleagues[64]).

Additionally, a large, pooled analysis of a national cohort of patients with many autoimmune diseases including SSc, antisynthetase syndrome, mixed-CTD was screened for the presence of subclinical ILD and found that 67/525 (13%) of patients with autoimmune diseases had radiographic evidence of subclinical ILD.[67] Recent expert consensus statements were published regarding screening for ILD and early intervention within SSc populations, which will be an important step toward understanding these important questions.[9,68]

A more exhaustive discussion of all observational data in subclinical CTD-ILD is beyond the scope of this review; however, these prospective studies highlight one very important principle: subclinical ILD is common in autoimmune disease states and is readily identifiable via HRCT scans of the chest.

Screening in Autoimmune Disease

Although data have been presented in this review of subclinical ILD rates in autoimmune disease, there remains no clear data to guide the *clinical* utility of screening in autoimmune disease, that is to say, there remains no clear proven benefit to identifying subclinical ILD in this population. One might surmise that an early intervention in these states would be beneficial; however, this remains only a hypothesis without clinical data to support this decision. As highlighted in the treatment section of this review, there are only 4 RCTs of therapy in CTD-ILD and none of those 4 are focused on a subclinical state. The same is true in the field of pulmonary fibrosis or ILD writ large, where no interventional trials have been undertaken in preclinical or subclinical states.

Therefore, for now, the primary utility of approaching subclinical states of ILD in autoimmunity remains within the realm of translational and clinical research. However, there are several reasons highlighted in this review, which point out the potential benefits of ongoing research in this field, which could even translate beyond autoimmune disease into all realms of subclinical ILD.

RESEARCH AGENDA

In recent years, there have been many important advances in our understanding of CTD-ILD pathogenesis and clinical management but there remain many gaps in this area that need further study. The authors of this review think that the following areas of research focus during the coming years are likely to have the biggest impact on the field and the biggest impact on patient outcomes.

- Establish clinical screening and monitoring guidelines for CTD-ILD such that patients can be identified at the earliest stage of disease.
- Understand the pathogenesis of subclinical ILD such that patients can be identified who are most likely to benefit from earlier treatment.
- Identify shared and distinct pathogenic pathways across CTD-ILDs such that therapeutics targeting disease-specific pathways can improve the efficacy of CTD-ILD treatments.

SUMMARY

ILD is a common manifestation of several autoimmune diseases, and its association with poor quality of life and mortality warrant further study that can lead to more effective screening and treatment. There have been advances in the treatment of CTD-ILD in recent years but many unanswered questions remain. The pathogenesis of CTD-ILDs likely have both shared and distinct pathways, and understanding how genetics, environmental factors, and immune responses in each CTD contribute to ILD development will likely improve our understanding of pathogenesis and the effectiveness of our treatments for patients with CTD-ILD.

CLINICS CARE POINTS

- Prevalent ILD and ILD prognosis are associated with disease activity scores in CTD; therefore, a pillar of effective CTD-ILD treatment management remains adequate baseline DMARD treatment to control primary CTD manifestations.

- Methotrexate neither causes fibrotic ILD nor does it exacerbate the underlying ILD in RA; therefore, it is safe to continue as an effective DMARD in patients with adequate disease control.

- Added immunosuppression or alterations of the immunosuppression regimen for new ILD manifestations (or ILD progression) in patients with underlying autoimmune disease should be carefully considered between pulmonary and rheumatology physicians with experience balancing these entities.

- Three therapies have randomized, placebo-controlled level evidence in SSc-ILD, which supports their safety, improvement in lung function over placebo, and, in the case of mycophenolate and cyclophosphamide, improvement in health-related quality of life (mycophenolate, cyclophosphamide, and tocilizumab).

- Antifibrotic therapy seems to have a role as adjunctive therapy for patients with CTD-ILD with progressive fibrotic features in patients with adequate CTD disease activity control.

- There are high rates of subclinical ILD in autoimmune disease populations but there remains unclear clinical benefit to early intervention in screened populations.
- Randomized, placebo-controlled studies are urgently needed in both subclinical and clinical CTD-ILD with fibrotic features to determine the safety of added immunosuppression and to determine the clinical efficacy of early intervention in subclinical ILD states.

DECLARATION OF INTERESTS

S.M. Matson is supported by P20GM130423 and the Joseph A. Cates Pulmonary Fibrosis Research fund at the University of Kansas Medical Center. M.K. Demoruelle has investigator-initiated research funding from Pfizer, United States and Boehringer Ingelheim, United States.

REFERENCES

1. Bongartz T, Nannini C, Medina-Velasquez YF, et al. Incidence and mortality of interstitial lung disease in rheumatoid arthritis: a population-based study. Arthritis Rheum 2010;62:1583–91.
2. Hoffmann-Vold AM, Fretheim H, Halse AK, et al. Tracking impact of interstitial lung disease in systemic sclerosis in a complete nationwide cohort. Am J Respir Crit Care Med 2019;200:1258–66.
3. Marie I, Hachulla E, Cherin P, et al. Interstitial lung disease in polymyositis and dermatomyositis. Arthritis Rheum 2002;47:614–22.
4. Park JH, Kim DS, Park IN, et al. Prognosis of fibrotic interstitial pneumonia: idiopathic versus collagen vascular disease-related subtypes. Am J Respir Crit Care Med 2007;175:705–11.
5. Solomon JJ, Ryu JH, Tazelaar HD, et al. Fibrosing interstitial pneumonia predicts survival in patients with rheumatoid arthritis-associated interstitial lung disease (RA-ILD). Respir Med 2013;107:1247–52.
6. Solomon JJ, Chung JH, Cosgrove GP, et al. Predictors of mortality in rheumatoid arthritis-associated interstitial lung disease. Eur Respir J 2016;47:588–96.
7. Fujisawa T, Hozumi H, Kono M, et al. Prognostic factors for myositis-associated interstitial lung disease. PLoS One 2014;9:e98824.
8. Volkmann ER, Tashkin DP, Sim M, et al. Short-term progression of interstitial lung disease in systemic sclerosis predicts long-term survival in two independent clinical trial cohorts. Ann Rheum Dis 2019;78:122–30.
9. Hoffmann-Vold A-M, Maher TM, Philpot EE, et al. The identification and management of interstitial lung disease in systemic sclerosis: evidence-based European consensus statements. The Lancet Rheumatology 2020;2:e71–83.
10. Raghu G, Remy-Jardin M, Richeldi L, et al. Idiopathic pulmonary fibrosis (an update) and progressive pulmonary fibrosis in adults: an official ATS/ERS/JRS/ALAT clinical practice guideline. Am J Respir Crit Care Med 2022;205:e18–47.
11. Fraenkel L, Bathon JM, England BR, et al. 2021 American college of rheumatology guideline for the treatment of rheumatoid arthritis. Arthritis Rheumatol 2021;73:1108–23.
12. Cannon GW, Ward JR, Clegg DO, et al. Acute lung disease associated with low-dose pulse methotrexate therapy in patients with rheumatoid arthritis. Arthritis Rheum 1983;26:1269–74.
13. Juge P-A, Lee JS, Lau J, et al. Methotrexate and rheumatoid arthritis associated interstitial lung disease. Eur Respir J 2020;57(2):2000337.

14. Mehta P, Redhead G, Nair A, et al. Can we finally exonerate methotrexate as a factor in causing or exacerbating fibrotic interstitial lung disease in patients with rheumatoid arthritis? Clin Rheumatol 2022;41:2925–8.

15. Schnabel A, Richter C, Bauerfeind S, et al. Bronchoalveolar lavage cell profile in methotrexate induced pneumonitis. Thorax 1997;52:377–9.

16. Nakashita T, Ando K, Kaneko N, et al. Potential risk of TNF inhibitors on the progression of interstitial lung disease in patients with rheumatoid arthritis. BMJ Open 2014;4:e005615.

17. Wolfe F, Caplan L, Michaud K. Rheumatoid arthritis treatment and the risk of severe interstitial lung disease. Scand J Rheumatol 2007;36:172–8.

18. Huang Y, Lin W, Chen Z, et al. Effect of tumor necrosis factor inhibitors on interstitial lung disease in rheumatoid arthritis: angel or demon? Drug Des Dev Ther 2019;13:2111–25.

19. Panopoulos ST, Sfikakis PP. Biological treatments and connective tissue disease associated interstitial lung disease. Curr Opin Pulm Med 2011;17:362–7.

20. Rojas-Serrano J, Mejía M, Rivera-Matias PA, et al. Rheumatoid arthritis-related interstitial lung disease (RA-ILD): a possible association between disease activity and prognosis. Clin Rheumatol 2022;41:1741–7.

21. Sparks JA, He X, Huang J, et al. Rheumatoid arthritis disease activity predicting incident clinically apparent rheumatoid arthritis-associated interstitial lung disease: a prospective cohort study. Arthritis Rheumatol 2019;71:1472–82.

22. Khanna D, Lin CJF, Furst DE, et al. Tocilizumab in systemic sclerosis: a randomised, double-blind, placebo-controlled, phase 3 trial. Lancet Respir Med 2020;8:963–74.

23. Tashkin DP, Elashoff R, Clements PJ, et al. Cyclophosphamide versus placebo in scleroderma lung disease. N Engl J Med 2006;354:2655–66.

24. Tashkin DP, Roth MD, Clements PJ, et al. Mycophenolate mofetil versus oral cyclophosphamide in scleroderma-related interstitial lung disease (SLS II): a randomised controlled, double-blind, parallel group trial. Lancet Respir Med 2016;4:708–19.

25. Raghu G, Anstrom KJ, King TE Jr, et al. Prednisone, azathioprine, and N-acetylcysteine for pulmonary fibrosis. N Engl J Med 2012;366:1968–77.

26. Matson S, Lee J, Eickelberg O. Two sides of the same coin? A review of the similarities and differences between idiopathic pulmonary fibrosis and rheumatoid arthritis associated interstitial lung disease. Eur Respir J 2021;57(5):2002533.

27. Mukhopadhyay S. Usual interstitial pneumonia (UIP): a clinically significant pathologic diagnosis. Mod Pathol 2022;35:580–8.

28. Richeldi L, du Bois RM, Raghu G, et al. Efficacy and safety of nintedanib in idiopathic pulmonary fibrosis. N Engl J Med 2014;370:2071–82.

29. King TE Jr, Bradford WZ, Castro-Bernardini S, et al. A phase 3 trial of pirfenidone in patients with idiopathic pulmonary fibrosis. N Engl J Med 2014;370:2083–92.

30. Distler O, Highland KB, Gahlemann M, et al. Nintedanib for systemic sclerosis-associated interstitial lung disease. N Engl J Med 2019;380:2518–28.

31. Solomon JJ, Danoff SK, Woodhead FA, et al. Safety, tolerability, and efficacy of pirfenidone in patients with rheumatoid arthritis-associated interstitial lung disease: a randomised, double-blind, placebo-controlled, phase 2 study. Lancet Respir Med 2023;11(1):87–96.

32. Flaherty KR, Wells AU, Cottin V, et al. Nintedanib in progressive fibrosing interstitial lung diseases. N Engl J Med 2019;381:1718–27.

33. Wuyts WA, Agostini C, Antoniou KM, et al. The pathogenesis of pulmonary fibrosis: a moving target. Eur Respir J 2013;41:1207–18.

34. Laurent GJ, McAnulty RJ, Hill M, et al. Escape from the matrix: multiple mechanisms for fibroblast activation in pulmonary fibrosis. Proc Am Thorac Soc 2008; 5:311–5.
35. Juge PA, Lee JS, Ebstein E, et al. MUC5B promoter variant and rheumatoid arthritis with interstitial lung disease. N Engl J Med 2018;379:2209–19.
36. Palomaki A, FinnGen Rheumatology Clinical Expert G, Palotie A, et al. Lifetime risk of rheumatoid arthritis-associated interstitial lung disease in MUC5B mutation carriers. Ann Rheum Dis 2021;80:1530–6.
37. Seibold MA, Wise AL, Speer MC, et al. A common MUC5B promoter polymorphism and pulmonary fibrosis. N Engl J Med 2011;364:1503–12.
38. Shao T, Shi X, Yang S, et al. Interstitial lung disease in connective tissue disease: a common lesion with heterogeneous mechanisms and treatment considerations. Front Immunol 2021;12:684699.
39. Doyle TJ, Patel AS, Hatabu H, et al. Detection of Rheumatoid Arthritis-Interstitial Lung Disease Is Enhanced by Serum Biomarkers. Am J Respir Crit Care Med 2015;191:1403–12.
40. Kelly CA, Saravanan V, Nisar M, et al. British Rheumatoid Interstitial Lung N. Rheumatoid arthritis-related interstitial lung disease: associations, prognostic factors and physiological and radiological characteristics–a large multicentre UK study. Rheumatology 2014;53:1676–82.
41. Nihtyanova SI, Schreiber BE, Ong VH, et al. Prediction of pulmonary complications and long-term survival in systemic sclerosis. Arthritis Rheumatol 2014;66: 1625–35.
42. Zhang L, Wu G, Gao D, et al. Factors associated with interstitial lung disease in patients with polymyositis and dermatomyositis: a systematic review and meta-analysis. PLoS One 2016;11:e0155381.
43. Nihtyanova SI, Sari A, Harvey JC, et al. Using Autoantibodies and Cutaneous Subset to Develop Outcome-Based Disease Classification in Systemic Sclerosis. Arthritis Rheumatol 2020;72:465–76.
44. Khanna D, Tashkin DP, Denton CP, et al. Etiology, risk factors, and biomarkers in systemic sclerosis with interstitial lung disease. Am J Respir Crit Care Med 2020; 201:650–60.
45. Teel A, Lu J, Park J, et al. The role of myositis-specific autoantibodies and the management of interstitial lung disease in idiopathic inflammatory myopathies: a systematic review. Semin Arthritis Rheum 2022;57:152088.
46. Giles JT, Darrah E, Danoff S, et al. Association of cross-reactive antibodies targeting peptidyl-arginine deiminase 3 and 4 with rheumatoid arthritis-associated interstitial lung disease. PLoS One 2014;9:e98794.
47. Brinkmann V, Reichard U, Goosmann C, et al. Neutrophil extracellular traps kill bacteria. Science 2004;303:1532–5.
48. Kuley R, Stultz RD, Duvvuri B, et al. N-Formyl methionine peptide-mediated neutrophil activation in systemic sclerosis. Front Immunol 2021;12:785275.
49. Khandpur R, Carmona-Rivera C, Vivekanandan-Giri A, et al. NETs are a source of citrullinated autoantigens and stimulate inflammatory responses in rheumatoid arthritis. Sci Transl Med 2013;5:178ra140.
50. Seto N, Torres-Ruiz JJ, Carmona-Rivera C, et al. Neutrophil dysregulation is pathogenic in idiopathic inflammatory myopathies. JCI Insight 2020;5(3):e134189.
51. Saffarzadeh M, Juenemann C, Queisser MA, et al. Neutrophil extracellular traps directly induce epithelial and endothelial cell death: a predominant role of histones. PLoS One 2012;7:e32366.

52. Chrysanthopoulou A, Mitroulis I, Apostolidou E, et al. Neutrophil extracellular traps promote differentiation and function of fibroblasts. J Pathol 2014;233: 294–307.
53. Zhang S, Jia X, Zhang Q, et al. Neutrophil extracellular traps activate lung fibroblast to induce polymyositis-related interstitial lung diseases via TLR9-miR-7-Smad2 pathway. J Cell Mol Med 2020;24(2):1658–69.
54. Carmona-Rivera C, Zhao W, Yalavarthi S, et al. Neutrophil extracellular traps induce endothelial dysfunction in systemic lupus erythematosus through the activation of matrix metalloproteinase-2. Ann Rheum Dis 2015;74:1417–24.
55. Takemasa A, Ishii Y, Fukuda T. A neutrophil elastase inhibitor prevents bleomycin-induced pulmonary fibrosis in mice. Eur Respir J 2012;40:1475–82.
56. Okamoto Y, Devoe S, Seto N, et al. Association of Sputum Neutrophil Extracellular Trap Subsets With IgA Anti-Citrullinated Protein Antibodies in Subjects at Risk for Rheumatoid Arthritis. Arthritis Rheumatol 2022;74:38–48.
57. Kinder BW, Brown KK, Schwarz MI, et al. Baseline BAL neutrophilia predicts early mortality in idiopathic pulmonary fibrosis. Chest 2008;133:226–32.
58. Gerlag DM, Safy M, Maijer KI, et al. Effects of B-cell directed therapy on the preclinical stage of rheumatoid arthritis: the PRAIRI study. Ann Rheum Dis 2019;78: 179–85.
59. Krijbolder DI, Verstappen M, van Dijk BT, et al. Intervention with methotrexate in patients with arthralgia at risk of rheumatoid arthritis to reduce the development of persistent arthritis and its disease burden (TREAT EARLIER): a randomised, double-blind, placebo-controlled, proof-of-concept trial. Lancet (London, England) 2022;400:283–94.
60. Matson SM, Deane KD, Peljto AL, et al. Prospective Identification of Subclinical Interstitial Lung Disease in Rheumatoid Arthritis Cohort is Associated with the MUC5B Promoter Variant. Am J Respir Crit Care Med 2022;205(4):473–6.
61. Juge PA, Granger B, Debray MP, et al. A risk score to detect subclinical rheumatoid arthritis-associated interstitial lung disease. Arthritis Rheumatol 2022;74(11): 1755–65.
62. Juge PA, Borie R, Kannengiesser C, et al. Shared genetic predisposition in rheumatoid arthritis-interstitial lung disease and familial pulmonary fibrosis. Eur Respir J 2017;49(5):1602314.
63. Turesson C, O'Fallon WM, Crowson CS, et al. Extra-articular disease manifestations in rheumatoid arthritis: incidence trends and risk factors over 46 years. Ann Rheum Dis 2003;62:722–7.
64. Hoffmann-Vold AM, Aaløkken TM, Lund MB, et al. Predictive value of serial high-resolution computed tomography analyses and concurrent lung function tests in systemic sclerosis. Arthritis Rheumatol 2015;67:2205–12.
65. Launay D, Remy-Jardin M, Michon-Pasturel U, et al. High resolution computed tomography in fibrosing alveolitis associated with systemic sclerosis. J Rheumatol 2006;33:1789–801.
66. Reyes-Long S, Gutierrez M, Clavijo-Cornejo D, et al. Subclinical interstitial lung disease in patients with systemic sclerosis. A pilot study on the role of ultrasound. Reumatol Clínica 2021;17:144–9.
67. Hoffmann-Vold AM, Andersson H, Reiseter S, et al. Subclinical ILD is frequent and progresses across different connective tissue diseases. Eur Respir J 2021; 58:OA2973.
68. Rahaghi FF, Hsu VM, Kaner RJ, et al. Expert consensus on the management of systemic sclerosis-associated interstitial lung disease. Respir Res 2023;24:6.

69. Suissa S, Hudson M, Ernst P. Leflunomide use and the risk of interstitial lung disease in rheumatoid arthritis. Arthritis Rheum 2006;54:1435–9.
70. Perez-Alvarez R, Perez-de-Lis M, Diaz-Lagares C, et al. Interstitial lung disease induced or exacerbated by TNF-targeted therapies: analysis of 122 cases. Semin Arthritis Rheum 2011;41:256–64.
71. Tomioka R, King TE Jr. Gold-induced pulmonary disease: clinical features, outcome, and differentiation from rheumatoid lung disease. Am J Respir Crit Care Med 1997;155:1011–20.
72. Goodwin SD, Glenny RW. Nonsteroidal anti-inflammatory drug-associated pulmonary infiltrates with eosinophilia. Review of the literature and Food and Drug Administration adverse drug reaction reports. Arch Intern Med 1992;152:1521–4.
73. Parry SD, Barbatzas C, Peel ET, et al. Sulphasalazine and lung toxicity. Eur Respir J 2002;19:756–64.
74. Cassone G, Manfredi A, Vacchi C, et al. Treatment of rheumatoid arthritis-associated interstitial lung disease: lights and shadows. J Clin Med 2020;9:1082.
75. Oldham JM, Lee C, Valenzi E, et al. Azathioprine response in patients with fibrotic connective tissue disease-associated interstitial lung disease. Respir Med 2016;121:117–22.
76. Md Yusof MY, Kabia A, Darby M, et al. Effect of rituximab on the progression of rheumatoid arthritis-related interstitial lung disease: 10 years' experience at a single centre. Rheumatology 2017;56:1348–57.
77. Mena-Vázquez N, Rojas-Gimenez M, Fuego-Varela C, et al. Safety and effectiveness of abatacept in a prospective cohort of patients with rheumatoid arthritis-associated interstitial lung disease. Respir Med 2019;154:6–11.
78. Huapaya JA, Hallowell R, Silhan L, et al. Long-term treatment with human immunoglobulin for antisynthetase syndrome-associated interstitial lung disease. Respir Med 2019;154:6–11.
79. Witt LJ, Demchuk C, Curran JJ, et al. Benefit of adjunctive tacrolimus in connective tissue disease-interstitial lung disease. Pulm Pharmacol Ther 2016;36:46–52.
80. Volkmann ER, Tashkin DP, LeClair H, et al. Treatment with mycophenolate and cyclophosphamide leads to clinically meaningful improvements in patient-reported outcomes in scleroderma lung disease: results of scleroderma lung study II. ACR Open Rheumatol 2020;2:362–70.

Hypersensitivity Pneumonitis

Updates in Evaluation, Management, and Ongoing Dilemmas

Sahil M. Pandya, MD, FCCP[a],*, Aarti P. Pandya, MD[b],
Daffolyn Rachael Fels Elliott, MD, PhD, FRCPC[c],
Mark J. Hamblin, MD, FCCP[a]

KEYWORDS

- Hypersensitivity pneumonitis • Fibrotic • Lymphocytosis • Interstitial lung disease
- Exposure

KEY POINTS

- Hypersensitivity pneumonitis (HP) requires thorough exposure evaluation to assess pre-test probability, establish radiologic correlates, and determine the role of pathologic data.
- The utility of bronchoalveolar lavage lymphocytosis in fibrotic HP remains a dilemma and may add value in atypical cases.
- Immunomodulation may have a role in early disease modification but requires serial assessment to balance risk and benefit of ongoing treatment.
- Identifying advanced fibrotic phenotypes (progressive decline, honeycombing, usual interstitial pneumonia pattern) may signal early introduction of antifibrotic therapy given similar clinical trajectories to idiopathic pulmonary fibrosis.

INTRODUCTION

Hypersensitivity pneumonitis (HP) is a heterogenous disease entity characterized by an aberrant immune response to inhalational antigens. Pathologically, the pulmonary interstitium encompasses the alveolar epithelium, capillary endothelium, basement membrane, peri lymphatic, and perivascular tissues.[1] Radiographically, it is divided into the axial (bronchovascular tree adjacent), parenchymal, and peripheral (pleura adjacent) zones.[2] Given the spectrum of inflammatory immune response and fibrotic cascade in severe cases, patients can be affected at all pathologic and radiographic zones. Disease modification hinges on early antigen remediation with a goal to atten-uate immune dysregulation. Disease severity and progression are mediated by an

[a] University of Kansas Medical Center, 4000 Cambridge Street, Mail Stop 3007, Kansas City, KS 66160, USA; [b] Children's Mercy Hospital, 3101 Broadway Boulevard, Kansas City, MO 64111, USA; [c] University of Kansas Medical Center, 3901 Rainbow Boulevard, Mail Stop 3045, Kansas City, KS 66160, USA
* Corresponding author.
E-mail address: Spandya2@kumc.edu

Immunol Allergy Clin N Am 43 (2023) 245–257
https://doi.org/10.1016/j.iac.2023.01.011
0889-8561/23/Published by Elsevier Inc.
immunology.theclinics.com

interface between degree, type and chronicity of exposure, genetic predisposition, and biochemical properties of the inducing agent.[3]

EPIDEMIOLOGY

The incidence and prevalence of HP is variable based on geographic location, local industry, and practices that can create environmental culprits.[4] Given that HP is often misdiagnosed,[5] true incidence and prevalence is likely underreported. In the United States yearly incidence approaches 1.7 to 2.7 per 100,000. Japanese data report an incidence 0.3 to 0.9 per 100,000 yearly. In the United Kingdom, data approximate 0.9 per 100,000.[6] These data capture heterogenous populations; therefore, incidence in specific regions (eg, farming communities, areas of heavy rain) may be much higher.[7]

PATHOGENESIS
Immune Response

HP results from an abnormal cell-mediated or humoral immune response to antigens. Antigens derived from organic matter can be avian, vegetable, grains, bacterial, or fungal in origin. Antigens from inorganic matter can include haptens derived from isocyanates, zinc, nickel, and so forth. These haptens can complex with human serum albumin to become antigens that will trigger the pathogenesis in HP. In acute HP, the patient will develop immunoglobulin G (IgG) antibodies to an antigen; this can lead to the development of immune complex formation, resulting in direct complement activation and recruitment of macrophages that will secrete neutrophil recruiting cytokines including CXCL8, CCL5, and CCL3.[8] Macrophages also secrete CCL18, which can recruit lymphocytes to the alveoli. Neutrophils, through their released mediators, lead to tissue damage and fibrosis. In addition, apoptosis of lymphocytes is inhibited and can lead to alveolar lymphocytosis. Chronic HP occurs largely from CD4+ Th1, Th2, and Th17 lymphocytes. Th1 and Th17 lymphocytes promote lung inflammation. A Th2 response skewing can also occur in later stages of HP.

When exposed to antigens causing HP, most individuals develop immune tolerance. Inhalation can lead to alveolar lymphocytosis without development of an inflammatory response. Therefore the "two-hit" hypothesis has been proposed for individuals who develop disease.[9]

Genetics

Each case of HP carries significant interpatient variability in both clinical symptoms and radiographic manifestations. This variability is a complex interaction between inciting antigen and genetic predisposition. Often, patients with the same degree and duration of antigen exposure experience marked differences in severity.[10] Shortened telomere length is one genetic feature that has been shown to worsen survival in patients with HP and is associated with an increased presence of radiographic and pathologic fibrosis.[11] The MUC5B polymorphism is associated with traction bronchiectasis and fibrotic changes,[12] and telomere-related genes (TERT, RTEL1, PARN) have been associated with worse transplant-free survival. Screening for features of short telomere syndrome (familial pulmonary fibrosis, premature graying, aplastic anemia, cryptogenic cirrhosis, myelodysplasia/leukemia) is crucial to early identification of progressive phenotypes.[13]

CLINICAL CHARACTERISTICS
History and Diagnosis

The diagnosis of HP assumes an initial insult in the form of antigen exposure. Despite established diagnostic criteria, nearly 50% of cases fail to have an exposure identified.[3,14,15] With insidious, continuous exposures, patients experience disease progression with transition to difficult to control inflammation and fibrosis.[16,17] The consequences of unidentified exposures are seen by the differences in median survival between these 2 cohorts (8.75 years vs 4.9 years for those without identified antigen).[14,18] The removal of a single antigen may not be sufficient to slow disease progression if multiple inciting agents exist. This lack of clarity has a significant impact on efficacy of therapy, prognosis, risk of relapse, and symptom control.[19]

Multiple questionnaires exist for history assessment with varying degrees of validity. The presence of an exposure heavily affects management strategy, even in the absence of radiographic and laboratory correlates. The converse scenario, in which the radiographic features suggest HP in the absence of identified exposure, creates low confidence in a suspected diagnosis.[3,17,20]

Barnes and colleagues[20] performed a Delphi assessment to characterize interclinician agreement on most common inciting antigens. Highest confidence exposures were grouped into 3 major categories: microbial particulate matter (water and mold based), plant/animal proteins (avian), and chemical agents. Jenkins and colleagues[21] demonstrated via retrospective review that serum IgG had high sensitivity and specificity to distinguish those with HP from healthy exposed and unexposed individuals. Serum IgG was not helpful to distinguish HP from other non-HP interstitial lung diseases (ILDs).

Imaging Features

The ATS/JRS/ALAT guidelines have classified HP into 2 categories: nonfibrotic and fibrotic.[3] Nonfibrotic HP represents an inflammatory profile with diffuse distribution of the parenchyma and interstitium (ground glass opacities). This definition requires radiographic evidence of small airway involvement, which includes inspiratory centrilobular nodules and expiratory air trapping. Nonfibrotic HP demonstrates areas of lobular mosaic attenuation, representing areas of pneumonitis in affected lobules neighboring unaffected lobules with normal attenuation.[3,22] Chung and colleagues[23] demonstrated that the presence of air trapping and mosaic attenuation conferred a reduced risk of mortality regardless of the presence of fibrosis. This raises the hypothesis that these features signal ongoing immune dysregulation that may be responsive to immunomodulation. In some cases, airspace consolidation/organizing pneumonia and cysts can be appreciated.

Fibrotic HP has features of architectural distortion including coarse or fine reticulation, traction bronchiectasis, and septal thickening in the background of ground glass opacities.[3,24,25] In severe cases, honeycombing can be seen. Salisbury and colleagues[26] compared radiographic phenotypes to predict clinical trajectory and transplant-free survival. They found that the presence of honeycombing conferred the worst prognosis and mirrored survival for honeycombing found in idiopathic pulmonary fibrosis (IPF). Patients with HP with nonhoneycomb fibrosis had intermediate survival that was an average of 2 years greater than those with IPF. Finally, the cohort with nonfibrotic HP had the best survival and greatest degree of forced vital capacity (FVC) improvement at 12 months. Mooney and colleagues[27] demonstrated that in nonusual interstitial pneumonia (UIP) patterns, with similar degrees of fibrosis, survival in HP was higher than those with IPF. UIP can be seen in fibrotic HP; however, Perez-Padilla and colleagues[28] compared bird exposed UIP patients and nonexposed UIP patients and found an identical survival time in these patients; this suggests that this cohort of patients with HP often follow a similar trajectory to those with IPF.

The Lymphocytosis Dilemma

The role of bronchioalveolar lavage (BAL) lymphocytosis has been a dilemma in the evaluation of HP. Nonfibrotic HP cases may show BAL lymphocyte counts greater than 60%, but elevated lymphocyte counts can be seen in other ILDs.[29] The absence of lymphocytosis in nonfibrotic disease lowers the probability enough to exclude the possibility of HP.

Fibrotic HP poses additional challenges related to BAL lymphocytosis. It should be noted that lymphocytosis is not reliably present even with pathologically confirmed fibrotic HP. Ohshimo and colleagues[30] demonstrated that in those with BAL lymphocytosis greater than 30% with a UIP pattern favors HP over IPF. De Sadeleer and colleagues[31] stratified survival in fibrotic HP with BAL lymphocytosis greater than 20% versus less than 20% and found improved survival in those in the former group. Adderley and colleagues[32] reported in a large, pooled estimate for BAL lymphocyte percentage from 42 studies that male sex, history of smoking, and age were independently associated with lower lymphocyte counts. In this meta-analysis the lymphocyte count was estimated at 42.8% for chronic HP, 23.4% in connective tissue disease-associated ILD (CTD-ILD), 31.2% in sarcoidosis, and 10.0% in IPF. Sensitivity and specificity vary depending on the threshold of BAL lymphocytosis used, as well as the main alternative diagnosis under consideration. Ultimately, higher thresholds of lymphocytosis have the potential to provide greater specificity at the cost of lower sensitivity.[32] A recent cohort analysis by Hill and colleagues[33] worked to eliminate incorporation bias in understanding the role of BAL lymphocytosis; this was attempted by choosing patients with high to moderate confidence in HP diagnosis without the incorporation of BAL lymphocytosis. It demonstrated that only 28% of fibrotic HP and 41% of nonfibrotic HP met consensus criteria for diagnostic BAL lymphocytosis. Consequently, the real value of BAL lymphocytosis depends on the pretest probability of HP. The CHEST HP guidelines recommend multidisciplinary discussion of exposures and high-resolution computed tomography (HRCT) pattern before considering BAL, and in patients with an exposure history and HRCT pattern typical for HP, BAL is unlikely to add additional diagnostic value.[34] In patients with fibrotic ILD, the absence of lymphocytosis does not exclude HP as a diagnostic consideration; thus lung biopsy should be considered.

Modality of Lung Biopsy

Transbronchial cryobiopsy (TBLC) and surgical lung biopsy (SLB) are considerations in patients with discordant radiographic and historical features. Obtaining lung tissue is most important when the diagnostic confidence from multidisciplinary discussion (MDD) is low. Studies have revealed in-hospital mortality as high as 1.7% associated with SLB.[35] These studies, however, analyze older studies that used the open surgical technique. In current practice, most surgical biopsies are completed via a video-assisted thoracoscopic approach, which carries one-third of the risk of open lung approach. Recent data suggest that high volume centers have lower risk of postoperative complications.[36,37] Factors that increase risk include age greater than 75 years, obesity, diffusion capacity for carbon monoxide (DLCO) less than 50%, and presence of pulmonary hypertension.[38] TBLC has average in-hospital mortality reported at 0.5% to 0.8% and can be performed on an outpatient basis.[39] The COLD-DICE data demonstrated high concordance between SLB and TBLC (95%) and showed that SLB did not add significant additional information during MDD.[40] The utility of cryobiopsy, when performed in a high-volume center, is in a patient who is at higher risk for surgical approach and carries low preprocedural diagnostic confidence.[41]

There has been increasing interest in the role of genomic classifiers because patients with a UIP pattern often follow a similar trajectory regardless of classification.[42] Results from the BRAVE study using the Envisia Genomic Classifier for unidentified interstitial lung disease showed that patients with a positive UIP result who received both corticosteroids and a nonsteroidal immunosuppressant showed a 1-year decline in FVC of 9.4% compared with a decline of 1.9% in patients not taking both ($P = .01$).[43] It should be noted that the study did not specifically look at patients with fibrotic HP but rather included a broad range of suspected fibrotic ILDs.

Pathology

According to the ATS/JRS/ALAT and CHEST guidelines, histopathological features are categorized into nonfibrotic and fibrotic HP.[3] Nonfibrotic (cellular) HP is characterized by a cellular interstitial pneumonia that begins in the peribronchiolar interstitium and may extend to diffusely involve the lung parenchyma. Nonfibrotic HP requires 3 major histologic features per ATS/JRS/ALAT guidelines: cellular interstitial pneumonia, cellular bronchiolitis, and poorly formed nonnecrotizing granulomas. The CHEST guidelines add a fourth criterion that the inflammatory infiltrate should be predominantly composed of lymphocytes.[44] Both guidelines require absence of additional features that suggest an alternative diagnosis, including excessive plasma cells or lymphoid hyperplasia that is often seen in CTD-ILD. Other granulomatous lung diseases that can mimic HP histologically (**Fig. 1, Table 1**) include granulomatous infections (especially atypical mycobacterial or fungal), sarcoidosis, chronic aspiration, adverse drug reaction, common variable immunodeficiency, and Crohn disease manifestations in the lung.

Typical fibrotic HP also requires 3 major features per both guidelines[3,44]: chronic fibrosing interstitial pneumonia, airway-centered fibrosis, and poorly formed nonnecrotizing granulomas. Similar to the radiographic dilemmas that arise, the analysis of histopathology is often used to differentiate predominantly fibrotic processes from ongoing inflammatory processes that can be modified with immunomodulatory therapy. Grunes and colleagues[45] demonstrated that bridging fibrosis (areas between bronchioles and lobular septa) and peribronchiolar metaplasia are key findings to assist in differentiation between IPF and fibrotic HP. Inflammation is airway centered and can often have associated lymphocytic infiltration, organizing pneumonia, and multinucleated giant cells.

MANAGEMENT
Environmental Testing/Remediation

Regardless of fibrotic or nonfibrotic disease, identification of the inciting antigen is a key part of management.[18] Unfortunately, this can be challenging detective work. The source of exposure may come from the home, workplace, a secondary home, a

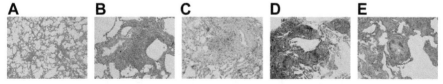

Fig. 1. Pathologic mimics of hypersensitivity pneumonitis. (*A*) At low magnification, a chronic inflammatory infiltrate expands the interstitium with accentuation around bronchioles (*stars*) in hypersensitivity pneumonitis. (*B*) A loose aggregate of epithelioid histiocytes adjacent to a bronchiole in hypersensitivity pneumonitis. (*C*) A tight cluster of multinucleated giant cells and epithelioid histiocytes adjacent to a blood vessel in sarcoidosis. (*D*) Clusters of multinucleated giant cells associated with an interstitial chronic inflammatory infiltrate in drug-induced lung injury due to sulfasalazine. (*E*) Foreign-body giant cells surround an organic particulate in chronic aspiration (200X magnification, hematoxylin and eosin [H&E] stain).

Table 1
Pathologic mimics of hypersensitivity pneumonitis

Histologic Feature	HP	Granulomatous Infection	Sarcoidosis	Chronic Aspiration	Adverse Drug Reaction
Granulomas (distribution)	Poorly-formed, nonnecrotizing (peribronchiolar interstitium)	Well-formed, often necrotizing (peribronchiolar interstitium and airspaces)	Well-formed, coalescing, rarely necrotizing (lymphangitic interstitium)	Foreign-body giant cells, aspirated particulates (peribronchiolar airspaces)	Poorly formed, nonnecrotizing (interstitium and airspaces)
Interstitial pneumonia	Characteristic airway-centered	Focal	Absent	Absent	Common, may be diffuse
Fibrosis	Airway-centered, peribronchiolar metaplasia	Uncommon localized fibrosis may be present in chronic infection	Hyalinizing, lymphangitic distribution	Airway-centered, peribronchiolar metaplasia	Variable
Organizing pneumonia	Common, focal	Common, may be prominent	Absent	Common, may have fibrinous exudate with neutrophils	Common, may be prominent

frequently visited family member, church, place of recreation, or it may even be an industrial or local agricultural operation. For many ILD specialists, this in-depth exposure tracking is routine but may take several visits to identify an occult exposure.

Commercially available mold test kits may be a fiscally reasonable option but using an environmental hygienist to assess quantitative mold levels may be more likely to lead to identification.[46] Even this professional level of assessment may miss a hidden exposure, later uncovered during a home renovation, proving just how challenging this aspect of management can be.

Immunosuppression

In a patient with mild disease, antigen remediation may be the only necessary intervention. However, for patients with respiratory compromise, pharmacologic therapy is advisable, but with no established treatment algorithm. Corticosteroid therapy provides short-term efficacy, specifically in terms of DLCO in the first month of treatment.[31] Sustained impact on lung stabilization and symptom improvement has never been reliably demonstrated.[47] Retrospective studies have shown improvement in lung function (FVC, DLCO) after a year of treatment with mycophenolate mofetil (MMF) or azathioprine (AZA).[48–50] However, a retrospective study evaluating fibrotic HP outcomes with immunosuppressive agents found no difference in lung function decline or survival when treated with AZA or MMF plus prednisone versus prednisone alone.[51] Immunosuppressives added on to prednisone did change the slope of FVC decline, but patients receiving any immunosuppressive therapy, as compared with those who were not treated with medications, had worse FVC decline over 36 months (-10.0% vs -1.3%, $P = .042$). Rituximab has also been seen in a small retrospective study to stabilize or improve FVC and DLCO in select patients.[52,53] The decision for immunomodulation hinges on the goal for early modification in the context of aggressive disease while weighing risk and benefit ratio of treatment-related side effects.

Hypersensitivity Pneumonitis with a Progressive Pulmonary Fibrosis Phenotype

Currently no guidelines outline the management of fibrotic HP.[25] Many radiographic phenotypes demonstrate similar clinical trajectories, raising the question whether advanced fibrotic disease requires differentiation in treatment strategies. Honeycombing in fibrotic HP, for example, follows a similar mortality curve to UIP in IPF.[24,26,27,54] Therefore, treating these 2 processes similarly is a therapeutic consideration. The INBUILD trial demonstrated reduction in rate of FVC decline for progressive disease other than IPF with the addition of nintedanib.[55] This effect was consistent despite baseline ILD diagnosis with 26% of patient previously diagnosed with fibrotic HP, and a follow-up subgroup analysis confirmed the beneficial effect of nintedanib on HP (PMID: 32145830). This ultimatley has led to the update in the progressive pulmonary fibrosis guidelines that assist with identification of rapidly progressive phenoptyes that may benefit from early introduction of anti-fibrotic therapies.

Pirfenidone has also been considered for use in fibrotic HP, with small retrospective studies demonstrating decreased rate of FVC decline at 6 months compared with placebo.[56] Mateos-Toledo and colleagues[57] demonstrated small improvement in quality-of-life outcomes with addition of pirfenidone to corticosteroid therapy over addition of azathioprine. Unfortunately, nature of this disease process is aggressive, and small observational cohort studies have demonstrated significant decline in FVC and DLCO despite antifibrotic therapy at 3 years.[58]

Many HP cases display a mix of fibrotic and nonfibrotic disease clouding the management algorithm and raising the question of whether to consider combination

Table 2
Clinical dilemmas in hypersensitivity pneumonitis

Clinical Question	Associated Considerations
Treatment of HP in the absence of antigen exposure	• Nearly 50% of cases of clinical HP are without distinctly identified antigen • Immune dysregulation may accelerate inflammation that can become difficult to control without early intervention • Treatment carries significant side effects and requires an individualized approach
Role of BAL lymphocytosis	• The presence of lymphocytosis has the potential to have prognostic significance; however, the thresholds to provide discriminatory power remains with variable sensitivity, specificity, and predictive value • Fibrotic HP often demonstrates lower degree of lymphocytosis, and its absence does not rule out HP as a diagnosis • Will BAL change posttest probability of decision for treatment?
Modality of tissue biopsy	• In-hospital mortality of surgical lung biopsy reported as high as 1.7%—however, these studies included open lung approach that does not reflect most of the current practices • Transbronchial biopsy may be an additional consideration for higher risk patients and has been shown to have high concordance with surgical lung biopsy in high volume centers • Genomic classifier may identify UIP patterns that deserve earlier antifibrotic therapy over immunosuppression
Choice of adjunct therapy	• Patients who receive immunosuppression have worse survival than those who do not—does immunosuppression change the clinical trajectory? • Does early transition to immunosuppressive therapy reduce treatment emergent adverse events?
Role of antifibrotic therapy	• Advanced fibrotic disease often shares a similar clinical trajectory to IPF—should we treat the same? • Role of dual immunosuppressive and antifibrotic therapy with mixed inflammatory and fibrotic phenotypes

immunosuppression and antifibrotic therapy. Future studies will be needed to help define optimal management.

Lung transplant evaluation should be completed early to optimize eligibility for listing. Patients with HP have better medium-term outcomes and reduced risk for death relative to IPF.[59] Long-term oxygen therapy should be used to prevent resting hypoxemia with adjunct exertional oxygen to assist with exertional capacity. Screening for group 3 pulmonary hypertension is an important prognostic factor, as survival curves in fibrotic lung disease seem to converge after DLCO declines less than 35%. It is hypothesized that at this point pulmonary hypertension becomes an additional driving factor of mortality.[60,61]

Nonpharmacologic interventions such as vaccinations, pulmonary rehabilitation, and patient support groups are key patient-centered initiatives that hold equal weight to pharmacologic therapies.[3,7,10,15]

	Radiology	Radiology Features	Pathology	Pathology Features	Treatment Considerations	Special Considerations
Non-Fibrotic Hypersensitivity Pneumonitis		Features of parenchymal infiltration AND small airway disease Ground Glass Opacities Expiratory Air Trapping Centrilobular Nodules		A cellular chronic interstitial pneumonia expands the interstitum with accentuation around bronchioles	Phenotype that is most often responsive to therapy Antigen remediation can be treatment alone Consideration of corticosteroid treatment ± immunosuppression	
Fibrotic Hypersensitivity Pneumonitis		Features of Lung Fibrosis AND small airway disease Coarse Reticulation/ Traction Bronchiectasis/ Non-Dominant Honeycombing Centrilobular Nodules, Expiratory Air Tapping, "Three-Density Sign"		There is patchy fibrosis with architectural distortion resembling usual interstitial pneumonia, peribronchiolar metaplasia, and rare multinucleated giant cells with cholesterol clefts and	Consideration for immunosuppression with features of ongoing alveolitis (expiratory air trapping, BAL lymphocytosis, strong ground glass features) Consideration for anti-fibrotic therapy for progressive pulmonary fibrosis, predominant fibrotic profiles, high risk for immunosuppression complications	

SUMMARY

HP remains a challenging disease to classify and manage. Diagnostic modalities provide variable confidence, with classification heavily reliant on the identification of an inciting antigen. Guidelines have provided a standardized approach; however, decision-making remains with many clinical dilemmas (**Table 2**). MDD remains the gold standard in the management of HP, which allows for the appropriate synthesis of history, radiographic, and pathologic data. The delineation of fibrotic and nonfibrotic HP is crucial to identify the differences in clinical trajectories, and further clinical trials are needed to understand optimal therapeutic strategies.

CLINICS CARE POINTS

- When assessing HP as a potential diagnosis, it is important to use a systematic and thorough approach to exposure evaluation. Occult exposure identification may take several visits.
- It is important to evaluate pretest probability of HP diagnosis before considering further diagnostic to avoid obtaining information that will not affect management.
- A careful risk–benefit assessment must be taken before initiating immunomodulatory therapy to weigh the burden of treatment related with the chance for disease modification.
- Clinical dilemmas in HP should be reviewed via MDD to ensure comprehensive synthesis of data and avoidance of anchoring on one data point.

DISCLOSURES

None of the authors have any commercial or financial disclosures.

REFERENCES

1. Leslie KO. Pathology of interstitial lung disease. Clin Chest Med 2004;25(4): 657–703, vi.
2. Bergin CJ, Müller NL. CT of interstitial lung disease: a diagnostic approach. AJR Am J Roentgenol 1987;148(1):9–15.
3. Raghu G, Remy-Jardin M, Ryerson CJ, et al. Diagnosis of Hypersensitivity Pneumonitis in Adults. An Official ATS/JRS/ALAT Clinical Practice Guideline. Am J Respir Crit Care Med 2020;202(3):e36–69.
4. Coultas DB, Zumwalt RE, Black WC, et al. The epidemiology of interstitial lung diseases. Am J Respir Crit Care Med 1994;150(4):967–72.
5. Fink JN, Ortega HG, Reynolds HY, et al. Needs and opportunities for research in hypersensitivity pneumonitis. Am J Respir Crit Care Med 2005;171(7):792–8.
6. Fernandez Perez ER, Kong AM, Raimundo K, et al. Epidemiology of Hypersensitivity Pneumonitis among an Insured Population in the United States: A Claims-based Cohort Analysis. Ann Am Thorac Soc 2018;15(4):460–9.
7. Costabel U, Bonella F, Guzman J. Chronic hypersensitivity pneumonitis. Clin Chest Med 2012;33(1):151–63.
8. Watts MM, Grammer LC. Hypersensitivity pneumonitis. Allergy Asthma Proc 2019;40(6):425–8.
9. Pereira CA, Gimenez A, Kuranishi L, et al. Chronic hypersensitivity pneumonitis. J Asthma Allergy 2016;9:171–81.
10. Alberti ML, Rincon-Alvarez E, Buendia-Roldan I, et al. Hypersensitivity Pneumonitis: Diagnostic and Therapeutic Challenges. Front Med 2021;8:718299.

11. Ley B, Torgerson DG, Oldham JM, et al. Rare Protein-Altering Telomere-related Gene Variants in Patients with Chronic Hypersensitivity Pneumonitis. Am J Respir Crit Care Med 2019;200(9):1154–63.

12. Ley B, Newton CA, Arnould I, et al. The MUC5B promoter polymorphism and telomere length in patients with chronic hypersensitivity pneumonitis: an observational cohort-control study. Lancet Respir Med 2017;5(8):639–47.

13. Kropski JA, Young LR, Cogan JD, et al. Genetic Evaluation and Testing of Patients and Families with Idiopathic Pulmonary Fibrosis. Am J Respir Crit Care Med 2017;195(11):1423–8.

14. Creamer AW, Barratt SL. Prognostic factors in chronic hypersensitivity pneumonitis. Eur Respir Rev 2020;29(156). https://doi.org/10.1183/16000617.0167-2019.

15. Hamblin M, Prosch H, Vasakova M. Diagnosis, course and management of hypersensitivity pneumonitis. Eur Respir Rev 2022;31(163). https://doi.org/10.1183/16000617.0169-2021.

16. de Gracia J, Morell F, Bofill JM, et al. Time of exposure as a prognostic factor in avian hypersensitivity pneumonitis. Respir Med 1989;83(2):139–43.

17. Vasakova M, Selman M, Morell F, et al. Hypersensitivity Pneumonitis: Current Concepts of Pathogenesis and Potential Targets for Treatment. Am J Respir Crit Care Med 2019;200(3):301–8.

18. Fernandez Perez ER, Swigris JJ, Forssen AV, et al. Identifying an inciting antigen is associated with improved survival in patients with chronic hypersensitivity pneumonitis. Chest 2013;144(5):1644–51.

19. Silva CI, Müller NL, Lynch DA, et al. Chronic hypersensitivity pneumonitis: differentiation from idiopathic pulmonary fibrosis and nonspecific interstitial pneumonia by using thin-section CT. Radiology 2008;246(1):288–97.

20. Barnes H, Morisset J, Molyneaux P, et al. A Systematically Derived Exposure Assessment Instrument for Chronic Hypersensitivity Pneumonitis. Chest 2020; 157(6):1506–12.

21. Jenkins AR, Chua A, Chami H, et al. Questionnaires or Serum Immunoglobulin G Testing in the Diagnosis of Hypersensitivity Pneumonitis among Patients with Interstitial Lung Disease. Ann Am Thorac Soc 2021;18(1):130–47.

22. Tateishi T, Ohtani Y, Takemura T, et al. Serial high-resolution computed tomography findings of acute and chronic hypersensitivity pneumonitis induced by avian antigen. J Comput Assist Tomogr 2011;35(2):272–9.

23. Chung JH, Zhan X, Cao M, et al. Presence of Air Trapping and Mosaic Attenuation on Chest Computed Tomography Predicts Survival in Chronic Hypersensitivity Pneumonitis. Ann Am Thorac Soc 2017;14(10):1533–8. https://doi.org/10.1513/AnnalsATS.201701-035OC.

24. Hanak V, Golbin JM, Hartman TE, et al. High-resolution CT findings of parenchymal fibrosis correlate with prognosis in hypersensitivity pneumonitis. Chest 2008;134(1):133–8.

25. Salisbury ML, Myers JL, Belloli EA, et al. Diagnosis and Treatment of Fibrotic Hypersensitivity Pneumonia. Where We Stand and Where We Need to Go. Am J Respir Crit Care Med 2017;196(6):690–9.

26. Salisbury ML, Gu T, Murray S, et al. Hypersensitivity Pneumonitis: Radiologic Phenotypes Are Associated With Distinct Survival Time and Pulmonary Function Trajectory. Chest 2019;155(4):699–711.

27. Mooney JJ, Elicker BM, Urbania TH, et al. Radiographic fibrosis score predicts survival in hypersensitivity pneumonitis. Chest 2013;144(2):586–92.

28. Pérez-Padilla R, Salas J, Chapela R, et al. Mortality in Mexican patients with chronic pigeon breeder's lung compared with those with usual interstitial pneumonia. Am Rev Respir Dis 1993;148(1):49–53.

29. Lacasse Y, Girard M, Cormier Y. Recent advances in hypersensitivity pneumonitis. Chest 2012;142(1):208–17.

30. Ohshimo S, Bonella F, Cui A, et al. Significance of bronchoalveolar lavage for the diagnosis of idiopathic pulmonary fibrosis. Am J Respir Crit Care Med 2009; 179(11):1043–7.

31. De Sadeleer LJ, Hermans F, De Dycker E, et al. Effects of Corticosteroid Treatment and Antigen Avoidance in a Large Hypersensitivity Pneumonitis Cohort: A Single-Centre Cohort Study. J Clin Med 2018;8(1). https://doi.org/10.3390/jcm8010014.

32. Adderley N, Humphreys CJ, Barnes H, et al. Bronchoalveolar lavage fluid lymphocytosis in chronic hypersensitivity pneumonitis: a systematic review and meta-analysis. Eur Respir J 2020;56(2). https://doi.org/10.1183/13993003.00206-2020.

33. Hill M, Petnak T, Moua T. Bronchoalveolar lavage lymphocytosis in hypersensitivity pneumonitis: a retrospective cohort analysis with elimination of incorporation bias. BMC Pulm Med 2022;22(1):49.

34. Fernández Pérez ER, Travis WD, Lynch DA, et al. Diagnosis and Evaluation of Hypersensitivity Pneumonitis: CHEST Guideline and Expert Panel Report. Chest 2021;160(2):e97–156.

35. Hutchinson JP, Fogarty AW, McKeever TM, et al. In-Hospital Mortality after Surgical Lung Biopsy for Interstitial Lung Disease in the United States. 2000 to 2011. Am J Respir Crit Care Med 2016;193(10):1161–7.

36. Nagano M, Miyamoto A, Kikunaga S, et al. Outcomes of Video-Assisted Thoracic Surgical Lung Biopsy for Interstitial Lung Diseases. Ann Thorac Cardiovasc Surg 2021;27(5):290–6.

37. Fisher JH, Shapera S, To T, et al. Procedure volume and mortality after surgical lung biopsy in interstitial lung disease. Eur Respir J 2019;53(2):1801164.

38. Cottin V. Lung biopsy in interstitial lung disease: balancing the risk of surgery and diagnostic uncertainty. Eur Respir J 2016;48(5):1274–7.

39. Maldonado F, Danoff SK, Wells AU, et al. Transbronchial Cryobiopsy for the Diagnosis of Interstitial Lung Diseases: CHEST Guideline and Expert Panel Report. Chest 2020;157(4):1030–42.

40. Troy LK, Grainge C, Corte T, et al. Cryobiopsy versus open lung biopsy in the diagnosis of interstitial lung disease (COLDICE): protocol of a multicentre study. BMJ Open Respir Res 2019;6(1):e000443.

41. Ravaglia C, Poletti V. Transbronchial lung cryobiopsy for the diagnosis of interstitial lung diseases. Curr Opin Pulm Med 2022;28(1):9–16.

42. Richeldi L, Scholand MB, Lynch DA, et al. Utility of a Molecular Classifier as a Complement to High-Resolution Computed Tomography to Identify Usual Interstitial Pneumonia. Am J Respir Crit Care Med 2021;203(2):211–20.

43. Raghu G, Flaherty KR, Lederer DJ, et al. Use of a molecular classifier to identify usual interstitial pneumonia in conventional transbronchial lung biopsy samples: a prospective validation study. Lancet Respir Med 2019;7(6):487–96.

44. Yang SR, Beasley MB, Churg A, et al. Diagnosis of Hypersensitivity Pneumonitis: Review and Summary of American College of Chest Physicians Statement. Am J Surg Pathol 2022;46(4):e71–93.

45. Grunes D, Beasley MB. Hypersensitivity pneumonitis: a review and update of histologic findings. J Clin Pathol 2013;66(10):888–95.

46. Johannson KA, Barnes H, Bellanger AP, et al. Exposure Assessment Tools for Hypersensitivity Pneumonitis. An Official American Thoracic Society Workshop Report. Ann Am Thorac Soc 2020;17(12):1501–9.
47. Kokkarinen JI, Tukiainen HO, Terho EO. Effect of corticosteroid treatment on the recovery of pulmonary function in farmer's lung. Am Rev Respir Dis 1992;145(1):3–5.
48. Fiddler CA, Simler N, Thillai M, et al. Use of mycophenolate mofetil and azathioprine for the treatment of chronic hypersensitivity pneumonitis-A single-centre experience. Clin Respir J 2019;13(12):791–4.
49. Terras Alexandre A, Martins N, Raimundo S, et al. Impact of Azathioprine use in chronic hypersensitivity pneumonitis patients. Pulm Pharmacol Ther 2020;60:101878.
50. Morisset J, Johannson KA, Vittinghoff E, et al. Use of Mycophenolate Mofetil or Azathioprine for the Management of Chronic Hypersensitivity Pneumonitis. Chest 2017;151(3):619–25.
51. Adegunsoye A, Oldham JM, Fernandez Perez ER, et al. Outcomes of immunosuppressive therapy in chronic hypersensitivity pneumonitis. ERJ Open Res 2017;3(3). https://doi.org/10.1183/23120541.00016-2017.
52. Ferreira M, Borie R, Crestani B, et al. Efficacy and safety of rituximab in patients with chronic hypersensitivity pneumonitis (cHP): A retrospective, multicentric, observational study. Respir Med 2020;172:106146.
53. Ojanguren I, Villar A, Ramón MA, et al. Rituximab for the treatment of chronic hypersensitivity pneumonitis. Eur Respir J 2015;46(suppl 59):PA815.
54. Takemura T, Akashi T, Kamiya H, et al. Pathological differentiation of chronic hypersensitivity pneumonitis from idiopathic pulmonary fibrosis/usual interstitial pneumonia. Histopathology 2012;61(6):1026–35.
55. Flaherty KR, Brown KK, Wells AU, et al. Design of the PF-ILD trial: a double-blind, randomised, placebo-controlled phase III trial of nintedanib in patients with progressive fibrosing interstitial lung disease. BMJ Open Respir Res 2017;4(1): e000212.
56. Shibata S, Furusawa H, Inase N. Pirfenidone in chronic hypersensitivity pneumonitis: a real-life experience. Sarcoidosis Vasc Diffuse Lung Dis 2018;35(2):139–42.
57. Mateos-Toledo H, Mejía-Ávila M, Rodríguez-Barreto Ó, et al. An Open-label Study With Pirfenidone on Chronic Hypersensitivity Pneumonitis. Arch Bronconeumol (Engl Ed) 2020;56(3):163–9.
58. Tzilas V, Tzouvelekis A, Bouros E, et al. Clinical experience with antifibrotics in fibrotic hypersensitivity pneumonitis: a 3-year real-life observational study. ERJ Open Res 2020;6(4). https://doi.org/10.1183/23120541.00152-2020.
59. Kern RM, Singer JP, Koth L, et al. Lung transplantation for hypersensitivity pneumonitis. Chest 2015;147(6):1558–65.
60. Nathan SD. Hypersensitivity pneumonitis and pulmonary hypertension: how the breeze affects the squeeze. Eur Respir J 2014;44(2):287–8.
61. Rose L, Prins KW, Archer SL, et al. Survival in pulmonary hypertension due to chronic lung disease: Influence of low diffusion capacity of the lungs for carbon monoxide. J Heart Lung Transplant 2019;38(2):145–55.

Sarcoidosis

Paolo Spagnolo, MD, PhD*, Nicol Bernardinello, MD

KEYWORDS

- Sarcoidosis • Diagnosis • Clinical manifestations • Treatment • Management

KEY POINTS

- Sarcoidosis is a systemic granulomatous disorder of unknown cause that results from a complex interplay between infectious/environmental triggers and genetic factors leading to an aberrant immune response.
- There is no diagnostic gold standard and the diagnosis is most likely in the presence of compatible clinical and radiological features coupled with evidence of noncaseating granulomatous inflammation at disease sites and after exclusion of other diseases that may present similarly.
- The majority of patients have a remitting disease with or without treatment. However, about one-third of the patients develop chronic disease, with extrapulmonary manifestations representing a major cause of morbidity and mortality.
- Corticosteroids are the mainstay of treatment but they do not cure the disease and are associated with significant side effects.
- Patients with refractory or life/organ-threatening diseases should be referred to expert centers.

INTRODUCTION

Sarcoidosis is a highly variable and unpredictable systemic disorder characterized by granulomatous inflammation in affected organs. Disease pathogenesis involves a complex interplay between a putative triggering antigen (or antigens), which remains unknown, and the host's genetic makeup. The incidence, severity, and clinical manifestations of sarcoidosis highly depend on race and ethnicity. Indeed, African Americans are afflicted more often and more severely than Caucasians, although prediction of disease behavior is difficult. The complex multidimensional nature of sarcoidosis coupled with its wide range of clinical manifestations underscores the need for a multidisciplinary approach to patient care.

EPIDEMIOLOGY

Sarcoidosis occurs worldwide with an overall prevalence ranging between 50 and 160 per 100,000 population.[1] Although traditionally regarded as a disease of young people,

Respiratory Disease Unit, Department of Cardiac, Thoracic, Vascular Sciences and Public Health, University of Padova, via Giustiniani 2, Padova 35128, Italy
* Corresponding author.
E-mail address: paolo.spagnolo@unipd.it

Immunol Allergy Clin N Am 43 (2023) 259–272
https://doi.org/10.1016/j.iac.2023.01.008
0889-8561/23/© 2023 Elsevier Inc. All rights reserved.
immunology.theclinics.com

recent data shows that more than half of the patients are older than 40 years at diagnosis.[2] The disease affects both sexes with a slight predilection for women, particularly among African Americans. Sarcoidosis is more common in Black Americans than in White Americans, with an estimated lifetime disease risk of 2.4% and 0.85%, respectively.[3] Northern Europeans are another ethnic group at particularly high risk for the disease, with a prevalence as high as 160 per 100,000 in Sweden.[4] Disease presentation and patterns of organ involvement differ substantially across ethnicities. Indeed, sarcoidosis tends to affect black people more acutely and more severely than people of other races.[3,5] In addition, some extra-thoracic manifestations are more prevalent in certain populations, such as chronic uveitis in African Americans and Japanese, lupus pernio in African Americans, and erythema nodosum in Scandinavians.[5] The observation that the prevalence of sarcoidosis follows a rough north–south gradient along with seasonal clustering of cases in winter and early spring suggests that sarcoidosis results from a complex (and poorly understood) interaction between environmental and genetic factors.[5,6] Finally, a lower disease prevalence in smokers has been reported but the evidence is inconsistent.

PATHOLOGY, PATHOGENESIS, AND POTENTIAL ETIOLOGIC FACTORS
Histopathology

Nonnecrotizing granulomas, the histopathological hallmark of sarcoidosis, are discrete aggregates of chronic inflammatory cells (ie, macrophages, epithelioid cells, multinucleated giant cells, and CD4$^+$ T lymphocytes), which tend to merge to form nodules in the mm size range.[7] Sarcoid granulomas are "epithelioid cell granulomas," as the epithelioid cells, which derive from mononuclear phagocytes (ie, monocytes and macrophages), are the dominant cell type.[7] They are located at the center of the granuloma surrounded by a mantle of lymphocytes, tissue macrophages, and giant cells, which also derive from mononuclear phagocytes. The granuloma is surrounded by fibroblasts and lamellar rings of hyaline collagen.

According to the general paradigm of disease immunopathogenesis, sarcoid granulomas result from a T-cell-mediated response to an (yet unknown) antigen that is processed by antigen-presenting cells—such as macrophages or dendritic cells—and presented to antigen-specific CD4$^+$ T cells in the context of class I or class II Human Leukocyte Antigen (HLA) molecules.[8] Specifically, the antigenic peptide and the HLA class II molecule activate antigen-specific CD4$^+$ T cells by binding to the T-cell receptor (TCR) on the T-cell surface. Once activated, the CD4$^+$ T cells orchestrate the immune response that culminates with granuloma formation.[8] A multitude of cytokines are involved in this process, including interleukin (IL)-2, tumor necrosis factor (TNF)-α, and interferon (IFN)-γ, which amplify the immune response by triggering macrophages to secrete, among others, TNF-α, IL-1, IL-6, IL-8, IL-12, IL-15, and IL-18.[9] In sarcoidosis, granulomatous inflammation is a highly polarized Th1 type cytokine response. However, in cases evolving from granulomatous inflammation to fibrosis, a shift from a Th1- to a Th2-type cytokine pattern is likely to occur.[9–11]

Genetic Factors

Several lines of evidence support a major role of host susceptibility in the pathogenesis of sarcoidosis. They include the familial occurrence of the disease, with a pooled prevalence as high as 7.3% in a meta-analysis based on 12 populations,[12] ethnic variations in its epidemiology and clinical manifestations as well as genetic studies showing consistent associations between a variety of variants, mostly within the HLA region, and sarcoidosis susceptibility, phenotypes, and prognosis.[13] However, subsets of patients sharing the same HLA associations may display different clinical manifestations based on their ethnic and racial background, suggesting that multiple factors are involved in the phenotypic expressions of sarcoidosis. Nevertheless, the HLA-DRB1*1101 allele is a risk factor for sarcoidosis in both Caucasians and African Americans,[14] whereas Löfgren's syndrome is strongly associated with the HLA-DRB1*0301 allele, particularly in Scandinavians.[15,16] Additional variants that confer susceptibility to sarcoidosis are located within butyrophilin-like 2 (BTNL2)[17] and annexin A11 (ANXA11)[18] genes.

Potential Etiologies

Numerous microorganisms have been implicated as possible causes of sarcoidosis.[19] Several studies have explored the etiological role of Mycobacterium tuberculosis based on the histologic similarities between sarcoidosis and mycobacterial infection.[20,21] Song and colleagues[22] identified M tuberculosis catalase-peroxidase (mKatG), a mycobacterial antigen, in 5 of 9 sarcoidosis tissues but in none of 14 control tissues. Moreover, T cells reactive to mKatG were found at increased levels in both peripheral blood and bronchoalveolar lavage (BAL) fluid from sarcoidosis patients compared with healthy controls.[21] Propionibacterium acnes and P granulosum have also been isolated in a significantly higher proportion of sarcoidosis specimens compared with control specimens.[19] Although the infectious theory is intriguing, a definitive conclusion as to whether microorganisms play a role in the pathogenesis of sarcoidosis will require more extensive investigations. Certain occupational exposures, most notably beryllium, can induce sarcoid-like granulomatous inflammation,[23] thus suggesting that occupational or environmental agents might also trigger the disease, at least in a subset of cases. In this regard, firefighters exposed to World Trade Center (WTC) "dust" were at significantly increased risk of developing sarcoidosis-like pulmonary disease during the 5 years following the disaster.[24]

DIAGNOSTIC APPROACH

There is no diagnostic gold standard for sarcoidosis. However, the diagnosis is highly probable in the presence of compatible clinical-radiological features supported by histologic evidence of non-necrotizing granulomas in one or more affected tissues and after the exclusion of alternative causes of granulomatous inflammation.[25] Yet, there are scenarios in which a confident diagnosis of sarcoidosis can be made without histologic confirmation, such as patients presenting with Löfgren's syndrome (ie, bilateral hilar lymph adenopathy [BHL], fever, erythema nodosum, and arthralgia), Heerfordt's syndrome (ie, facial nerve paralysis, parotid or salivary glands enlargement and anterior uveitis), lupus pernio (ie, indurated purplish papules or plaques that involve the nose, cheeks, lips, ears, and eyelids) as well as in asymptomatic individuals presenting with symmetric BHL.[5,6,25] In this latter case, however a close clinical follow-up to ensure stability or resolution is recommended.[25] Biopsies should be obtained from the most accessible affected sites such as the skin, or palpable lymph nodes. If none of these sites is affected, the next step is sampling intrathoracic lymph nodes or the lung parenchyma. Serum levels of angiotensin-converting enzyme (ACE) are increased in up to 75% of untreated patients with sarcoidosis. However, its poor sensitivity and insufficient specificity make it ACE of limited value as a diagnostic tool.[26]

BAL supports the diagnosis of sarcoidosis when it shows a moderate (20% to 50%) lymphocytosis with a T lymphocyte CD4:CD8 ratio greater than 3.5.[26,27] BAL is also useful in excluding alternative diagnoses such as infections and malignancy.

Endobronchial mucosal biopsy reveals non-necrotizing granulomas in about 70% of cases in the presence of visible abnormalities (ie, cobblestone appearance of the mucosa) as well as in around 30% of cases with a normal-appearing mucosa. Transbronchial lung biopsy has a diagnostic yield of 50% to 75% in patients with BHL or compatible parenchymal abnormalities on chest high-resolution computed tomography (HRCT) (ie, micronodules with a perilymphatic distribution clustered along the bronchovascular bundles, interlobular septa, and interlobar fissures).[11] Alternatively, transbronchial needle aspiration (TBNA) with or without ultrasound guidance can be used to sample mediastinal lymph nodes or pulmonary lesions. Notably, in patients with mediastinal lymphadenopathy and a clinical suspicion of sarcoidosis, endoscopic ultrasound-guided needle aspiration of intrathoracic lymph nodes via esophageal endoscopic ultrasound (EUS) or endobronchial ultrasound (EBUS) has a diagnostic yield of 80% to 90%.[28] If diagnostic uncertainty persists, mediastinal lymph node biopsy via mediastinoscopy is the preferred diagnostic modality. Lung biopsy via thoracoscopy is rarely needed.

CLINICAL MANIFESTATIONS

The spectrum of clinical manifestations of sarcoidosis is highly heterogeneous. Although pulmonary involvement is almost universal, any organ can be affected. The presenting symptoms are generally related to the organs involved, but patients may also present with nonspecific systemic symptoms, such as low-grade fever, weight loss, and fatigue.

Respiratory Tract

Sarcoidosis affects the lungs and mediastinal lymph nodes in more than 90% of cases.[5,6,25] Accordingly, the main respiratory complaints are cough, shortness of breath, and chest pain. However, 30% to 60% of patients with pulmonary disease are asymptomatic, and are diagnosed incidentally.[25] BHL is the most common radiographic presentation, and when accompanied by erythema nodosum and arthralgia, defines Löfgren syndrome, an acute, self-limiting, and genetically distinct form of the disease.[9,13,16,29] Historically, pulmonary involvement has been classified using the Scadding system, which, by relying on chest radiograph, provides a rough estimate of the likelihood of resolution at 5 years[30] (Figs. 1–4). The Scadding system is simple and reproducible, but does not correlate with the likelihood of cutaneous or ocular disease and correlates only poorly with lung function tests and need for treatment in individual patients. HRCT is generally performed to evaluate abnormalities seen on chest radiograph and typically reveals hilar and mediastinal lymphadenopathy, bronchovascular bundle thickening, nodules with a perilymphatic distribution (ie, along bronchi, vessels, and subpleural regions), and ground glass opacity[11,31,32] (Fig. 5). Pulmonary fibrosis, which develops in about 20% of cases, predominates in the middle and upper zones and manifests as masses, cysts, distortion of the airways and lung parenchyma, and traction bronchiectasis[11,31,32] (Fig. 6). Fluorine-18-fluorodeoxyglucose-positron emission tomography (FDG-PET) may be helpful in identifying occult lesions more accessible to biopsy, but does not differentiate sarcoidosis from other inflammatory conditions, infection, or malignancy. When abnormal, pulmonary function tests (PFTs) generally reveal a restrictive ventilatory defect associated with a reduced diffusing capacity of the lung for carbon monoxide (DL_{CO}) whereas distortion of the airways and endobronchial disease may lead to an obstructive pattern.[33] PFTs may also allow to assess the severity of respiratory impairment and to monitor the disease course.[33]

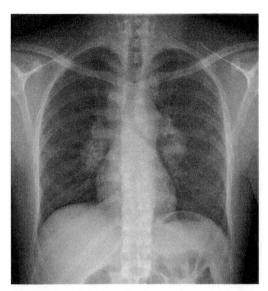

Fig. 1. Scadding stage I: bilateral hilar lymphadenopathy.

EXTRAPULMONARY MANIFESTATIONS

Extrapulmonary involvement is seen in up to 50% of sarcoidosis patients,[34] with isolated extrapulmonary disease occurring in less than 10% of total cases.[35] Such cases generally represent a diagnostic dilemma. The most common sites of disease outside the lung are skin, peripheral lymph nodes, eyes, and liver.[36]

Skin

The most common cutaneous manifestation of sarcoidosis is erythema nodosum (EN), a form of panniculitis characterized by painful lesions on the anterior surface of the

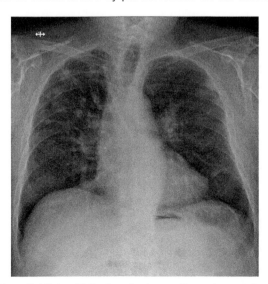

Fig. 2. Scadding stage II: bilateral hilar lymphadenopathy and parenchymal infiltrates.

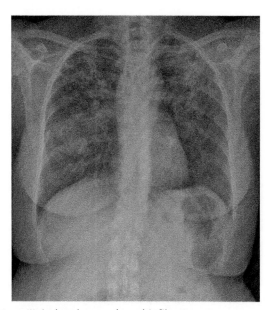

Fig. 3. Scadding stage III: isolated parenchymal infiltrates.

lower limbs. EN occurs in approximately 25% of cases and is typically associated with Löfgren's syndrome.[29,37] Notably, EN should not be biopsied, as it does not contain granulomas. Several types of skin lesions can occur, including diffuse erythematous papules, subcutaneous nodules, and plaques.[38] Lupus pernio, the most characteristic cutaneous manifestation of sarcoidosis, is characterized by red-to-purple indurated plaques, papules, or nodules that primarily affect the nose, cheeks, and ears. Early recognition and treatment are paramount, as lupus pernio can infiltrate the underlying tissues and cause disfigurement. Typically, skin sarcoidosis involves scars and tattoos.[37,38]

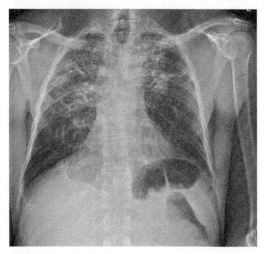

Fig. 4. Scadding stage IV: pulmonary fibrosis.

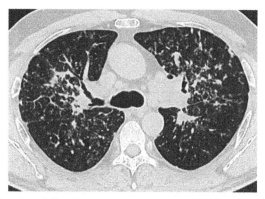

Fig. 5. Chest CT showing diffuse micronodules prevalent in the upper zones and with a typical peribronchovascular distribution. This pattern is typical, though not pathognomonic, of sarcoidosis.

Eyes

Ocular involvement occurs in 10% to 50% of sarcoidosis patients and is the presenting manifestation in about 5% of cases.[39] The prevalence is higher in females as well as in African American and Japanese patients.[40] Any part of the eye can be involved, although the anterior and posterior ocular segments, conjunctiva, and lacrimal glands are mostly commonly affected. Uveitis is the most common form of ocular sarcoidosis, with anterior uveitis (defined as iritis and/or iridocyclitis) accounting for up to 75% of all sarcoid uveitis cases.[40] Symptoms include blurry vision, redness, photophobia, dry

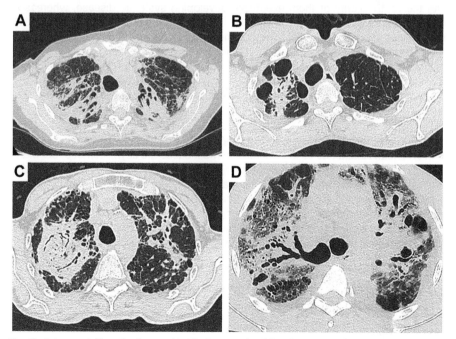

Fig. 6. Advanced fibrotic disease (*A–D*) characterized by distortion of the airways (*D*) and lung parenchyma (*A*); fibrocystic disease (*B*); pulmonary fibrosis colonized by *Aspergillum fumigatus* (*C*).

eyes, and ocular pain, whereas posterior or intermediate uveitis generally causes floaters. As ocular involvement can be asymptomatic, all patients with newly diagnosed sarcoidosis should undergo ophthalmologic screening. Refractory and sight-threatening forms require a multi-disciplinary approach and aggressive treatment.

Heart

Cardiac sarcoidosis (CS) is clinically evident in about 5% of patients, although the prevalence of subclinical involvement is significantly higher (20% to 70%), as suggested by autopsy and cardiac imaging studies.[41] Similarly, CS can be benign and discovered incidentally or cause sudden death due to ventricular tachyarrhythmia or bradyarrhythmia.[41] Of note, cardiac disease accounts for as many as 85% of deaths among Japanese patients with sarcoidosis.[42] Heart block and arrhythmias (due to involvement of the conducting system) are the most common manifestations of CS.[43] Cardiac Magnetic Resonance (CMR) and/or FDG-PET are generally used to confirm the diagnosis of CS, as endomyocardial biopsy has a low sensitivity due to the patchy distribution of the disease and exposes patients to risks.[44] No single tool can reliably detect early and asymptomatic disease and the best approach remains clinical suspicion of cardiac involvement.

Nervous system

Historically, neurosarcoidosis (NS) has been reported to occur in 5% to 10% of all sarcoidosis patients, although these prevalence rates derive from pulmonary sarcoidosis-focused cohorts. Indeed, autopsy studies have identified clinically occult NS in as many as 34% of patients with systemic sarcoidosis.[45] Notably, only about 30% of patients with NS have systemic manifestations of the disease at presentation, with the vast majority of them eventually developing systemic disease, whereas in 10% to 20% of case NS remains isolated.[46] Any part of the nervous system can be involved but the cranial nerves, hypothalamus, meninges, spinal cord, and peripheral nerves are most commonly affected.[47] Optic neuritis and optic neuropathy caused by infiltrating or mass-like lesions may also occur. The diagnosis—which is particularly challenging when NS occurs in isolation—is usually straightforward when neurologic symptoms develop in patients with an established diagnosis of sarcoidosis.

Liver, spleen, and kidney

Hepatic sarcoidosis has been reported in up to 70% of patients and is twice as common in African Americans as in Caucasians. Most cases are asymptomatic, but many have liver function test abnormalities or hepatomegaly.[48] Portal hypertension and cirrhosis are a rare complication of long-standing hepatic disease.[49] Splenic involvement is also common in patients with sarcoidosis, although most cases are asymptomatic.[50] Splenomegaly is usually homogeneous, but multiple low-attenuating nodular lesions indistinguishable from a metastatic disease may also be seen. Renal involvement is a rare but potentially serious complication of sarcoidosis. It ranges from disordered calcium homeostasis leading to hypercalcemia and hypercalciuria, the most common manifestations, to tubulointerstitial nephritis.[51] Severe hypercalcemia and/or hypercalciuria are indications for treatment, as they may lead to renal failure.

SYSTEMIC MANIFESTATIONS

Fatigue, is the most common systemic symptom of sarcoidosis being reported in up to 80% of patients,[52] with fever, sleep disorders, irritability, weight loss, anorexia, and flushing representing additional common complaints. Small fiber neuropathy (SFN) is another common complication of sarcoidosis that manifests as numbness, pain, and migratory and intermittent paraesthesia.[53] In a study, burning pain was the most severe and disabling symptom and was present in about one-third of patients.[54] SFN is more common in Caucasians and in women, and is often refractory to standard therapies used for systemic disease.[55]

TREATMENT

In sarcoidosis, a "wait and watch strategy" is often justified, as the disease frequently remits with or without therapy. In addition, corticosteroids, the cornerstone of treatment, do not cure the disease and are associated with serious side effects. Therefore, treatment is indicated in patients with progressive and organ/life-threatening disease or significantly impaired quality of life, weighed carefully the pros and cons of initiating therapy.[56]

Pulmonary sarcoidosis

Most patients with pulmonary sarcoidosis do not require systemic therapy.[56,57] When treatment is needed, corticosteroids are the first-line agents, although the recommendation for their use is based on low-quality evidence.[56] The 2021 guideline document on treatment recommends corticosteroid treatment for patients at high risk of mortality or permanent disability to improve and/or preserve FVC and quality of life.[56] Specific indications for treatment include bothersome or worsening pulmonary symptoms (ie, cough, dyspnea, and chest pain), worsening lung function, or progression of radiographic abnormalities.[56] The optimal dose and duration of corticosteroid treatment are unknown, but most authors use an initial dose equivalent to prednisone 20 to 40 mg/ daily continued for four to 6 weeks then slowly tapered and weaned over 9 to 12 months. For patients experiencing disease progression despite treatment or intolerable side effects of corticosteroids, escalation to immunosuppressive agents is suggested, with methotrexate being the preferred second-line agent ("Conditional recommendation, very low quality of evidence").[56] Less commonly used second-line drugs include azathioprine, leflunomide, hydroxychloroquine, and mycophenolate mofetil.[56] Patients with persistently active/progressive disease despite immunosuppressive therapy may respond to TNF-α antagonists (ie, infliximab or adalimumab), but their use is associated with an increased risk of infection.[56,58] Patients with end-stage pulmonary disease should be considered for lung transplantation.[59]

Skin sarcoidosis

Erythema nodosum is generally self-limiting and does not require specific therapy; however, short-course corticosteroids or nonsteroidal anti-inflammatory drugs may be needed to alleviate pain and discomfort. Systemic corticosteroids are generally reserved for patients with disfiguring or cosmetically distressing lesions, rapidly progressive disease, or following failure of local treatment.[37] Patients with refractory disease may benefit from a second-line agent, such as hydroxychloroquine or methotrexate, whereas in patients with active skin disease despite corticosteroids and/or immunosuppressive therapy the addition of infliximab should be considered.[56]

Ocular sarcoidosis

Owing to the risk of sight-threatening sequelae, ocular sarcoidosis almost invariably requires treatment, which generally starts with local corticosteroids.[60] Systemic corticosteroid treatment is required if local therapy fails to induce remission, whereas in patients who fail to respond to or do not tolerate corticosteroids escalation to second-line agents, mainly methotrexate, should be considered. Similar to pulmonary sarcoidosis, biologic agents are reserved for patients with recalcitrant disease.[56]

Cardiac sarcoidosis

The treatment of clinically overt CS consists of both suppression of cardiac inflammation—with the aim of preventing irreversible organ damage or conduction abnormalities—and appropriate care of arrhythmia and heart failure. Treatment is invariably required, as spontaneous remission does not occur.[61] Corticosteroids are the first-line treatment; prednisone (or equivalent) is generally initiated at a daily dose of 40 to 60 mg with a taper regimen similar to that for pulmonary sarcoidosis.[61] If corticosteroids fail to induce remission or are associated with an intolerable side effect, methotrexate is the preferred second-line agent,[13] whereas infliximab is reserved to refractory or progressive disease.[56] The anti-CD20 rituximab is a potential alternative to infliximab.[62] The standard indications for a permanent pacemaker or for an implantable cardioverter defibrillator apply also to CS. Heart transplantation is the definitive treatment for patients with refractory ventricular arrhythmias or end-stage heart failure.[63]

Neurosarcoidosis

NS almost invariably requires treatment, as spontaneous remission is rare. High-dose corticosteroids (equivalent to 1 mg/kg/d of prednisone) are the first-line treatment,[64] but severe manifestations, such as visual loss or altered mental status, or rapidly progressive disease may require intravenous methylprednisolone at a dose of 1 g per day for 3 to 5 days.[64,65] Methotrexate is the most commonly used second-line agents, but some experts suggest the early association of methotrexate to corticosteroids to prevent symptoms recurrence, as corticosteroids are gradually tapered.[64] As with pulmonary and extrapulmonary sarcoidosis, refractory disease requires biological treatment (ie, infliximab)[66] due to potentially catastrophic consequences of progressive disease. SFN generally responds poorly to standard therapy whereas intravenous immunoglobulin and biological agents appear to be more efficacious treatment options.[54]

FOLLOW-UP AND PROGNOSIS

The optimal modality of follow-up of patients with sarcoidosis has not been established. Most experts monitor symptoms, lung function, and imaging at 3 to 6 month intervals, but asymptomatic patients are evaluated less frequently. The clinical course of sarcoidosis is highly variable and unpredictable. However, in approximately half of the patients the disease resolves spontaneously within 2 to 3 years, whereas chronic disease (ie, disease lasting for ≥ 3 years) carries an increased risk of pulmonary and extrapulmonary fibrosis and impaired quality of life.[67] Patients with sarcoidosis have a lower survival compared with the general population,[68] with pulmonary fibrosis being the most common cause of death in western countries, whereas cardiac involvement is the main cause of mortality in Japan.[5,6]

SUMMARY

Sarcoidosis remains an enigmatic disease without a diagnostic gold standard, effective treatments, and reliable predictors of disease behavior. The disease is generally benign but a large minority of patients experience chronic progressive disease. Such diversity makes it difficult to classify patients into homogeneous subgroups, which contributes to the paucity of clinical trials of novel treatments. Patients with sarcoidosis of the heart, brain, and eyes and those with advanced and progressive/refractory disease should be referred to expert centers.

CLINICS CARE POINTS

- With very rare exceptions, the diagnosis of sarcoidosis should always be histologically confirmed.
- In the presence of noncaseating granuloma on biopsy, mycobacterial and fungal infection, foreign body reaction, and drug toxicity, among others, should be excluded.
- The easily accessible skin lesions and superficial lymph nodes should be the preferred sites for a biopsy.
- Elevation of serum angiotensin-converting enzyme level has a low sensitivity and poor specificity for sarcoidosis and should not be used as diagnostic tool.
- In patients with pulmonary sarcoidosis always look for extrapulmonary localizations of the disease.
- All patients diagnosed with sarcoidosis should be screened for cardiac involvement using clinical history, physical examination, and 12-lead electrocardiogram, as cardiac sarcoidosis can be life-threatening.
- The main indications for treatment are progressive granulomatous inflammation leading to life- or organ-threatening disease and disabling symptoms causing severe impairment of quality of life
- Second-line agents (ie, methotrexate) should be considered for cases of corticosteroid
- Failure, intolerance, or dependence.
- Consider biological agents (ie, infliximab) in refractory disease.

DISCLOSURE

P. Spagnolo reports personal fees from Novartis, Behring and Chiesi outside the submitted work. N. Bernardinello has nothing to disclose.

REFERENCES

1. Arkema EV, Cozier YC. Sarcoidosis epidemiology: recent estimates of incidence, prevalence and risk factors. Curr Opin Pulm Med 2020;26:527–34.
2. Sikjær MG, Hilberg O, Ibsen R, et al. Sarcoidosis: A nationwide registry-based study of incidence, prevalence and diagnostic work-up. Respir Med 2021;187:106548.
3. Rybicki BA, Major M, Popovich J, et al. Racial Differences in Sarcoidosis Incidence: A 5-Year Study in a Health Maintenance Organization. Am J Epidemiol 1997;145:234–41.
4. Arkema EV, Grunewald J, Kullberg S, et al. Sarcoidosis incidence and prevalence: a nationwide register-based assessment in Sweden. Eur Respir J 2016; 48:1690–9.
5. Drent M, Crouser ED, Grunewald J. Challenges of Sarcoidosis and Its Management. N Engl J Med 2021;385:1018–32.
6. Valeyre D, Prasse A, Nunes H, et al. Sarcoidosis. Lancet 2014;383:1155–67.

7. Rossi G, Cavazza A, Colby TV. Pathology of Sarcoidosis. Clin Rev Allergy Immunol 2015;49:36–44.
8. Moller DR, Chen ES. Genetic basis of remitting sarcoidosis: triumph of the trimolecular complex? Am J Respir Cell Mol Biol 2002;27:391–5.
9. Grunewald J, Spagnolo P, Wahlström J, et al. Immunogenetics of Disease-Causing Inflammation in Sarcoidosis. Clin Rev Allergy Immunol 2015;49:19–35.
10. Agostini C, Adami F, Semenzato G. New pathogenetic insights into the sarcoid granuloma. Curr Opin Rheumatol 2000;1271–6.
11. Spagnolo P, Rossi G, Trisolini R, et al. Pulmonary sarcoidosis. Lancet Respir Med 2018;6:389–402.
12. Terwiel M, van Moorsel CHM. Clinical epidemiology of familial sarcoidosis: A systematic literature review. Respir Med 2019;149:36–41.
13. Spagnolo P, Maier LA. Genetics in sarcoidosis. Curr Opin Pulm Med 2021;27: 423–9.
14. Rossman MD, Thompson B, Frederick M, et al. HLA-DRB1*1101: a significant risk factor for sarcoidosis in blacks and whites. Am J Hum Genet 2003;73:720–35.
15. Berlin M, Fogdell-Hahn A, Olerup O, et al. HLA-DR predicts the prognosis in Scandinavian patients with pulmonary sarcoidosis. Am J Respir Crit Care Med 1997;156:1601–5.
16. Spagnolo P, Renzoni EA, Wells AU, et al. C-C chemokine receptor 2 and sarcoidosis: association with Lofgren's syndrome. Am J Respir Crit Care Med 2003;168: 1162–6.
17. Valentonyte R, Hampe J, Huse K, et al. Sarcoidosis is associated with a truncating splice site mutation in BTNL2. Nat Genet 2005;37:357–64.
18. Hofmann S, Franke A, Fischer A, et al. Genome-wide association study identifies ANXA11 as a new susceptibility locus for sarcoidosis. Nat Genet 2008;40: 1103–6.
19. Chen ES, Moller DR. Etiologies of Sarcoidosis. Clin Rev Allergy Immunol 2015; 49:6–18.
20. Drake WP, Pei Z, Pride DT, et al. Molecular analysis of sarcoidosis tissues for mycobacterium species DNA. Emerg Infect Dis 2002;8:1334–41.
21. Chen ES, Wahlström J, Song Z, et al. T cell responses to mycobacterial catalase-peroxidase profile a pathogenic antigen in systemic sarcoidosis. J Immunol 2008; 181:8784–96.
22. Song Z, Marzilli L, Greenlee BM, et al. Mycobacterial catalase-peroxidase is a tissue antigen and target of the adaptive immune response in systemic sarcoidosis. J Exp Med 2005;201:755–67.
23. Rosen Y. Pathology of sarcoidosis. Semin Respir Crit Care Med 2007;28:36–52.
24. Izbicki G, Chavko R, Banauch GI, et al. World Trade Center "sarcoid-like" granulomatous pulmonary disease in New York City Fire Department rescue workers. Chest 2007;131:1414–23.
25. Crouser ED, Maier LA, Wilson KC, et al. Diagnosis and Detection of Sarcoidosis. An Official American Thoracic Society Clinical Practice Guideline. Am J Respir Crit Care Med 2020;201:e26–51.
26. Bernardinello N, Petrarulo S, Balestro E, et al. Pulmonary Sarcoidosis: Diagnosis and Differential Diagnosis. Diagnostics 2021;11:1558.
27. Costabel U, Bonella F, Ohshimo S, et al. Diagnostic modalities in sarcoidosis: BAL, EBUS, and PET. Semin Respir Crit Care Med 2010;31:404–8.
28. Agarwal R, Srinivasan A, Aggarwal AN, et al. Efficacy and safety of convex probe EBUS-TBNA in sarcoidosis: A systematic review and meta-analysis. Resp Med 2012;106:883–92.

29. Grunewald J, Eklund A. Sex-specific manifestations of Löfgren's syndrome. Am J Respir Crit Care Med 2007;175:40–4.
30. Scadding JG. Prognosis of intrathoracic sarcoidosis in England. A review of 136 cases after five years' observation. Br Med J 1961;2:1165–72.
31. Spagnolo P, Sverzellati N, Wells AU, et al. Imaging aspects of the diagnosis of sarcoidosis. Eur Radiol 2014;24:807–16.
32. Criado E, Sánchez M, Ramírez J, et al. Pulmonary sarcoidosis: typical and atypical manifestations at high-resolution CT with pathologic correlation. Radiographics 2010;30:1567–86.
33. Gupta R, Judson MA, Baughman RP. Management of Advanced Pulmonary Sarcoidosis. Am J Respir Crit Care Med 2022;205:495–506.
34. Mañá J, Rubio-Rivas M, Villalba N, et al. Multidisciplinary approach and long-term follow-up in a series of 640 consecutive patients with sarcoidosis: Cohort study of a 40-year clinical experience at a tertiary referral center in Barcelona, Spain. Medicine (Baltim) 2017;96:e7595.
35. Inoue Y, Inui N, Hashimoto D, et al. Cumulative incidence and predictors of progression in corticosteroid- naive patients with sarcoidosis. PLoS One 2015;10: e0143371.
36. Valeyre D, Jeny F, Rotenberg C, et al. How to Tackle the Diagnosis and Treatment in the Diverse Scenarios of Extrapulmonary Sarcoidosis. Adv Ther 2021;38: 4605–27.
37. Haimovic A, Sanchez M, Judson MA, et al. Sarcoidosis: a comprehensive review and update for the dermatologist, part I: Cutaneous disease. J Am Acad Dermatol 2012;66:699.e1-18.
38. Wu JH, Imadojemu S, Caplan AS. The Evolving Landscape of Cutaneous Sarcoidosis: Pathogenic Insight, Clinical Challenges, and New Frontiers in Therapy. Am J Clin Dermatol 2022;23:499–514.
39. Sève P, Jamilloux Y, Tilikete C, et al. Ocular Sarcoidosis. Semin Respir Crit Care Med 2020;41:673–88.
40. Patel S. Ocular sarcoidosis. Int Ophthalmol Clin 2015;55:15–24.
41. Birnie DH, Nery PB, Ha AC, et al. Cardiac sarcoidosis. J Am Coll Cardiol 2016;68: 411–21.
42. Iwai K, Sekiguti M, Hosoda Y, et al. Racial difference in cardiac sarcoidosis incidence observed at autopsy. Sarcoidosis 1994;11:26–31.
43. Serei VD, Fyfe B. The Many Faces of Cardiac Sarcoidosis. Am J Clin Pathol 2020; 153:294–302.
44. Trivieri MG, Spagnolo P, Birnie D, et al. Challenges in Cardiac and Pulmonary Sarcoidosis: JACC State-of-the-Art Review. J Am Coll Cardiol 2020;76:1878–901.
45. Joubert B, Chapelon-Abric C, Biard L, et al. Association of prognostic factors and immunosuppressive treatment with long-term outcomes in neurosarcoidosis. JAMA Neurol 2017;74:1336–44.
46. Fritz D, van de Beek D, Brouwer MC. Clinical features, treatment and outcome in neurosarcoidosis: systematic review and meta-analysis. BMC Neurol 2016; 16:220.
47. Bradshaw MJ, Pawate S, Koth LL, et al. Neurosarcoidosis: Pathophysiology, Diagnosis, and Treatment. Neurol Neuroimmunol Neuroinflamm 2021;8:e1084.
48. Tadros M, Forouhar F, Wu GY. Hepatic Sarcoidosis. J Clin Transl Hepatol 2013;1: 87–93.
49. Ungprasert P, Crowson CS, Simonetto DA, et al. Clinical Characteristics and Outcome of Hepatic Sarcoidosis: A Population-Based Study 1976-2013. Am J Gastroenterol 2017;112:1556–63.

50. Judson MA. Extrapulmonary sarcoidosis. Semin Respir Crit Care Med 2007;28: 83–101.
51. Bergner R, Löffler C. Renal sarcoidosis: approach to diagnosis and management. Curr Opin Pulm Med 2018;24:513–20.
52. de Kleijn WP, De Vries J, Lower EE, et al. Fatigue in sarcoidosis: a systematic review. Curr Opin Pulm Med 2009;15:499–506.
53. Hoitsma E, Marziniak M, Faber CG, et al. Small fiber neuropathy in sarcoidosis. Lancet 2002;359:2085–6.
54. Tavee JO, Karwa K, Ahmed Z, et al. Sarcoidosis-associated small fiber neuropathy in a large cohort: clinical aspects and response to IVIG and anti-TNF alpha treatment. Respir Med 2017;126:135–8.
55. Heij L, Dahan A, Hoitsma E. Sarcoidosis and pain caused by Small-fiber neuropathy, 2012. Pain Res Treat; 2012. p. 256024.
56. Baughman RP, Valeyre D, Korsten P, et al. ERS clinical practice guidelines on treatment of sarcoidosis. Eur Respir J 2021;58:2004079.
57. Gibson GJ, Prescott RJ, Muers MF, et al. British Thoracic Society Sarcoidosis study: effects of long term corticosteroid treatment. Thorax 1996;51:238–47.
58. Ungprasert P, Ryu JH, Matteson EL. Clinical Manifestations, Diagnosis, and Treatment of Sarcoidosis. Mayo Clin Proc Innov Qual Outcomes 2019;3:358–75.
59. Meyer KC. Lung transplantation for pulmonary sarcoidosis. Sarcoidosis Vasc Diffuse Lung Dis 2019;36:92–107.
60. Pasadhika S, Rosenbaum JT. Ocular Sarcoidosis. Clin Chest Med 2015;36: 669–83.
61. Sadek MM, Yung D, Birnie DH, et al. Corticosteroid therapy for cardiac sarcoidosis: a systematic review. Can J Cardiol 2013;29:1034–41.
62. Krause ML, Cooper LT, Chareonthaitawee P, et al. Successful use of rituximab in refractory cardiac sarcoidosis. Rheumatology 2016;55:189–91.
63. Jackson KC, Youmans QR, Wu T, et al. Heart transplantation outcomes in cardiac sarcoidosis. J Heart Lung Transplant 2022;41:113–22.
64. Ungprasert P, Matteson EL. Neurosarcoidosis. Rheum Dis Clin North Am 2017; 43:593–606.
65. Nozaki K, Judson MA. Neurosarcoidosis: clinical manifestations, diagnosis and treatment. Presse Med 2012;41:e331–48.
66. Cohen Aubart F, Bouvry D, Galanaud D, et al. Long-term outcomes of refractory neurosarcoidosis treated with infliximab. J Neurol 2017;264:891–7.
67. Judson MA, Boan AD, Lackland DT. The clinical course of sarcoidosis: presentation, diagnosis, and treatment in a large white and black cohort in the United States. Sarcoidosis Vasc Diffuse Lung Dis 2012;29:119–27.
68. Swigris JJ, Olson AL, Huie TJ, et al. Sarcoidosis-related mortality in the United States from 1988 to 2007. Am J Respir Crit Care Med 2011;183:1524–30.

Smoking-Related Interstitial Lung Diseases

Amarilys Alarcon-Calderon, MD[a], Robert Vassallo, MD[a], Eunhee S. Yi, MD[b], Jay H. Ryu, MD[a],*

KEYWORDS

- Desquamative interstitial pneumonia • Respiratory bronchiolitis
- Acute eosinophilic pneumonia • Pulmonary Langerhans cell histiocytosis
- Combined pulmonary fibrosis and emphysema

KEY POINTS

- Smoking is associated with several forms of interstitial lung disease (ILD), including pulmonary Langerhans cell histiocytosis, respiratory bronchiolitis-associated ILD, desquamative interstitial pneumonia, acute eosinophilic pneumonia, and combined pulmonary fibrosis and emphysema; some are diagnosed almost exclusively in smokers.
- High-resolution computed tomography shows various patterns depending on the specific type of smoking-related ILD.
- Although histopathologic confirmation via lung biopsy may be indicated in some situations, it is not always necessary.
- Smoking cessation is a major component of the management strategy for patients with smoking-related ILDs.

INTRODUCTION

Cigarette smoke is associated with the development of several diffuse parenchymal lung diseases, known collectively as smoking-related interstitial lung diseases (ILDs) **Box 1**.[1,2] These disease entities include (a) pulmonary Langerhans cell histiocytosis (PLCH), (b) respiratory bronchiolitis (RB) ILD, (c) desquamative interstitial pneumonia, (d) acute eosinophilic pneumonia (AEP), and (e) combined pulmonary fibrosis and emphysema (CPFE). This review describes the characteristics of the diseases mentioned above, their clinical manifestations, pathogenesis, diagnosis, and treatment strategies.

[a] Division of Pulmonary and Critical Care Medicine, Mayo Clinic College of Medicine and Science, 200 1st Street, Southwest, Rochester, MN 55905, USA; [b] Department of Laboratory Medicine & Pathology, Mayo Clinic College of Medicine and Science, 200 1st Street, Southwest, Rochester, MN 55905, USA
* Corresponding author.
E-mail address: Ryu.jay@mayo.edu

Immunol Allergy Clin N Am 43 (2023) 273–287
https://doi.org/10.1016/j.iac.2023.01.007
0889-8561/23/© 2023 Elsevier Inc. All rights reserved.
immunology.theclinics.com

PULMONARY LANGERHANS CELL HISTIOCYTOSIS

Langerhans cell histiocytosis (LCH) is a rare disease characterized by tissue infiltration of CD1a + myeloid cells that share many features with Langerhans cells and can present with a broad spectrum of clinical manifestations, from a self-limited process localized to a single organ to severe, life-threatening multiorgan involvement.[3] It commonly affects bone, skin, pituitary, spleen, and liver.[3,4] Most cases of PLCH involve the lung alone, but coexistence with extrapulmonary sites of involvement can also occur.[5–7] Initially, the pathogenesis was mainly attributed to a reactive process secondary to tobacco smoke exposure. However, the paradigm shifted with the description of mutation BRAF V600E and mutations in other genes resulting in constitutive activation of the MAPK (mitogen-activated protein kinase) pathway.[8,9] A combination of cigarette smoke and MAPK signaling pathway mutations results in a PLCH-like process in animal models.[10] Although the precise role of smoking in disease pathogenesis remains to be determined, it is likely that smoking acts as a pro-inflammatory trigger in susceptible individuals.[11]

PLCH is typically diagnosed in young adults, and over 90% of patients are current or former smokers at the time of diagnosis.[6,7,12] Occasionally, patients are asymptomatic and present with incidental radiographic changes.[6] Common respiratory symptoms include chronic dry cough and dyspnea; less commonly, patients report wheezing or hemoptysis. Systemic symptoms, such as asthenia, chest pain, fever, and weight loss can also be present.[7,12] Fifteen to twenty percent develop pneumothorax related to cystic lung process,[13,14] with recurrence in about half of the affected patients.[15]

Pulmonary function tests (PFTs) reveal a decreased diffusing capacity in approximately 90% of patients, and both restrictive and obstructive patterns are seen.[6,16] Chest radiography typically shows a micronodular, reticular, or cystic pattern involving both lungs with basilar sparing.[17] The classic description of PLCH on high-resolution computed tomography (HRCT) scans is the coexistence of nodules and cysts in the upper and middle lobes, with relative sparing of the lung bases (**Fig. 1**).[18] However, nodular opacities alone (including cavitating nodules) are more common in early disease.[6,16] Bronchoscopy with bronchoalveolar lavage (BAL) can help establish the diagnosis, with more than 5% of CD1a + cells being consistent with PLCH.[19] According to current consensus guidelines, histopathologic confirmation is recommended, accompanied by analysis for mutations in the BRAF or MAPK-ERK pathways.[20] Typical cases, with characteristic HRCT features of PLCH, in the appropriate clinical context, may be an exception.[20] Bronchoscopic or surgical lung biopsies provide a definitive diagnosis, with increased diagnostic yield with surgical biopsies.[21,22] Alternatively, a positive biopsy

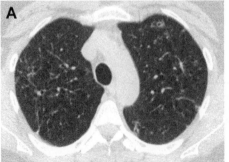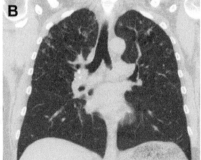

Fig. 1. PLCH. (*A*) Axial CT image showing nodules, cavitating nodules, and cysts in both upper lungs. (*B*) Coronal CT image showing predominantly upper lung distribution of abnormalities with relative sparing of the lower lungs.

of an extrapulmonary site, accompanied by compatible imaging, is diagnostic of PLCH. Echocardiography is helpful in screening for pulmonary hypertension (PH), a prevalent complication.[23] Histopathology shows multiple nodules with abundant Langerhans cells, which stain positive for S100 protein and the more specific markers CD1a and Langerin (CD207) (**Fig. 2**). In early disease, there is a predominance of cellular inflammation, with destructive bronchiolitis.[24] In advanced cases, scarring, such as stellate scars, is more common, and Langerhans cells might not be detectable.[24] Vascular medial thickening is commonly reported.[12,24]

The natural history of the disease is variable. Two years after diagnosis, 40% of patients have evidence of worsening pulmonary function.[5] Ongoing tobacco use and lower PaO2 are associated with the risk of lung function deterioration.[5] A recent study reported an estimated ten-year survival of 93%,[25] implying an improvement compared to the median survival of 12.5 years reported previously.[6,26] The presence of PH, abnormal diffusion capacity for carbon monoxide (DLCO), air trapping, decreased forced expiratory volume in one second (FEV1), and persistent smoking are markers of poor prognosis.[6,23,26] Therefore, counseling patients with PLCH about smoking cessation is essential. Oral glucocorticoids, immunosuppressive and chemotherapeutic agents are options in progressive disease, albeit with limited evidence. Cladribine has been reported to improve symptoms and spirometry in several small case series, and it is recommended as first-line systemic therapy in cases of progressive disease or persistent respiratory dysfunction, including those patients unable to quit smoking.[20,27] In patients with pulmonary arterial hypertension, PH-targeted therapy has been shown to improve hemodynamics.[28] Finally, lung transplantation should be considered in advanced disease when appropriate.[29]

RESPIRATORY BRONCHIOLITIS-INTERSTITIAL LUNG DISEASE

RB is a histopathologic term used to describe the presence of brown-pigmented macrophages in the respiratory bronchioles and was initially described as an incidental finding on autopsies of smokers.[30] It is a finding present in virtually all lung biopsies of smokers and many former smokers and is not necessarily a marker of clinical disease.[30–33] On the contrary, when there is clinical and radiological evidence of ILD associated with RB, it is classified as RB-ILD.[34] Myers and colleagues[34] described RB-ILD in 1987, with cases of heavy cigarette smokers presenting with respiratory symptoms and abnormal chest radiographs. Surgical-lung biopsy showed a mild

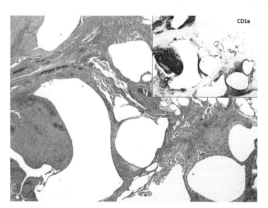

Fig. 2. PLCH. Lung biopsy showing cystic changes associated with collections of Langerhans cells highlighted by CD1a immunohistochemical staining (*inset*).

chronic inflammatory cell infiltration and thickening of the alveolar septa, in addition to RB. The initial report was followed by several case series describing similar findings[1,35–37]

Typically, patients with RB-ILD present in the third to the sixth decade of life (**Table 1**). Almost all the cases correspond to smokers or former smokers.[35,37,38] Symptoms include dyspnea, cough, and chest pain, and about half complain of sputum production.[34,35,37] On auscultation, patients often present with crackles and wheezing. Examination of the extremities reveals clubbing in 10% to 30% of cases.[1,35,39] Pulmonary function is variable, with normal PFTs in 10% to 20%.[35,39] The most consistent finding is a decrease in the DLCO, but it can be normal in up to 30%.[35,39]

Chest radiography shows reticular or reticulonodular interstitial patterns.[34,38] The most common findings on high-resolution computerized tomography (HRCT) are bronchial wall thickening, ground-glass opacities, and centrilobular nodules in both upper and lower lobes (**Fig. 3**). Two-thirds of patients also have centrilobular emphysema with upper lobe predominance.[40] A reticular pattern is identified in close to 30%: however, significant fibrosis, traction bronchiectasis, and honeycombing are typically absent.[40] Of note, hypersensitivity pneumonitis (HP) may present with similar radiologic findings, but a history of smoking makes the diagnosis of RB-ILD more likely, as smoking is associated with a lower incidence of HP compared to the general population.[41]

Findings on BAL are nonspecific and can yield the pigment-laden macrophages associated with smoking, with no abnormal increase of other leukocyte types suggestive of an alternative diagnosis.[34,42] A biopsy is not always needed for the diagnosis. However, when obtained, surgical lung biopsy is the method of choice, given the patchy distribution of the disease, which could result in sampling error with bronchoscopic biopsies. Histopathology reveals pigmented macrophages in alveolar ducts, alveoli, and respiratory bronchioles, interstitial inflammation, and mild fibrosis of the alveolar septa. There is a patchy, peribronchiolar, and periarterial distribution of the interstitial abnormalities[34,37,38] (see **Fig. 3**). Whether RB and RB-ILD can be separated based on histopathological criteria alone is controversial.

Table 1
Clinical characteristics of respiratory bronchiolitis-associated interstitial lung diseases and desquamative interstitial pneumonitis

	RB-ILD	Desquamative Interstitial Pneumonitis
Demographics	Age: 30 to 60 years old	Age: 40 to 50 years old Slight male predominance
Associations	Smoking >95%	Smoking 80% Occupational exposures Connective tissue Infection
Imaging	Centrilobular nodules Bronchial wall thickening	Ground glass opacities, lower lobe predominant. Reticular pattern
Pulmonary function tests	Variable. May be normal Decreased diffusion capacity (mild)	Restriction is more common, although other patterns can be present. Decreased diffusion capacity (moderate-severe)
Treatment	Smoking cessation	Smoking cessation Corticosteroids

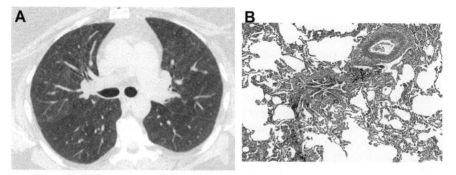

Fig. 3. RB-ILD. (*A*) Axial CT image showing hazy ground-glass opacities involving anterior portions of the upper lobes. (*B*) RB-ILD shows less prominent collections of alveolar macrophages than in DIP, mainly localized to bronchiolar lumens and adjacent centriacinar alveolar spaces, with little or no interstitial fibrosis.

Smoking cessation is the mainstay of treatment of RB-ILD and may bring on stability or improvement of symptoms after a few years.[34,37] A small series showed improvement in centrilobular ground-glass opacities and DLCO in all patients (n = 5) after quitting smoking, with a mean follow-up of 46 months.[43] However, many patients experience worsening symptoms despite smoking cessation.[39] Therefore, clinicians often prescribe oral glucocorticoids or immunosuppressant drugs to treat RB-ILD, but the evidence is limited. In general, the prognosis of RB-ILD is good, and mortality is rare.[39]

DESQUAMATIVE INTERSTITIAL PNEUMONIA

Liebow first described desquamative interstitial pneumonia (DIP) in 1965.[44] It was initially thought that the characteristic lesions corresponded to the desquamation of the alveolar cells into the distal air spaces. However, in reality, the lesion is caused by the accumulation of pigment-laden macrophages in the alveoli. In 2001, the American Thoracic Society and European Respiratory Society discussed changing the name to "alveolar macrophage pneumonia", but they elected to preserve the historic nomenclature.[45] There is a significant clinical and histopathologic overlap between RB-ILD and DIP, and although the pathogenesis has not been entirely elucidated, they likely share some common mechanisms. Approximately 20% of cases are encountered in never-smokers, as opposed to RB-ILD, which virtually always presents in tobacco users.[46] Approximately one-third of patients have a history of environmental exposure to dust and fumes, and high levels of inorganic particles have been found on biopsies of patients with DIP,[46,47] suggesting that occupational exposures may play a role in the development of the disease. Indeed, DIP has been reported from exposure to copper, beryllium, fire extinguisher powder, diesel fumes, solder fumes and nylon filaments[48] Additional possible associations include connective tissue disorders such as scleroderma and rheumatoid arthritis, drugs such as sirolimus, nitrofurantoin, tocainide, sulfasalazine, and viral infections.[46,49–54]

On average, patients are middle-aged at presentation, although cases in children have also been described.[55,56] Most series report a male predominance.[35–37,46,57] The most common symptom in DIP is dyspnea (86%), followed by cough (65%), which is usually nonproductive. Chest pain and constitutional symptoms, such as weight loss, fatigue, and weakness, can also occur.[46] One-fifth of patients have a normal physical exam, whereas crackles and clubbing are common findings. The predominant pattern on PFTs is restrictive in 70% of cases, with impaired gas exchange, as evidenced by a decreased diffusion capacity.[35,46] The functional abnormalities tend to be more severe in DIP than in RB-ILD (**Table1**).[37]

Chest radiography generally shows bilateral interstitial markings. HRCT is characteristic for ground glass opacities with lower lobe and slight peripheral predominance; consolidative opacities are less commonly seen (**Fig. 4**). Reticular opacities are present in half of the cases, but findings of fibrosis like architectural distortion and honeycombing are unusual. In some, thin-walled cysts may be noted in the parenchyma and are usually small.[58,59] BAL can show eosinophilia (mean eosinophil count of 18% in one study) in a minority of cases.[60] As in other ILDs, confirmation of the diagnosis often requires a surgical lung biopsy, although cryobiopsy is an emerging option.[22] The cardinal feature of DIP is the uniform filling of the alveolar spaces with mononuclear cells (see **Fig. 4**), as opposed to the patchy, bronchiolocentric distribution of RB-ILD.[61] However, the distinction between these processes is not always clear and may represent a continuous spectrum of smoking-related reactions. Lymphoid follicles, interstitial fibrosis, and eosinophils are more common in DIP compared to those with RB.[36] Varying degrees of fibrosis have been reported, but typically not as prominent as in usual interstitial pneumonia (UIP),[62] the histopathologic pattern seen in idiopathic pulmonary fibrosis and fibrotic forms of connective tissue-associated ILD, hypersensitivity pneumonitis, and drug-induced lung disease.

DIP may manifest fibrotic changes when progressive, although the proportion of patients with progression of their disease is much smaller than with UIP.[58] Smoking and other inhalational exposures should be avoided. Most patients are treated with corticosteroids or immunosuppressants with variable responses, although with scarce evidence supporting their therapeutic efficacy. Two-thirds of patients have clinical improvement, whereas close to 25% decline.[46] Without treatment, the proportion of clinical worsening is higher.[57] A minority of patients require lung transplantation.[50]

ACUTE EOSINOPHILIC PNEUMONIA

AEP is an acute respiratory illness presenting with hypoxemia, diffuse pulmonary infiltrates, and a markedly elevated eosinophil count on BAL.[63,64] Typically, it presents in young males in the third to fifth decades of life, especially in those initiating or

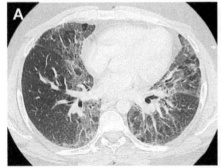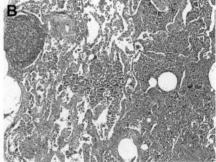

Fig. 4. DIP. (*A*) Axial CT image showing bilateral ground-glass opacities along with some reticular opacities and few regions of hyperlucency (air-trapping). (*B*) Diffuse accumulation of pigmented alveolar macrophages with mild interstitial thickening due to fibrosis. Lymphoid follicles with a prominent germinal center (shown in the upper left field) are often present in DIP.

increasing the amount of tobacco smoked.[65] Secondhand smoke, electronic cigarettes, recreational drugs, dust, and other occupational exposures have also been reported to precipitate this disorder.[66–70] AEP can also be associated with medication use, including daptomycin, minocycline, mesalamine, and other antimicrobials, antidepressants, and anti-inflammatory and chemotherapeutics.[71–73]

In patients with smoking-related AEP, an acutely evolving (days to few weeks) presentation occurs with cough, fever, chest pain, and dyspnea. Peripheral eosinophilia is often absent on initial presentation and develops later in the course.[74,75] Chest radiography shows alveolar and interstitial opacities, Kerley B-lines; bilateral pleural effusions are seen in approximately half of patients.[75] CT typically shows ground-glass, nodular and consolidative opacities, interlobular septal thickening, and pleural effusions (**Fig. 5**A).[76] A BAL with an eosinophil count of >25% is usually diagnostic in the appropriate clinicoradiologic setting (**Fig. 5**B). Interestingly, eosinophilia on BAL has been reported to be associated with less hypoxemia.[75] If a biopsy is performed, it shows interstitial edema and infiltration of alveolar, bronchiolar, and interstitial spaces by eosinophils and diffuse alveolar damage (**Fig. 5**C).[77]

Although the presentation can be severe, including respiratory failure requiring mechanical ventilation, the prognosis is generally good, and most patients experience complete resolution with steroid treatment when diagnosed promptly.[78,79] Typically, the treatment includes intravenous or oral steroids in the acute setting, followed by a taper over 2 to 4 weeks.[78] Review of potential exposures and subsequent avoidance of the offending agent is crucial.

COMBINED PULMONARY FIBROSIS AND EMPHYSEMA

CPFE is a clinical syndrome that classifies a subgroup of patients with emphysema with coexistent pulmonary fibrosis (**Fig. 6**).[80–83] It remains controversial whether CPFE is a distinct entity or merely the coexistence of two separate processes. **Box 1** presents a summary of the clinical, physiologic, and radiologic characteristics associated with CPFE. PFTs may show normal lung volumes and spirometry despite the profoundly abnormal physiology due to two opposing pathophysiologic processes. Reduced gas exchange capacity occurs with both emphysematous and fibrotic disorders; therefore, decreased DLCO may be the sole abnormality on PFTs.[82,83]

Unfortunately, CPFE is associated with a high mortality rate, with a clinical course characterized by frequent exacerbations and gradual progression to chronic respiratory failure.[84–87] In addition, the incidence of lung cancer and PH is high.[85,88,89] The outcomes of patients with CPFE are worse than in COPD alone but comparable to idiopathic pulmonary fibrosis when adjusting for the degree of fibrosis.[81] There is no specific treatment of CPFE other than optimizing the treatment of the emphysema and fibrosis. Management includes general measures such as smoking cessation, supplemental oxygen if required, and pulmonary rehabilitation. Bronchodilators may be useful in patients with airflow limitations. Antifibrotics can be considered in cases with progressive fibrosis. However, patients with significant emphysema have been generally excluded from clinical trials assessing the efficacy of antifibrotic therapy.[81] Identification of PH and specific treatment thereof can be considered for these patients.[88,90]

OTHER INTERSTITIAL LUNG DISORDERS

There is growing recognition of parenchymal abnormalities in smokers that do not meet the criteria for distinct smoking-related ILDs described above. With the

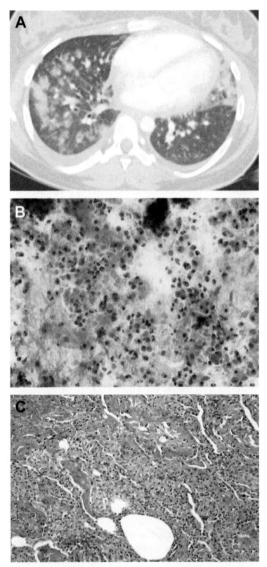

Fig. 5. AEP. (*A*) Axial CT image showing patchy consolidative opacities bilaterally with small pleural effusions, right greater than left. (*B*) Cytology specimen showing numerous eosinophils with occasional Charcot Leyden crystals (right middle field). (*C*) Lung biopsy with numerous intraalveolar eosinophils accompanied by features of diffuse alveolar damage including hyaline membranes and alveolar fibrinous exudates.

implementation of lung cancer screening for smokers, it has been reported that many have interstitial lung abnormalities (ILAs), even in the absence of respiratory symptoms.[91,92] Although the clinical significance is unclear, ILAs have been associated with decreased functional capacity, lung function, quality of life, and increased mortality.[93–95] In addition, the histopathologic term "smoking-related interstitial fibrosis" (SRIF) describes a common finding in smokers' lungs, with interstitial fibrosis in the subpleural lung tissue showing prominent collagen deposition.[96] Some patients may

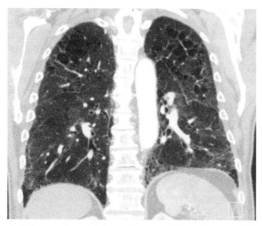

Fig. 6. CPFE. Coronal CT image showing emphysematous changes predominantly in the upper lungs with a bibasilar and peripheral distribution of fibrotic changes.

manifest mild-moderate changes in lung function measurement, but long-term follow-up data are lacking.[96,97] In contrast, hypersensitivity pneumonitis is less prevalent in smokers for reasons that are still not fully defined but may involve the effect of nicotine on immune responses to inhaled antigens.[98] Sarcoidosis also has a decreased prevalence in tobacco smokers, and some studies suggest that smoking could modify the effect of genetic predisposition.[99,100]

Box 1
Clinical characteristics of combined pulmonary fibrosis and emphysema (CPFE)

Clinical characteristics of combined pulmonary fibrosis and emphysema (CPFE)

Demographics
  Age: Commonly 60 to 80 years old
  Sex: Over 70% male

Symptoms
  Dyspnea on exertion
  Cough
  Recurrent exacerbations

Associated comorbidities
  Pulmonary hypertension
  Lung cancer

Physical examination
  Inspiratory basal crackles
  Clubbing

Radiographic findings
  Fibrotic changes: honeycombing, reticular opacities, traction bronchiectasis, ground-glass opacities, and architectural distortion; more prominent in lower lung zones
  Emphysema and bullae, more prominent in upper lung zones (see **Fig. 6**)

Pulmonary function tests
  Severely reduced diffusion capacity
  FEV1/FVC ratio is normal or slightly reduced
  Spirometry and lung volumes may be normal or near normal

Data from Refs.[81,82]

SUMMARY

Smoking-related ILDs encompass a heterogeneous group of pulmonary diseases diagnosed in association with tobacco use, including RB-ILD, DIP, PLCH, AEP, and CPFE. Their pathogenesis is not entirely understood, and the contribution from cigarette smoke itself versus other environmental and genetic factors is a current area of investigation. Prognosis varies among these disorders, but smoking cessation is a major component of management for affected patients.

CLINICS CARE POINTS

- Smoking induces a broad spectrum of pathologic processes in the lung and includes interstitial lung diseases (ILDs).
- Currently recognized forms of smoking-related ILDs include pulmonary Langerhans cell histiocytosis, respiratory bronchiolitis-interstitial lung disease, desquamative interstitial pneumonia, acute eosinophilic pneumonia, and combined pulmonary fibrosis and emphysema.
- Smoking cessation is an essential component of management for patients with smoking-related ILDs.
- The coexistence of emphysema and pulmonary fibrosis often escapes clinical recognition but is frequently associated with the occurrence of pulmonary hypertension and lung cancer.

DISCLOSURE

The Authors declare nothing to disclose.

REFERENCES

1. Moon J, du Bois RM, Colby TV, et al. Clinical significance of respiratory bronchiolitis on open lung biopsy and its relationship to smoking related interstitial lung disease. Thorax 1999;54(11):1009–14.
2. Ryu JH, Colby TV, Hartman TE, et al. Smoking-related interstitial lung diseases: a concise review. Eur Respir J 2001;17(1):122.
3. Emile JF, Abla O, Fraitag S, et al. Revised classification of histiocytoses and neoplasms of the macrophage-dendritic cell lineages. Blood 2016;127(22): 2672–81.
4. Kobayashi M, Ando S, Kawamata T, et al. Clinical features and outcomes of adult Langerhans cell histiocytosis: a single-center experience. Int J Hematol 2020;112(2):185–92.
5. Tazi A, de Margerie C, Naccache JM, et al. The natural history of adult pulmonary Langerhans cell histiocytosis: a prospective multicentre study. Orphanet J Rare Dis 2015;10:30.
6. Vassallo R, Ryu JH, Schroeder DR, et al. Clinical outcomes of pulmonary langerhans'-cell histiocytosis in adults. N Engl J Med 2002;346(7):484–90.
7. Colby TV, Lombard C. Histiocytosis X in the lung. Hum Pathol 1983;14(10): 847–56.
8. Badalian-Very G, Vergilio J-A, Degar BA, et al. Recurrent BRAF mutations in Langerhans cell histiocytosis. Blood 2010;116(11):1919–23.
9. Roden AC, Hu X, Kip S, et al. BRAF V600E expression in Langerhans cell histiocytosis: clinical and immunohistochemical study on 25 pulmonary and 54 extrapulmonary cases. Am J Surg Pathol 2014;38(4):548–51.

10. Liu H, Osterburg AR, Flury J, et al. MAPK mutations and cigarette smoke promote the pathogenesis of pulmonary Langerhans cell histiocytosis. JCI Insight 2020;5(4). https://doi.org/10.1172/jci.insight.132048.

11. Vassallo R, Harari S, Tazi A. Current understanding and management of pulmonary Langerhans cell histiocytosis. Thorax 2017;72(10):937–45.

12. Travis WD, Borok Z, Roum JH, et al. Pulmonary Langerhans cell granulomatosis (histiocytosis X). A clinicopathologic study of 48 cases. Am J Surg Pathol 1993; 17(10):971–86.

13. Mendez JL, Nadrous HF, Vassallo R, et al. Pneumothorax in pulmonary Langerhans cell histiocytosis. Chest 2004;125(3):1028–32.

14. Radzikowska E, Błasińska-Przerwa K, Wiatr E, et al. Pneumothorax in Patients with Pulmonary Langerhans Cell Histiocytosis. Lung 2018;196(6):715–20.

15. Le Guen P, Chevret S, Bugnet E, et al. Management and outcomes of pneumothorax in adult patients with Langerhans cell Histiocytosis. Orphanet J Rare Dis 2019;14(1):229.

16. Tazi A, Marc K, Dominique S, et al. Serial computed tomography and lung function testing in pulmonary Langerhans' cell histiocytosis. Eur Respir J 2012; 40(4):905.

17. Lacronique J, Roth C, Battesti JP, et al. Chest radiological features of pulmonary histiocytosis X: a report based on 50 adult cases. Thorax 1982;37(2):104–9.

18. Brauner MW, Grenier P, Mouelhi MM, et al. Pulmonary histiocytosis X: evaluation with high-resolution CT. Radiology 1989;172(1):255–8.

19. Auerswald U, Barth J, Magnussen H. Value of CD-1-positive cells in bronchoalveolar lavage fluid for the diagnosis of pulmonary histiocytosis X. Lung 1991; 169(6):305–9.

20. Goyal G, Tazi A, Go RS, et al. International expert consensus recommendations for the diagnosis and treatment of Langerhans cell histiocytosis in adults. Blood 2022;139(17):2601–21.

21. Baqir M, Vassallo R, Maldonado F, et al. Utility of bronchoscopy in pulmonary Langerhans cell histiocytosis. J Bronchology Interv Pulmonol 2013;20(4): 309–12.

22. Barata M, Caetano Mota P, Melo N, et al. Transbronchial lung cryobiopsy in smoking-related interstitial lung diseases. Sarcoidosis Vasc Diffuse Lung Dis 2020;37(4):e2020013.

23. Chaowalit N, Pellikka PA, Decker PA, et al. Echocardiographic and clinical characteristics of pulmonary hypertension complicating pulmonary langerhans cell histiocytosis. Mayo Clinic Proc 2004;79(10):1269–75.

24. Roden AC, Yi ES. Pulmonary langerhans cell histiocytosis: an update from the pathologists' perspective. Arch Pathol Lab Med 2016;140(3):230–40.

25. Benattia A, Bugnet E, Walter-Petrich A, et al. Long-term outcomes of adult pulmonary Langerhans cell histiocytosis: a prospective cohort. Eur Respir J 2022; 59(5). https://doi.org/10.1183/13993003.01017-2021.

26. Delobbe A, Durieu J, Duhamel A, et al. Determinants of survival in pulmonary Langerhans' cell granulomatosis (histiocytosis X). Groupe d'Etude en Pathologie Interstitielle de la Société de Pathologie Thoracique du Nord. Eur Respir J 1996;9(10):2002–6.

27. Grobost V, Khouatra C, Lazor R, et al. Effectiveness of cladribine therapy in patients with pulmonary Langerhans cell histiocytosis. Orphanet J Rare Dis 2014; 9:191.

28. Le Pavec J, Lorillon G, Jaïs X, et al. Pulmonary Langerhans cell histiocytosis-associated pulmonary hypertension: clinical characteristics and impact of pulmonary arterial hypertension therapies. Chest 2012;142(5):1150–7.

29. Dauriat G, Mal H, Thabut G, et al. Lung transplantation for pulmonary langerhans' cell histiocytosis: a multicenter analysis. Transplantation 2006;81(5):746–50.

30. Niewoehner DE, Kleinerman J, Rice DB. Pathologic changes in the peripheral airways of young cigarette smokers. N Engl J Med 1974;291(15):755–8.

31. Fraig M, Shreesha U, Savici D, et al. Respiratory bronchiolitis: a clinicopathologic study in current smokers, ex-smokers, and never-smokers. Am J Surg Pathol 2002;26(5):647–53.

32. Wright JL, Lawson LM, Pare PD, et al. Morphology of peripheral airways in current smokers and ex-smokers. Am Rev Respir Dis 1983;127(4):474–7.

33. Cosio MG, Hale KA, Niewoehner DE. Morphologic and morphometric effects of prolonged cigarette smoking on the small airways. Am Rev Respir Dis 1980; 122(2):265–71.

34. Myers JL, Veal CF Jr, Shin MS, et al. Respiratory bronchiolitis causing interstitial lung disease. A clinicopathologic study of six cases. Am Rev Respir Dis 1987; 135(4):880–4.

35. Ryu JH, Myers JL, Capizzi SA, et al. Desquamative interstitial pneumonia and respiratory bronchiolitis-associated interstitial lung disease. Chest 2005; 127(1):178–84.

36. Craig PJ, Wells AU, Doffman S, et al. Desquamative interstitial pneumonia, respiratory bronchiolitis and their relationship to smoking. Histopathology 2004; 45(3):275–82.

37. Yousem SA, Colby TV, Gaensler EA. Respiratory bronchiolitis-associated interstitial lung disease and its relationship to desquamative interstitial pneumonia. Mayo Clin Proc 1989;64(11):1373–80.

38. Yousem SA. Respiratory bronchiolitis-associated interstitial lung disease with fibrosis is a lesion distinct from fibrotic nonspecific interstitial pneumonia: a proposal. Mod Pathol 2006;19(11):1474–9.

39. Portnoy J, Veraldi KL, Schwarz MI, et al. Respiratory bronchiolitis-interstitial lung disease: long-term outcome. Chest 2007;131(3):664–71.

40. Park JS, Brown KK, Tuder RM, et al. Respiratory bronchiolitis-associated interstitial lung disease: radiologic features with clinical and pathologic correlation. J Comput Assist Tomogr 2002;26(1):13–20.

41. Solaymani-Dodaran M, West J, Smith C, et al. Extrinsic allergic alveolitis: incidence and mortality in the general population. QJM: An Int J Med 2007; 100(4):233–7.

42. Agius RM, Rutman A, Knight RK, et al. Human pulmonary alveolar macrophages with smokers' inclusions: their relation to the cessation of cigarette smoking. Br J Exp Pathol 1986;67(3):407–13.

43. Nakanishi M, Demura Y, Mizuno S, et al. Changes in HRCT findings in patients with respiratory bronchiolitis-associated interstitial lung disease after smoking cessation. Eur Respir J 2007;29(3):453–61.

44. Liebow AA, Steer A, Billingsley JG. Desquamative Interstitial Pneumonia. Am J Med 1965;39:369–404.

45. American Thoracic Society/European Respiratory Society International Multidisciplinary Consensus Classification of the Idiopathic Interstitial Pneumonias. Am J Resp Crit Care 2002;165(2):277–304.

46. Hellemons ME, Moor CC, von der Thusen J, et al. Desquamative interstitial pneumonia: a systematic review of its features and outcomes. Eur Respir Rev 2020;29(156). https://doi.org/10.1183/16000617.0181-2019.

47. Abraham JL, Hertzberg MA. Inorganic particulates associated with desquamative interstitial pneumonia. Chest 1981;80(1 Suppl):67–70.

48. Godbert B, Wissler MP, Vignaud JM. Desquamative interstitial pneumonia: an analytic review with an emphasis on aetiology. Eur Respir Rev 2013;22(128): 117–23.

49. Ishii H, Iwata A, Sakamoto N, et al. Desquamative interstitial pneumonia (DIP) in a patient with rheumatoid arthritis: is DIP associated with autoimmune disorders? Intern Med 2009;48(10):827–30.

50. Ong S, Levy RD, Yee J, et al. Successful lung transplantation in an HIV seropositive patient with desquamative interstitial pneumonia: a case report. BMC Pulm Med 2018;18(1):162.

51. Hasegawa H, Nakamura Y, Kaida Y, et al. [A case of desquamative interstitial pneumonia associated with hepatitis C virus infection]. Nihon Kokyuki Gakkai Zasshi 2009;47(8):698–703.

52. Sung SA, Ko GJ, Kim JY, et al. Desquamative interstitial pneumonia associated with concurrent cytomegalovirus and Aspergillus pneumonia in a renal transplant recipient. Nephrol Dial Transpl 2005;20(3):635–8.

53. Schroten H, Manz S, Köhler H, et al. Fatal desquamative interstitial pneumonia associated with proven CMV infection in an 8-month-old boy. Pediatr Pulmonol 1998;25(5):345–7.

54. Iskandar SB, McKinney LA, Shah L, et al. Desquamative interstitial pneumonia and hepatitis C virus infection: a rare association. South Med J 2004;97(9): 890–3.

55. Buchino JJ, Keenan WJ, Algren JT, et al. Familial desquamative interstitial pneumonitis occurring in infants. Am J Med Genet Suppl 1987;3:285–91.

56. Stillwell PC, Norris DG, O'Connell EJ, et al. Desquamative interstitial pneumonitis in children. Chest 1980;77(2):165–71.

57. Carrington CB, Gaensler EA, Coutu RE, et al. Natural history and treated course of usual and desquamative interstitial pneumonia. N Engl J Med 1978;298(15): 801–9.

58. Hartman TE, Primack SL, Kang EY, et al. Disease progression in usual interstitial pneumonia compared with desquamative interstitial pneumonia. Assess serial CT. Chest 1996;110(2):378–82.

59. Akira M, Yamamoto S, Hara H, et al. Serial computed tomographic evaluation in desquamative interstitial pneumonia. Thorax 1997;52(4):333–7.

60. Kawabata Y, Takemura T, Hebisawa A, et al. Eosinophilia in bronchoalveolar lavage fluid and architectural destruction are features of desquamative interstitial pneumonia. Histopathology 2008;52(2):194–202.

61. Konopka KE, Myers JL. A Review of Smoking-Related Interstitial Fibrosis, Respiratory Bronchiolitis, and Desquamative Interstitial Pneumonia: Overlapping Histology and Confusing Terminology. Arch Pathol Lab Med 2018;142(10): 1177–81.

62. Carrington CB, Gaensler EA, Coutu RE, et al. Usual and desquamative interstitial pneumonia. Chest 1976;69(2 Suppl):261–3.

63. Allen JN, Pacht ER, Gadek JE, et al. Acute eosinophilic pneumonia as a reversible cause of noninfectious respiratory failure. N Engl J Med 1989;321(9): 569–74.

64. Badesch DB, King TE Jr, Schwarz MI. Acute eosinophilic pneumonia: a hyper-sensitivity phenomenon? Am Rev Respir Dis 1989;139(1):249–52.

65. Uchiyama H, Suda T, Nakamura Y, et al. Alterations in smoking habits are associated with acute eosinophilic pneumonia. Chest 2008;133(5):1174–80.

66. Chaaban T. Acute eosinophilic pneumonia associated with non-cigarette smoking products: a systematic review. Adv Respir Med 2020;88(2):142–6.

67. Rom WN, Weiden M, Garcia R, et al. Acute eosinophilic pneumonia in a New York City firefighter exposed to World Trade Center dust. Am J Respir Crit Care Med 2002;166(6):797–800.

68. Cherian SV, Sardinas G, Al Salihi SA, et al. A 62-year-old man with cough and dyspnea after crack cocaine inhalation. Ann Am Thorac Soc 2016;13(8):1416–8.

69. De Giacomi F, Vassallo R, Yi ES, et al. Acute eosinophilic pneumonia. causes, diagnosis, and management. Am J Respir Crit Care Med 2018;197(6):728–36.

70. Oh P, Balter M. Cocaine induced eosinophilic lung disease. Thorax 1992;47(6): 478–9.

71. Bartal C, Sagy I, Barski L. Drug-induced eosinophilic pneumonia: a review of 196 case reports. Medicine (Baltimore) 2018;97(4):e9688.

72. De Giacomi F, Decker PA, Vassallo R, et al. Acute eosinophilic pneumonia: correlation of clinical characteristics with underlying cause. Chest 2017;152(2): 379–85.

73. Higashi Y, Nakamura S, Tsuji Y, et al. Daptomycin-induced eosinophilic pneumonia and a review of the published literature. Intern Med 2018;57(2):253–8.

74. Buelow BJ, Kelly BT, Zafra HT, et al. Absence of Peripheral Eosinophilia on Initial Clinical Presentation Does Not Rule Out the Diagnosis of Acute Eosinophilic Pneumonia. J Allergy Clin Immunol Pract 2015;3(4):597–8.

75. Choi JY, Lim JU, Jeong HJ, et al. Association between peripheral blood/bronchoalveolar lavage eosinophilia and significant oxygen requirements in patients with acute eosinophilic pneumonia. BMC Pulm Med 2020;20(1):22.

76. Daimon T, Johkoh T, Sumikawa H, et al. Acute eosinophilic pneumonia: Thin-section CT findings in 29 patients. Eur J Radiol 2008;65(3):462–7.

77. Tazelaar HD, Linz LJ, Colby TV, et al. Acute eosinophilic pneumonia: histopathologic findings in nine patients. Am J Respir Crit Care Med 1997;155(1): 296–302.

78. Rhee CK, Min KH, Yim NY, et al. Clinical characteristics and corticosteroid treatment of acute eosinophilic pneumonia. Eur Respir J 2013;41(2):402–9.

79. Philit F, Etienne-Mastroianni B, Parrot A, et al. Idiopathic acute eosinophilic pneumonia: a study of 22 patients. Am J Respir Crit Care Med 2002;166(9): 1235–9.

80. Cottin V. Combined pulmonary fibrosis and emphysema: bad and ugly all the same? Eur Respir J 2017;50(1). https://doi.org/10.1183/13993003.00846-2017.

81. Cottin V, Selman M, Inoue Y, et al. Syndrome of Combined Pulmonary Fibrosis and Emphysema: An Official ATS/ERS/JRS/ALAT Research Statement. Am J Respir Crit Care Med 2022;206(4):e7–41.

82. Cottin V, Nunes H, Brillet PY, et al. Combined pulmonary fibrosis and emphysema: a distinct underrecognised entity. Eur Respir J 2005;26(4):586–93.

83. Nemoto M, Koo CW, Ryu JH. Diagnosis and Treatment of Combined Pulmonary Fibrosis and Emphysema in 2022. JAMA 2022;328(1):69–70.

84. Mejia M, Carrillo G, Rojas-Serrano J, et al. Idiopathic pulmonary fibrosis and emphysema: decreased survival associated with severe pulmonary arterial hypertension. Chest 2009;136(1):10–5.

85. Hage R, Gautschi F, Steinack C, et al. Combined Pulmonary Fibrosis and Emphysema (CPFE) Clinical Features and Management. Int J Chron Obstruct Pulmon Dis 2021;16:167–77.

86. Kim HJ, Snyder LD, Neely ML, et al. Clinical Outcomes of Patients with Combined Idiopathic Pulmonary Fibrosis and Emphysema in the IPF-PRO Registry. Lung 2022;200(1):21–9.

87. Ryerson CJ, Hartman T, Elicker BM, et al. Clinical features and outcomes in combined pulmonary fibrosis and emphysema in idiopathic pulmonary fibrosis. Chest 2013;144(1):234–40.

88. Cottin V, Le Pavec J, Prevot G, et al. Pulmonary hypertension in patients with combined pulmonary fibrosis and emphysema syndrome. Eur Respir J 2010; 35(1):105–11.

89. Goh NSL. Pulmonary hypertension in combined pulmonary fibrosis and emphysema: a tale of two cities. Respirology 2018;23(6):556–7.

90. Jacob J, Bartholmai BJ, Rajagopalan S, et al. Likelihood of pulmonary hypertension in patients with idiopathic pulmonary fibrosis and emphysema. Respirology 2018;23(6):593–9.

91. Chung JH, Richards JC, Koelsch TL, et al. Screening for lung cancer: incidental pulmonary parenchymal findings. AJR Am J Roentgenol 2018;210(3):503–13.

92. Tanner NT, Thomas NA, Ward R, et al. Association of cigarette type with lung cancer incidence and mortality: secondary analysis of the national lung screening trial. JAMA Intern Med 2019;179(12):1710–2.

93. Doyle TJ, Washko GR, Fernandez IE, et al. Interstitial lung abnormalities and reduced exercise capacity. Am J Respir Crit Care Med 2012;185(7):756–62.

94. Ash SY, Harmouche R, Putman RK, et al. Clinical and genetic associations of objectively identified interstitial changes in smokers. Chest 2017;152(4):780–91.

95. Washko GR, Hunninghake GM, Fernandez IE, et al. Lung Volumes and Emphysema in Smokers with Interstitial Lung Abnormalities. N Engl J Med 2011; 364(10):897–906.

96. Katzenstein AL, Mukhopadhyay S, Zanardi C, et al. Clinically occult interstitial fibrosis in smokers: classification and significance of a surprisingly common finding in lobectomy specimens. Hum Pathol 2010;41(3):316–25.

97. Katzenstein AL. Smoking-related interstitial fibrosis (SRIF), pathogenesis and treatment of usual interstitial pneumonia (UIP), and transbronchial biopsy in UIP. Mod Pathol 2012;25(Suppl 1):S68–78.

98. Blanchet MR, Israël-Assayag E, Cormier Y. Inhibitory effect of nicotine on experimental hypersensitivity pneumonitis in vivo and in vitro. Am J Respir Crit Care Med 2004;169(8):903–9.

99. Douglas JG, Middleton WG, Gaddie J, et al. Sarcoidosis: a disorder commoner in non-smokers? Thorax 1986;41(10):787–91.

100. Rivera NV, Patasova K, Kullberg S, et al. A gene-environment interaction between smoking and gene polymorphisms provides a high risk of two subgroups of sarcoidosis. Sci Rep 2019;9(1):18633.

Eosinophilic Lung Diseases

Vincent Cottin, MD, PhD[a,b,]*

KEYWORDS

- Eosinophil • Eosinophilic pneumonia • Interstitial lung disease
- Eosinophilic granulomatosis with polyangiitis • *Aspergillus*

KEY POINTS

- Eosinophilic lung diseases may present as eosinophilic pneumonia with chronic or acute onset, or as the more transient Löffler syndrome.
- The diagnosis of eosinophilic pneumonia is based on both characteristic clinical-imaging features and the demonstration of alveolar eosinophilia of 25% eosinophils or more at bronchoalveolar lavage.
- Peripheral blood eosinophilia can be absent at presentation.
- All possible causes of eosinophilia (especially fungus or parasitic infection, drug or toxic exposure) must be thoroughly investigated.
- Extra-thoracic manifestations with eosinophilic lung disease primarily suggest the diagnosis of eosinophilic granulomatosis with polyangiitis.

DEFINITION AND CLASSIFICATION
Definition

Eosinophilic lung diseases are a group of diffuse parenchymal lung diseases[1–3] characterized by the prominent infiltration of the lung interstitium and the alveolar spaces by polymorphonuclear eosinophils, with conservation of the lung architecture. Eosinophilic lung diseases therefore belong to the wider group of interstitial lung diseases, with the notable characteristic of a dramatic response to systemic corticosteroid therapy and healing without any sequelae in most cases.

Blood *eosinophilia* is defined by an eosinophil blood cell count greater than 0.5×10^9/L, and *hypereosinophilia* by an eosinophil blood cell count of greater than 1.5×10^9 on two examinations over at least a 1-month interval.[2,4,5] Alveolar eosinophilia is defined by a differential cell count of at least 25% eosinophils at bronchoalveolar lavage (BAL). Hypereosinophilia in the context of lung disease, and/or

Financial support: Hospices Civils de Lyon, Université Lyon 1.
[a] Service de pneumologie, Hospices Civils de Lyon, Hôpital Louis Pradel, Centre de référence coordonnateur des maladies pulmonaires rares (OrphaLung), 28 Avenue Doyen Lepine, Lyon Cedex 69677, France; [b] Université Lyon 1, INRAE, UMR754, Lyon, France
* Hospices Civils de Lyon, Hôpital Louis Pradel, Centre de référence coordonnateur des maladies pulmonaires rares (OrphaLung), Service de pneumologie, 28 Avenue Doyen Lepine, Lyon Cedex 69677, France.
E-mail address: vincent.cottin@chu-lyon.fr

Immunol Allergy Clin N Am 43 (2023) 289–322
https://doi.org/10.1016/j.iac.2023.01.002
0889-8561/23/© 2023 Elsevier Inc. All rights reserved.

immunology.theclinics.com

alveolar eosinophilia greater than 40%,[5] strongly suggest the diagnosis of eosinophilic lung disease.

Classification

Eosinophilic interstitial lung disorders can be classified according to (a) their mode of onset (acute or chronic pneumonia); (b) whether a cause or context has been identified; and (c) whether limited to the lungs or associated with systemic manifestation (**Table 1**). Acute eosinophilic pneumonia is frequently caused by exposure to drugs, tobacco smoking, fungal infection, or inhaled aerocontaminants, whereas eosinophilic pneumonia of chronic onset is most often idiopathic.

PATHOPHYSIOLOGY

Blood and tissue eosinophilia have long been identified as major players in immunity against parasites and in the pathogenesis of allergic diseases.[6] Following differentiation of precursor cells in the bone marrow under the action of several cytokines, including interleukin (IL)-5, IL-3, and granulocyte-macrophage colony-stimulating factor (GM-CSF),[7–9] eosinophils are recruited in the blood and tissue including the lung in response to circulating IL-5, eotaxins, and the C-C chemokine receptor-3 (CCR3). Because the recruitment of eosinophils to tissues is organ-specific, tissue and blood eosinophilia are not necessarily associated. The prominence of IL-5 in eosinophil differentiation and recruitment has led to the development of anti-IL-5 and anti-IL5 receptor (IL-5R) monoclonal antibodies to selectively target the eosinophil lineage in humans.[7,8,10] Although these drugs were developed in patients with an eosinophilic phenotype of asthma, they are now increasingly used in a variety of eosinophilic diseases.[11]

Reviews of the physiologic role of eosinophils in innate and adaptative immunity can be found elsewhere.[9,10] Eosinophils participate in host defense response, tissue regeneration, tissue repair after injury, metabolic homeostasis, immune homeostasis, angiogenesis, fibrosis, steady-state development of intestine and mammary gland, and tumor rejection.[7–10] Histopathologic lesions in eosinophilic pneumonias are formed by the recruitment of activated eosinophils and other inflammatory cells to tissues, and the release by eosinophils of numerous mediators, including pro-inflammatory cytokines, arachidonic acid–derived mediators, enzymes, reactive oxygen species, complement proteins, chemokines, chemoattractants, metalloproteases, and cationic proteins. The latter are released by degranulation in tissues of activated eosinophils,[8] which can be found in the BAL[12,13] and the lung tissue[14] of patients with eosinophilic pneumonias as degranulated ("hypodense") eosinophils.

Although most histopathologic abnormalities in eosinophilic pneumonia are largely reversible with corticosteroids, some tissue damage and remodeling with fibrosis may occur in the bronchial mucosa, as in allergic bronchopulmonary aspergillosis (ABPA) and in eosinophilic granulomatosis with polyangiitis (EGPA) (formerly Churg–Strauss syndrome), or in cardiac lesions that occur in the hypereosinophilic syndrome or in tropical eosinophilia.[15] Eosinophilic cationic proteins are largely considered responsible for tissue damage, as they exert direct cytotoxicity to the pulmonary epithelium, and enhance inflammation through upregulation of chemoattraction, expression of adhesion molecules, vascular permeability, and contraction of smooth muscle cells.[7–10]

IDIOPATHIC CHRONIC EOSINOPHILIC PNEUMONIA

First described in 1969 by Carrington and colleagues,[16] idiopathic chronic eosinophilic pneumonia (ICEP) is characterized by the onset over a few weeks of cough, dyspnea, malaise, and weight loss, with diffuse pulmonary infiltrates.

Table 1
Classification of the eosinophilic interstitial lung diseases in clinical practice

	Acute Onset	Chronic Onset
Only pulmonary manifestations		
Idiopathic	Idiopathic acute eosinophilic pneumonia	Idiopathic chronic eosinophilic pneumonia
Identified cause or trigger	Löffler syndrome Acute eosinophilic pneumonia induced by smoking or airborne dust Acute eosinophilic pneumonia due to medications Acute eosinophilic pneumonia due to illicit drugs Acute eosinophilic pneumonia due to infections	Allergic bronchopulmonary aspergillosis and related syndromes Eosinophilic pneumonias of parasitic origin Eosinophilic pneumonias of other infectious causes Eosinophilic pneumonias due to radiation therapy
With systemic manifestations		
Idiopathic	Eosinophilic granulomatosis with polyangiitis Eosinophilic vasculitis	Hypereosinophilic syndromes
Identified cause or trigger	DRESS (parasitic infection)	

Epidemiology and Risk Factors

Although it is a rare disease, ICEP is the most common of the eosinophilic pneumonias in nontropical areas where the prevalence of parasitic infection is low.[17] ICEP predominates in women (2:1 female/male ratio),[18,19] with a mean age at diagnosis of 45 years, but every age group can be affected.[18] No genetic predisposition has been reported. Two-thirds of ICEP patients have a prior history of asthma,[18,19] and about half a history of atopy, consisting of drug allergy, nasal polyposis, urticaria, and/or eczema,[18,19] therefore ICEP may occur predominantly in patients who are prone to develop a T-helper-2 response.[20] Most patients with ICEP are nonsmokers, in contrast with idiopathic acute eosinophilic pneumonia (IAEP).[18,19]

Clinical Description

The onset of ICEP is progressive or subacute, with several weeks or months between the onset of symptoms and the diagnosis.[18,19] Shortness of breath usually moderate is the prominent clinical manifestation. Cough (90%), rhinitis or sinusitis (20%), and rarely chest pain or hemoptysis (10% or less) may be present.[18,19] Wheezes or crackles are found in one-third of patients at auscultation. Respiratory failure requiring mechanical ventilation is exceptional in ICEP, in contrast to the frequent respiratory failure that occurs in IAEP.[21,22]

Approximately 75% of the patients with ICEP experience asthma at some time throughout the course of disease, generally before the onset of ICEP, but occasionally asthma occurs concomitantly with the diagnosis of ICEP.[23] Asthma in ICEP may be severe in the long term, with persistent airflow obstruction despite oral and inhaled corticosteroid therapy in approximatively 10% of patients,[23] warranting long-term follow-up of lung function.

Systemic manifestations are not present in ICEP, except for fatigue, malaise, fever, anorexia, night sweats, and weight loss.[18,19] Any significant extrathoracic manifestation should raise the suspicion of EGPA. However, limited extrathoracic manifestations have been reported in some series: pericardial effusion, arthralgias, nonspecific skin manifestations, and altered liver function tests.[16,18,24]

Chest Imaging

Albeit nonspecific, the imaging features of ICEP are often characteristic and suggestive of the diagnosis in approximately 75% of cases in the appropriate setting.[25] In most patients, the chest radiograph before initiation of treatment[16,18,19,25–27] shows bilateral alveolar infiltrates with ill-defined margins. The typical peripheral predominance is observed in approximately a quarter of patients.[19] Spontaneous migration of the opacities observed also in a quarter of the cases suggests the diagnosis of either ICEP or cryptogenic organizing pneumonia.[18]

On high-resolution computed tomography (HRCT), typical features consist of confluent consolidations and ground glass opacities (**Fig. 1**),[18,26,28] almost always bilateral[18] and predominating in the upper lobes and peripheral subpleural areas.[18,27,28] Imaging abnormalities rapidly regress upon corticosteroid therapy.[28] Septal line thickening, band-like opacities parallel to the chest, mediastinal lymph node enlargement, mild pleural effusion, and centrilobulary nodules may be found.[18,27,29] Cavitary lesions are exceedingly rare.

Laboratory Findings

It is crucial that blood cell analysis, and BAL if necessary, be performed in patients who have not yet received systemic corticosteroids, as both blood and alveolar eosinophilia are present in almost all untreated patients with ICEP. High-level peripheral blood eosinophilia[19] is the key to the diagnosis, with mean values of 5 to 6000/mm^3 in large series, representing 20% to 30% of blood leukocytes.[18] BAL eosinophilia, defined as 25% eosinophils or more at differential cell count and commonly greater than 40%, confirms the diagnosis of eosinophilic pneumonia especially when eosinophils represent the predominant cell in BAL. Sputum eosinophilia may be present but is less valuable for diagnosis. Increase in blood C-reactive protein and total immunoglobulin (Ig) E level are common but lack specificity.

Pathogenesis

The pathogenesis of ICEP is considered to be a direct consequence of lung infiltration by eosinophils and is reversible on corticosteroid treatment. Eosinophils from patients with ICEP release pro-inflammatory molecules and express a variety of activation markers.[1,8,30] Interestingly, a possible role has been suggested for clonal blood and lung tissue T cells,[31,32] similar to what is seen in the lymphocytic variant of the idiopathic hypereosinophilic syndrome.

Lung Function

Approximately half of the patients with ICEP have airflow obstruction, and the other half have a restrictive ventilatory defect related to pulmonary infiltration. In the latter case, multiple consolidations are apparent on imaging, and reduced carbon monoxide transfer factor and coefficient are present by pulmonary function testing. In addition, many patients present with mild hypoxemia.[18,19]

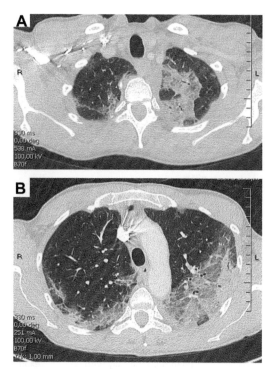

Fig. 1. Chest CT of a patient with idiopathic chronic eosinophilic pneumonia, showing peripheral airspace consolidation predominating in the upper lobes. (*A*) Upper lobes. (*B*) Mid-trachea level.

Pathology

The diagnosis of ICEP does not require a videothoracoscopic lung biopsy or a transbronchial cryobiopsy. Immunohistochemical and electron microscopic studies can show eosinophilic degranulation within the site of eosinophilic pneumonia;[13,33] however, these are not necessary for clinical practice. Transbronchial forceps lung biopsy may show characteristic features, but the small size of the specimen generally does not allow sufficient morphologic evidence for the differential diagnosis of eosinophilic pneumonias.

When available, pathology is characterized by prominent infiltration of the lung interstitium and the alveolar spaces by eosinophils[16,19] accompanied by a fibrinous exudate, with preservation of the lung architecture. Some histologic overlap is common with organizing pneumonia.[1] Eosinophilic microabscesses, a non-necrotizing non-granulomatous vasculitis, and occasional multinucleated giant cells (but no granuloma) can also be found in ICEP, and would lead to discuss overlap with EGPA.

Diagnosis

Diagnostic criteria are found in **Table 2**.[2,5] A thorough investigation for potential causes of eosinophilia should be conducted before the condition is considered idiopathic, including drug intake, infections with parasites or fungi, and exposure to toxins or illicit drugs. In the setting of a characteristic clinical and radiologic presentation, the presence of marked eosinophilia at BAL (at least 25% and usually >40% of BAL cells),

Table 2
Distinctive features and diagnostic criteria for idiopathic chronic eosinophilic pneumonia and for idiopathic acute eosinophilic pneumonia

	ICEP	IAEP
Onset	>2 to 4 wk	<1 mo
History of asthma	Yes	No
Smoking history	10% are smokers	2/3 smokers, often recent initiation
Respiratory failure	Rare	Usual
Initial blood eosinophilia	Yes	Often no (typically delayed)
BAL eosinophilia	>25%	>25%
Chest imaging	Homogeneous peripheral airspace consolidation	Bilateral patchy areas of ground glass attenuation, airspace consolidation, interlobular septal thickening, and bilateral pleural effusion
Relapse	Yes	No
Diagnostic criteria	1. Diffuse pulmonary alveolar consolidation with air bronchogram and/or ground glass opacities at chest imaging, especially with peripheral predominance; 2. Eosinophilia at BAL differential cell count $\geq$ 40% (or peripheral blood eosinophils $\geq$ 1000/mm3; 3. Respiratory symptoms present for at least 2 to 4 wk; 4. Absence of other known causes of eosinophilic lung disease (especially exposure to drug susceptible to induce pulmonary eosinophilia).	1. Acute onset with febrile respiratory manifestations ($\leq$1 mo, and especially $\leq$7 d duration before medical examination. 2. Bilateral diffuse opacities on imaging 3. Pao_2 on room air $\leq$60 mm Hg (8 kPa), or $Pao_2/Fio_2\leq$300 mm Hg (40 kPa), or oxygen saturation on room air <90% 4. Lung eosinophilia, with $\geq$25% eosinophils at BAL differential cell count (Or eosinophilic pneumonia at lung biopsy when done) 5. Absence of determined cause of acute eosinophilic pneumonia (including infection or exposure to drugs known to induce pulmonary eosinophilia). Recent onset of tobacco smoking or exposure to inhaled dusts may be present.

with eosinophils more numerous than neutrophils and lymphocytes,[5] confirms the diagnosis of eosinophilic pneumonia, and obviates the need for lung biopsy. Performing a BAL is generally indicated in patients with suspected eosinophilic pneumonia and those with diffuse alveolar opacities at imaging. However, the presence of markedly elevated peripheral blood eosinophilia together with typical clinical radiologic features also strongly suggests the diagnosis of ICEP. Diagnostic difficulties mainly arise in patients who are already receiving corticosteroid treatment, and therefore do not have peripheral or BAL eosinophilia at the time of clinical evaluation. BAL may not be required in patients who experience a relapse of clinical and radiological manifestations of ICEP and have elevated peripheral blood eosinophilia.

Treatment and Outcome

Although spontaneous resolution can occur, management of ICEP is based primarily on oral corticosteroids. The objective of therapy is to induce remission of disease and then to reduce the risk of relapse while balancing the intensity of treatment with the need to minimize the side effects of corticosteroids.

There are no established dose and duration of systemic corticosteroids in ICEP.[18,34] Because the response to corticosteroids is typically dramatic, with clinical improvement within 2 days,[19] and clearing of chest opacities within 1 week,[18,19] the initial dose can be limited to 0.5 mg/kg/d of oral prednisone for 2 weeks, followed by 0.25 mg/kg/d for 2 weeks, then corticosteroids are progressively reduced and stopped.[1,5] An open-label, parallel-group study found no difference in the relapse rate between a 3-month and a 6-month treatment regimen.[35] Whether inhaled corticosteroids may be useful in non-asthmatic patients with ICEP is unknown.

Relapses occur in more than half the patients while decreasing or after stopping corticosteroids; however, they respond very well to resumed corticosteroid treatment. Relapses can typically be treated with a dose of 20 mg/d of prednisone. Patients should therefore be informed of the possibility of relapse while the corticosteroids are progressively tapered and then stopped. Such an approach reduces the overall patient's exposure to long-term corticosteroids and anxiety.

Both chest imaging and lung function should return to normal with treatment.[18] Cases considered refractory to corticosteroids should lead the clinician to reconsider the diagnosis of ICEP. Potential morbidity is related to adverse events related to oral corticosteroids, and to possible persistent airflow obstruction that may develop despite bronchodilators and inhaled corticosteroids and often oral low-dose corticosteroids.[34] Successful off-label use of mepolizumab, a monoclonal antibody against IL-5, and benralizumab, an IL-5 receptor antagonist, were reported in ICEP with frequent relapses or severe asthma.[36] Such off-label use of medications targeting the IL-5 pathway should be carefully discussed on a case-by-case basis in an expert center, given the exquisite sensitivity of ICEP to corticosteroids.

IDIOPATHIC AND SMOKING-RELATED ACUTE EOSINOPHILIC PNEUMONIA

IAEP first described by Badesch and colleagues[37] and Allen and colleagues[38] in 1989 is both the most dramatic and the most frequently misdiagnosed of eosinophilic pneumonias,[39] because it mimics infectious pneumonia or acute respiratory distress syndrome in previously healthy young adults. It differs from ICEP by its acute onset, the severity of hypoxemia, the usual lack of increased blood eosinophils at the onset of disease, and the absence of relapse.

Epidemiology and Risk Factors

IAEP occurs acutely in previously healthy young adults, with male predominance and a mean age of approximately 30 years.[37–48] Two-thirds of patients are smokers, but there is usually no history of asthma. The disease can be triggered by various respiratory exposures, especially a recent initiation of tobacco smoking (as in military or new college student settings).[41] A change in smoking habits,[42,49] smoking large quantities of cigarettes (or cigars), reintroduction to smoking after a period of abstinence ("rechallenge"),[40,42,49] or even short-term passive smoking[49,50] can also trigger IAEP.

A variety of nonspecific environmental inhaled contaminants have also been shown to induce IAEP (reviewed in[1]), including parasites, fungi, viruses, red spiders, drugs, over-the-counter drugs, and illicit drugs. AEP may also occur after allogenic hematopoietic stem cell transplantation or in the context of acquired immunodeficiency virus infection.

Although some cases remain idiopathic, most cases correspond to acute eosinophilic pneumonia related to tobacco smoking or other respiratory exposures.[5,51,52]

Clinical Description

IAEP is characterized by acute onset of dyspnea (100% of patients), fever that is usually moderate (100%), cough (80% to 100%), and pleuritic thoracic pain (50% to 70%), myalgias (30% to 50%) or abdominal complaints (25%).[39–41,43–45,49,53] Acute onset is an important criterion for the diagnosis of IAEP (see **Table 2**), with a delay between the first symptoms and hospital admission of less than 1 month and usually less than 7 days.[39,40] Acute respiratory failure is frequent,[42] often meeting criteria for acute respiratory distress syndrome,[54] and admission to the intensive care unit and mechanical ventilation are often required.[40,41] Crackles are present in most patients at lung auscultation.

Chest Imaging

The chest radiograph shows bilateral, alveolar, and interstitial opacities, especially Kerley lines.[39,44,45] Chest HRCT shows the typical combination of poorly defined nodules of ground-glass attenuation (100%), often associated with airspace consolidation (55%), together with interlobular septal thickening (90%) and bilateral pleural effusion (76%) (**Fig. 2**).[25,40,44,55] Thickening of bronchovascular bundles, lymph node enlargement, and centrilobular nodules may be present. In the appropriate setting, and especially in the absence of heart failure, this imaging pattern suggests the diagnosis of IAEP.

Laboratory Findings

In contrast to other eosinophilic pneumonias, blood eosinophil count is *normal* at presentation in most cases of IAEP,[39,41] a feature that contributes to misdiagnosis of IAEP as infectious pneumonia. Within 1 to 7 days after presentation, the eosinophil count rises to high values,[39–41,43] which should suggest the diagnosis of IAEP. When present at presentation, peripheral eosinophilia may be associated with a milder disease status compared with those with normal eosinophil count.[46,56,57] Other serum biomarkers are not used in clinical practice.

BAL is often performed at admission, before blood eosinophilia is present, and therefore is often the key to the diagnosis of IAEP, showing more than 25% eosinophils (37% to 54% eosinophils on average).[39–41] BAL bacterial cultures are sterile. BAL eosinophilia usually resolves with corticosteroid therapy, but may persist for several weeks.[58] Thoracentesis when performed may show nonspecific pleural eosinophilia.

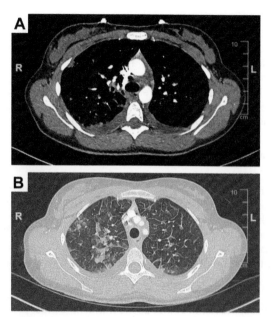

Fig. 2. Chest CT of a patient with idiopathic acute eosinophilic pneumonia. (*A*) Mediastinal window showing bilateral pleural effusion. (*B*) Lung window showing alveolar opacities, ground glass attenuation, and interlobular septal thickening.

Lung Function

Arterial blood gas shows hypoxemia, which can be severe due to right-to-left shunting in areas of alveolar consolidation.[38,40] Patients often meet diagnostic criteria for acute respiratory distress syndrome. Pulmonary function tests are only practical in less severe cases, but typically reveal a mild restrictive ventilatory defect, with reduced carbon monoxide transfer capacity, and increased alveolar-arterial oxygen tension difference.

Pathology

A lung biopsy is only performed in rare cases when the diagnosis of eosinophilic pneumonia has not been suspected. When performed, it shows acute and organizing diffuse alveolar damage together with interstitial, alveolar, and bronchiolar infiltration by eosinophils, intra-alveolar eosinophils, and interstitial edema.[39,53,59,60]

Diagnosis

BAL is mandatory to both establish the presence of alveolar eosinophilia and exclude infection. Working diagnostic criteria for AEP are listed in **Table 2**. Some patients with moderate disease severity may not fit established criteria.[42] As discussed above, possible causes of AEP must be sought for, and the etiologic inquiry should be repeated in case of poor response to corticosteroids.[52]

Treatment and Outcome

Most patients receive systemic corticosteroids, starting with 30 mg per day of oral prednisone.[42] The patient generally improves within 3 days,[42,61] and a total treatment duration of 2 weeks is sufficient. Imaging[39,40,42,45] and pulmonary function abnormalities[39,40] resolve within less than a month. Patients with respiratory failure may receive higher doses, that is, 1 to 2 mg/kg/d of intravenous methylprednisolone. Extrapulmonary organ failure, shock, or death, are exceptional.[41,60] Extracorporeal membrane oxygenation has been used occasionally.[62]

In contrast with ICEP, IAEP does not relapse, unless the patient resumes smoking. Patients should be informed about the etiologic role of tobacco (or of any other environmental exposure), and should be strongly encouraged to quit.

EOSINOPHILIC GRANULOMATOSIS WITH POLYANGIITIS
Definition

EGPA (formerly, Churg–Strauss syndrome) described in 1951[63] mainly from autopsied cases, is a systemic disease associated with asthma, eosinophilia, eosinophil-rich and granulomatous inflammation involving the respiratory tract, and a small-vessel, necrotizing small to medium-sized vessel necrotizing vasculitis.[64] Antineutrophil cytoplasmic antibodies (ANCA) are found in approximately 40% of cases, and therefore EGPA belongs to the group of pulmonary ANCA-associated vasculitides.[64]

Epidemiology and Risk Factors

EGPA predominates in the fourth or fifth decade, with no gender predominance.[65–81] It is a very rare condition, with an incidence of 0.5 to 6.8 cases/million inhabitants/y, and a prevalence of 10.7 to 13 cases/million inhabitants.[82] A genetic predisposition has been linked to the major histopathology complex DRB4 allele,[83] and the phenotype of EGPA may be affected by genetic predisposition. Familial EGPA has been reported.

Contrary to the initial terminology of the disease,[63] association with a history of allergy is weak, as allergy can be evidenced by specific serum IgE with corresponding clinical history in less than one-third of patients.[78,84] When present, allergy in EGPA mainly consists of perennial allergies especially to *Dermatophagoides*, whereas seasonal allergies are less frequent than in control asthmatics.[84]

EGPA is both a hypereosinophilic condition and an ANCA-associated systemic vasculitis, comprising two distinct yet overlapping pathogenic mechanisms.[85] Whether ANCA have a direct role in the pathogenesis of EGPA is still unclear.[82] Interestingly, EGPA can be triggered by several infectious agents (*Aspergillus*, *Candida*, *Ascaris*, *Actinomyces*), drugs (sulfonamides used together with antiserum, diflunisal, macrolides, diphenylhydantoin, and omalizumab), illicit drugs (cocaine), and bird exposure. Cases were reported more than 30 years ago in relation to allergic hyposensitization, and vaccinations or adjuvants (see[1] for review), however these observations were related to techniques and agents that are no longer used. Although the link between leukotriene-receptor antagonists (montelukast, zafirkukast, pranlukast) and the development of EGPA is controversial[86–90] and probably coincidental (EGPA arising while oral or inhaled corticosteroids are tapered in patients with smoldering EGPA[82,89]), it is reasonable to avoid these medications in asthmatics with eosinophilia and/or extrapulmonary manifestations compatible with smoldering EGPA. Clonal T cells may play a role.[91]

Clinical Description

The natural course of EGPA typically follows three phases,[65] with rhinosinusitis and asthma, blood and tissue eosinophilia, and eventually systemic vasculitis, but these often overlap in time. Asthma is always present in EGPA, although it may be missed in the absence of lung function tests, as many patients do not experience typical paroxysmal symptoms. Asthma occurs at a mean age of approximately 35 years in patients with EGPA. It is generally severe and rapidly requires oral corticosteroids.[65–71,78,79,92] Asthma precedes the onset of the vasculitis by 3 to 9 years,[65–68,71,72] and may become attenuated after the onset of the vasculitis,[65,67,78] likely reflecting the effect of systemic corticosteroids prescribed for EGPA.[78,93,94]

Eosinophilic pneumonia is the main pulmonary manifestation of EGPA other than asthma. It is often similar to ICEP in presentation, but may be acute in onset.[1] The frequency of eosinophilic pneumonia may be underestimated in some series of EGPA, because it rapidly resolves on corticosteroid treatment, may be limited to ground-glass attenuation on chest CT, and because extrathoracic manifestations may be prominent clinically. Pulmonary micronodules and other radiologic signs of bronchiolitis are also frequent features.[27]

Chronic rhinitis or rhinosinusitis is present in approximately 75% of cases. Although paraseptal sinusitis and nasal obstruction lack specificity, association with eosinophilic nasosinusal polyposis, often with eosinophilic infiltration at histopathology, may suggest the diagnosis.[95,96] Crusty rhinitis is frequent, but septal nasal perforation does not occur in EGPA as opposed to granulomatosis with polyangiitis.

General symptoms are present in two-thirds of patients (asthenia, weight loss, fever, arthralgias, myalgias). Any organ system can be affected by the systemic disease through eosinophilic infiltration and/or granulomatous vasculitis. Kidney involvement is frequently insidious[68,97] and must be systematically investigated due to potential morbidity. Cardiac involvement is often asymptomatic but can lead to sudden death or acute or chronic cardiac failure[65–68,71,98,99] due to eosinophilic myocarditis and less commonly from coronary arteritis.[100,101] Heart transplantation may be required.[102] Therefore, any patient with suspected EGPA should undergo a systematic cardiac evaluation with electrocardiogram, echocardiography,[103,104] N-terminal pro-brain natriuretic peptide, and serum level of troponin I. Magnetic resonance imaging of the heart is currently the preferred investigation when cardiac involvement is suspected;[99,104–106] however, it is not indicated in the absence of clinical suspicion, as the significance of subclinical abnormalities detected by magnetic resonance imaging is unknown. Patients with EGPA are also at greater risk of venous thromboembolic events.[107]

Chest Imaging

Chest imaging abnormalities in patients with EGPA are twofold.[25,27,108–111]

- Airspace consolidation and/or ill-defined ground glass opacities (50% to 70%) corresponding to eosinophilic pneumonia. Opacities may predominate in the periphery of the lung or have a random distribution and are sometimes migratory (**Fig. 3**). These abnormalities rapidly disappear upon corticosteroid therapy and therefore may be missed if treatment is initiated early.
- Airways abnormalities including centrilobular nodules, bronchial wall thickening, and bronchiectasis corresponding to eosinophilic involvement of bronchi and bronchioles.

Interlobular septal thickening, hilar or mediastinal lymphadenopathy, or pericardial effusion may also be seen.[25,27,109,110,112] Pleural effusion may correspond to eosinophilic pleural effusion or to a transudate caused by eosinophilic cardiomyopathy.

Laboratory Findings

Peripheral blood eosinophilia is a major feature of EGPA, with mean values generally between 5 and 20,000/mm^3 at diagnosis.[65,67,68,78] It is accompanied by BAL

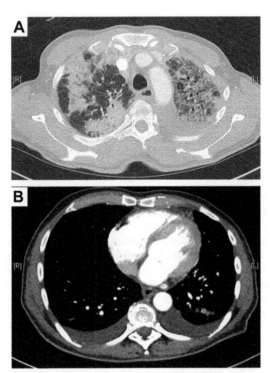

Fig. 3. Chest CT of a patient with eosinophilic granulomatosis with polyangiitis. (*A*) Lung window showing eosinophilic pneumonia with alveolar opacities and ground glass attenuation. (*B*) Mediastinal window showing bilateral pleural effusion due to eosinophilic myocarditis with heart failure. (*From* Cottin V. Eosinophilic Lung Diseases. Clin Chest Med. 2016;37(3):535-556.)

eosinophilia greater than 25% and usually greater than 40%.[78,113] Increase in serum IgE and C-reactive protein levels is nonspecific. Serum and urinary biomarkers to reflect eosinophil degranulation and disease activity in vivo await prospective validation.[114–116]

Although EGPA is one of the ANCA-associated pulmonary vasculitides, ANCA are found in only 40% of patients, and their absence does not exclude the diagnosis of EGPA. They are mainly perinuclear-ANCA with myeloperoxidase specificity.[68,71,73–76,79,117,118] When present, ANCA support the diagnosis of EGPA; however, their titer does not correlate with the activity of the disease. Different clinical phenotypes of the disease have been reported in ANCA-positive and ANCA-negative patients[73–76,79,117,118] (**Table 3**), possibly with a genetic correlate.[83,119] Patients with EGPA and ANCA more frequently present with clinical manifestations of genuine small vessel involvement, including palpable purpura, glomerulonephritis, alveolar hemorrhage, mononeuritis multiplex, and biopsy-proven vasculitis.

Lung Function

Airflow obstruction is present in 70% of patients at diagnosis despite inhaled bronchodilator and high-dose inhaled corticosteroid therapy for asthma.[78,93] Lung function improves with oral corticosteroid therapy given for the systemic disease.[78,93,94] Persistent airflow obstruction may be present in about a third of patients with long-

Table 3 Distinct subtypes of eosinophilic granulomatosis with polyangiitis		
	Vasculitic Phenotype	Eosinophilic Tissue Disease Phenotype
Respective frequency	~40%	~60%
ANCA	Present (mostly p-ANCA with anti-MPO specificity)	Absent
Predominant manifestations	Glomerular renal disease Peripheral neuropathy Purpura Biopsy-proven vasculitis	Cardiac involvement (eosinophilic myocarditis) Eosinophilic pneumonia Fever

Abbreviation: ANCA, antineutrophil cytoplasmic antibodies.

term follow-up.[78,93,94,120,121] Before the era of IL-5/IL-5R targeted therapies, many patients required low-dose, long-term oral corticosteroids in addition to inhaled therapy,[65,68,93] causing significant morbidity and susceptibility to infections.[77,78]

Pathology

The diagnosis of EGPA can frequently be made on the clinical presentation together with marked eosinophilia. Therefore, lung biopsy is seldom necessary. Biopsy of more accessible tissues, such as skin, nerve, or muscle, has a better safety profile and usually contributive; rhinosinusal biopsies can also be useful.[68] A single tissue specimen[122,123] rarely contains all three defining characteristics; vasculitis (necrotizing or not, involving mainly the medium-sized pulmonary arteries), granulomata, and eosinophilic tissue infiltration (with palisading histiocytes and giant cells). On rare occasions, EGPA limited to the lung may be diagnosed using lung biopsy, showing all histopathologic features of the disease.[124]

Diagnosis

The diagnosis of EGPA is based on the association of asthma, peripheral blood, and/or tissue eosinophilia, and the demonstration of involvement of organs outside of the respiratory system.[79] The diagnostic criteria proposed by Lanham and colleagues[65] include (1) asthma; (2) eosinophilia exceeding 1.5×10^9/L; and (3) systemic vasculitis of two or more extrapulmonary organs. However, they are not applicable to patients without a biopsy, those with the limited disease, for example, with the so-called *forme fruste* of EGPA, or in subjects receiving corticosteroid treatment.[92,125,126] Classification criteria of the American College of Rheumatology and the European Alliance of Associations for Rheumatology[127] can only be applied in cases with established systemic vasculitis, and therefore are often not applicable before severe organ involvement develops. Working diagnostic criteria are proposed (**Box 1**),[78] which include the diagnostic contribution of ANCA when present. Eligibility criteria used in recent international study[128] may also be used, although also requiring validation, and potentially overdiagnosing EGPA in patients with organ involvement limited to the respiratory system.

EGPA should be differentiated from idiopathic systemic eosinophilic vasculitis.[129] Although part of a common spectrum,[130] patients with idiopathic systemic eosinophilic vasculitis do not have a history of asthma, and systemic manifestations generally differ from those of EGPA.

Box 1
Pragmatic diagnostic criteria for eosinophilic granulomatosis with polyangiitis

- Diagnostic criteria used in trial NCT02020889[128]
  - History or presence of: asthma plus eosinophilia (>1.0 x 109/L and/or >10% of leukocytes) plus at least two of the following additional features of EGPA
    - A biopsy showing histopathological evidence of eosinophilic vasculitis, or perivascular eosinophilic infiltration, or eosinophil-rich granulomatous inflammation;
    - Neuropathy, mono or poly (motor deficit or nerve conduction abnormality);
    - Pulmonary infiltrates, nonfixed;
    - Sino-nasal abnormality;
    - Cardiomyopathy (established by echocardiography or MRI);
    - Glomerulonephritis (hematuria, red cell casts, proteinuria);
    - Alveolar hemorrhage (by bronchoalveolar lavage);
    - Palpable purpura;
    - ANCA positive (MPO or PR3).
- Working diagnostic criteria[2,3]

○ Asthma
  - Peripheral blood eosinophilia greater than 1500/mm^3 and/or alveolar eosinophilia greater than 25%
  - Extrapulmonary clinical manifestations of disease (other than rhinosinusitis), with at least one of the following:
    - Systemic manifestation typical of the disease: mononeuritis multiplex; or cardiomyopathy confidently attributed to the eosinophilic disorder; or palpable purpura;
    - Any extrapulmonary manifestation with histopathological evidence of vasculitis as shown especially by skin, muscle, or nerve biopsy;
    - Any extrapulmonary manifestation with evidence of ANCA with antimyeloperoxidase or antiproteinase 3 specificity.

NB: When a single extrarespiratory manifestation attributable to the systemic disease is present, disease may be called "forme fruste of EGPA."

Treatment and Outcome

Corticosteroids remain the mainstay of treatment of EGPA.[131–133] Oral prednisone is typically initiated at a dose of 1 mg/kg/d for 3 to 4 weeks, then tapered to reach 5 to 10 mg/d by 12 months of therapy.[82] An initial methylprednisolone bolus (15 mg/kg/d for 1 to 3 days) may be indicated in the most severe cases. Immunosuppressive therapy should be added to corticosteroids to induce remission in patients with manifestations that could result in mortality or severe morbidity,[134] especially heart failure,[135,136] with one or more of the following "poor prognostic" criteria: age over 65 years; cardiac symptoms; gastrointestinal involvement; renal insufficiency with serum creatinine greater than 150 μg/L; absence of ear, nose and throat manifestations.[134,137] Immunosuppression is generally based on cyclophosphamide therapy (0.6 to 0.7 g/m^2 intravenously at day 1, 15, 30, then every 3 weeks, reduced to 0.5 g/m^2 in individuals older than 65 years[138]); rituximab has been proposed as an alternative to cyclophosphamide[139] based on the results of a randomized control trial, not yet published, and observational data.[139–149]

Once remission has been achieved, prolonged maintenance therapy is necessary to prevent relapses. In patients with poor prognostic criteria, maintenance therapy for 18 to 24 months is generally based on azathioprine, which has a favorable risk/benefit ratio.[82] Patients without poor prognosis criteria are generally treated by corticosteroids alone[150]; azathioprine or methotrexate[151] are preferred to mycophenolate[152] as steroid-sparing agents in patients who require 10 mg/d of prednisone or more. Maintenance of corticosteroid treatment is often motivated by uncontrolled asthma despite optimal inhaled asthma therapy.[78,94,120]

The efficacy and safety of the anti-IL5 antibody mepolizumab was evaluated in a phase 3 randomized trial, as add-on therapy versus placebo in subjects with refractory or relapsing EGPA.[128] As compared with placebo, mepolizumab (300 mg every 4 weeks) led to an increased proportion of patients achieving remission, an increased duration of remission, a lower rate of relapse, and a lower average daily dose of oral corticosteroids.[128] Mepolizumab is indicated as an adjunct therapy in subjects with relapsing or refractory EGPA; however, many questions remain regarding its optimal use and timing in EGPA. Observational data confirm the efficacy of mepolizumab in EGPA,[140,153] and further suggest that mepolizumab (100 mg or 300 mg every 4 weeks) may further be beneficial in cases with persistent severe asthma when the vasculitis is in remission.[140,154] However, the optimal sequence and potential combinations of drugs for patients with EGPA remain to be determined.

A steroid-sparing effect has been shown with the anti-IL5 monoclonal antibody reslizumab and with the anti-IL5R monoclonal antibody benralizumab.[155,156] The anti-IgE monoclonal antibody omalizumab may also facilitate the reduction in doses of oral corticosteroids;[157,158] however, severe flares and new onset of EGPA were also reported,[158–163] therefore omalizumab is seldom used in patients diagnosed with EGPA. The anti-IL4/13 monoclonal antibody dupilimab should be used with caution when the diagnosis of EGPA is contemplated, as it may trigger hypereosinophilia with sudden deterioration of asthma, eosinophilic tissue infiltration, and EGPA-like symptoms.[164,165]

Approximately 25% of patients experience at least one relapse, generally with peripheral eosinophilia, with or without new-onset systemic manifestations.[79] The 5-year overall survival in EGPA is currently greater than 95%,[133,134,166] with most deaths occurring during the first year of treatment due to cardiac involvement.[167] Treatment-related side effects especially related to corticosteroids are the main cause of long-term morbidity. Uncontrolled asthma and persistent airflow obstruction also cause significant morbidity.[78,93,120,166] It is hoped that the use of monoclonal antibodies targeting the IL-5/IL-5R axis will contribute to reducing the burden of long-term persistent airflow obstruction and corticosteroid-related morbidity.

ALLERGIC BRONCHOPULMONARY ASPERGILLOSIS
Epidemiology and Pathogenesis

ABPA occurs almost exclusively in subjects with a prior history of the chronic bronchial disease. It may occur in up to 1% to 2% of asthmatic adults, 7% to 10% of patients with cystic fibrosis,[168,169] and only rarely in other settings (chronic obstructive pulmonary disease, workers in bagasse-containing sites in sugar-cane mills).[170] Chronic bronchial disease is associated with viscid mucus and mucus plugs in the airways, facilitating the growth of *Aspergillus*, impairing the mucociliary clearance, and causing complex chronic immune and inflammatory reactions and local damage in the bronchi and the surrounding lung parenchyma.[171] Both type I hypersensitivity mediated by IgE antibodies, and type III hypersensitivity responses (with the participation of IgG and IgA antibodies and of exaggerated Th2 CD4+ T-cell mediated immune response) are involved in the immunologic process. Excessive B-cell response, immunoglobulin production, high levels of circulating IL-4, and the release of eosinophil cationic proteins also play a key role.[172,173] Genetic predisposition may have a role in conjunction with environmental exposure.[174–181]

Clinical Description

Patients with ABPA experience chronic cough, dyspnea, expectoration of brown or tan sputum plugs, low-grade fever, and chronic rhinitis. Sputum production may be abundant in patients with bronchiectasis, with sputum cultures often positive for *Pseudomonas aeruginosa*, *Staphylococcus aureus*, *Aspergillus fumigatus*, and/or nontuberculous mycobacteria.[182] ABPA may be associated with allergic *Aspergillus* sinusitis,[183] resulting in a syndrome called sinobronchial allergic aspergillosis. The course of the disease is chronic with repeated exacerbations;[171] however, progression to chronic respiratory failure is rare. Pulmonary infiltrates or peripheral blood eosinophilia may only be present during the acute phase or recurrent exacerbations of the disease.

Chest Imaging

The diagnosis of ABPA is often suggested by HRCT abnormalities in a patient with uncontrolled asthma.[25] Bronchial abnormalities are prominent and include central cylindrical bronchiectasis (including in the upper lobes), bronchial wall thickening, mucous plugging (mucoid impaction) with "finger in glove" sign (ie, bronchial mucous impaction radiating from the hilum to the periphery),[184–187] ground glass attenuation and airspace consolidation.[25,186,188,189] Features of bronchiolitis are common, with centrilobular nodules and tree-in-bud pattern[188,189] (**Fig. 4**). Eosinophilic pneumonia can occur during the early course of the disease, but airspace consolidation should be differentiated from segmental or lobar atelectasis caused by mucus plugging.[171]

Laboratory Findings

Blood eosinophils are usually greater than $1000/mm^3$ in the absence of corticosteroid treatment. Serum levels of total IgE may be particularly high and lead to suspicion of ABPA in asthmatics[171]; conversely, a normal serum level IgE in the absence of oral corticosteroid therapy generally excludes active ABPA. Total IgE levels generally increase during exacerbations of ABPA.[190] Skin prick testing, and preferentially serum IgE reactions to *A fumigatus*, including antibodies specific for recombinant *Aspergillus* allergens (especially *Asp f4* and *Asp f6*), corroborate the diagnosis.[191,192] Serum IgG (precipitin) for *A fumigatus* are often positive, but high levels are more suggestive of chronic pulmonary aspergillosis than ABPA. Specific IgE against *A fumigatus* may be used to screen for ABPA in asthmatics.[193,194] Fungal mycelia can be found by direct examination of sputum plugs; however, sputum cultures are positive for *A fumigatus* in only 40% to 60% of the cases with ABPA, and may need to be repeated to increase the rate of positive results.[195–197]

Pathology

A lung biopsy is not necessary when the diagnosis of ABPA is suspected. Analysis of specimens from limited resection performed because of chronic pulmonary consolidation or atelectasis shows bronchiectasis with mucous or mucopurulent plugs containing fungal hyphae, granulomatous inflammation of the bronchiolar wall, peribronchiolar chronic eosinophilic infiltrate with areas of eosinophilic pneumonia, exudative bronchiolitis, and mucous impaction of bronchi.[198]

Diagnosis

Diagnostic criteria for ABPA were recently revised (**Box 2**).[197,199,200] Of note, allergic bronchopulmonary syndromes similar to ABPA can be associated with yeasts or other

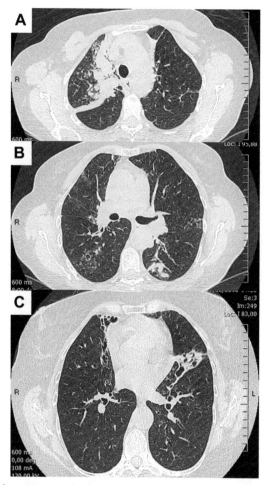

Fig. 4. Chest CT of a patient with allergic bronchopulmonary aspergillosis. (*A*) Eosinophilic pneumonia. (*B*) Bronchiolitis features, with tree-in-bud pattern, bronchial wall thickening, and centrilobular nodules. (*C*) Proximal bronchiectasis.

fungi,[1,201] and are particularly challenging to diagnose in the absence of available serology, although the new criteria may apply.[200]

Treatment and Outcome

Goals of treatment of ABPA includes the management of asthma exacerbations and prevention of progression to bronchiectasis and irreversible lung damage while minimizing corticosteroids side effects. The mainstay of treatment is the use of oral corticosteroid therapy during ABPA exacerbations. Treatment may be initiated using oral prednisolone 0.5 mg kg^{-1} day^{-1} for 2 weeks followed by 0.5 mg kg^{-1} on alternate days for 8 weeks, then taper by 5 mg every 2 weeks.[202] Corticosteroid therapy may be discontinued after 3 months (short regimen)[203] or 6 to 12 months (long regimen),[202] and is maintained only in patients with frequent symptomatic attacks or evidence of progressive lung damage. Intravenous pulses of high-dose methylprednisolone may be used in refractory ABPA exacerbations.[204] Conventional treatment of severe asthma is mandatory, that is, inhaled corticosteroids and long-acting bronchodilators.

Box 2
Diagnostic criteria of allergic bronchopulmonary aspergillosis

Modified ISHAM criteria
  for diagnosis
  of ABPA in asthma (2020)[199]
	Presence of the following:
	1. Asthma
	2. *A fumigatus*-specific IgE level > 0.35 KUA/L
	3. Serum total IgE levels > 500 IU/mL
	   and >2 of the following:
	   a. *A fumigatus*-specific IgG level > 0.35 kUA/L
	   b. Bronchiectasis on chest CT scan
	   c. Eosinophil count >500 cells/mL
	   d. Mucus impaction on chest CT scan

*Asano criteria for diagnosis
  of ABPM
in patients without cystic
  fibrosis (2021)[200]
	Presence of >6 of the following:
	1. Current or previous history of asthma or
	   asthmatic symptoms
	2. Peripheral eosinophilia >500 cells/mm^3
	3. Total IgE level > 417 IU/mL
	4. Positive result of immediate skin test or specific
	   IgE level for filamentous fungi§
	5. Presence of precipitins or specific IgE for
	   filamentous fungi
	6. Positive filamentous fungal sputum test or
	   bronchial lavage culture result
	7. Fungal hyphae in bronchial mucus plugs
	8. Central bronchiectasis on CT scan
	9. Mucus plugs detected by CT, bronchoscopy, or
	   expectoration
	10. High-attenuation bronchial mucus on CT scan

*The diagnosis "likely" if primary criteria 1 to 6 are present and "certain" if all primary criteria are present.

§Filamentous fungi in criteria 4 to 6 should be identical.

Abbreviations: ABPM, allergic bronchopulmonary mycosis; ISHAM, International Society of Animal and Human Mycology.

Treatment of episodes of pulmonary consolidation may prevent the progression of ABPA to fibrotic end-stage disease.[205]

Oral itraconazole prescribed for 16 to32 weeks to reduce the burden of fungal colonization in the lung is a useful adjunct to corticosteroids,[206,207] allowing steroid dose reductions, and decreasing the frequency of exacerbations.[206,207] Itraconazole can also be used as an alternative to corticosteroids.[208] Total serum IgE level is often used to monitor therapy.[171] Experience with voriconazole, posaconazole, and nebulized liposomal amphotericin B[209] in ABPA is moderate, and their use is generally limited to patients intolerant to itraconazole, or in itraconazole failures.

The anti-IgE recombinant antibody omalizumab may be useful, especially in subjects with difficult asthma in ABPA.[210–214] Persistent airflow obstruction may develop over years. Mepolizumab, benralizumab, and dupilumab have been used successfully in isolated cases.

OTHER EOSINOPHILIC LUNG DISEASES
Idiopathic Hypereosinophilic Syndrome

The idiopathic hypereosinophilic syndrome is defined by the association of three criteria.[4]

1. Absolute blood eosinophil count $\geq$1500/μL on two examinations (with an interval of 1 month or more) and/or tissue hypereosinophilia defined by the following:
   A. Percentage of eosinophils in bone marrow section exceeds 20% of all nucleated cells and/or
   B. Pathologist is of the opinion that tissue infiltration by eosinophils is extensive and/or
   C. Marked deposition of eosinophil granule proteins is found (in the absence or presence of major tissue infiltration by eosinophils).
2. Organ damage and/or dysfunction attributable to tissue hypereosinophilia, and
3. Exclusion of other disorders or conditions as a major reason for organ damage. The idiopathic hypereosinophilic syndrome is further divided into variants.[4]

Patients present with weakness and fatigue (26%), cough (24%), dyspnea (16%),[215] or asthmatic symptoms (25%).[216] Respiratory manifestations are generally of mild severity, with rare eosinophilic pneumonia if any.[216] Chest CT may show pleural effusion, pulmonary emboli, small nodules, occasionally a halo of ground-glass attenuation, and focal areas of ground-glass attenuation mainly in the lung periphery.[25,217] Notably, imaging features corresponding to eosinophilic lung involvement must be differentiated from those related to pulmonary edema resulting from cardiac involvement. Chronic dry cough can be remarkable and may be a presenting or the only feature.[218–220]

Eosinophilic Pneumonias in Parasitic Diseases

Parasitic infection is the main cause of eosinophilic pneumonia in the world, but is less common in Europe and North America. The diagnosis may be missed, because clinical and radiologic manifestations are nonspecific, and the disease rarely presents as a typical eosinophilic pneumonia.[1,221] A detailed description can be found elsewhere.[1,222,223] Briefly, infection with the nematode *Ascaris lumbricoides* mainly causes Löffler syndrome, for example, mild eosinophilic pneumonia with transient cough, wheezing, fever, high blood eosinophilia, and pulmonary infiltrates. Visceral larva migrans syndrome caused by *Toxocara canis* that occurs throughout the world causes fever, seizures, fatigue, blood eosinophilia, and transient pulmonary manifestations (cough, dyspnea, wheezes or crackles at pulmonary auscultation, and pulmonary infiltrates at chest X-ray). Hyperinfection syndrome caused by *Strongyloides stercoralis* is a severe disease in immunocompromised patients, which can affect all organs.[224] The filarial parasites *Wuchereria bancrofti* and *Brugia malayi* can cause tropical pulmonary eosinophilia,[222] characterized by chronic pulmonary and blood eosinophilia, with patchy bilateral opacities, small nodules, and/or consolidation corresponding to eosinophilic pneumonia at imaging.

Eosinophilic Pneumonias Induced by Drugs and Toxics

A diligent search for the etiology of eosinophilic lung diseases is of paramount importance, as the identification of a potential cause may have practical consequences, especially when the disease is caused by drugs.[1] When present, pleural effusion, and extrapulmonary manifestations including cutaneous rash, further suggest the possibility of drug-induced eosinophilic pneumonia.[1,225] Therefore, a thorough investigation must be conducted for drugs taken in the weeks or days before an eosinophilic lung disease.

Although many drugs have been incriminated, causality has been established for a limited number of agents.[225] The relative frequency of reports of drug-induced lung disease, and whether causality has been established (www.pneumotox.com), guide the diagnostic approach and evaluation of imputability.[225] Antibiotics and nonsteroid anti-inflammatory drugs are particularly frequent culprits.[225]

Presentation may be similar to that of ICEP or have an acute onset similar to IAEP. An acute onset similar to the presentation to IAEP is common, especially with minocycline[226] or nitrofurantoin,[227] but the differential often includes chronic eosinophilic pneumonia. Acute eosinophilic pneumonia may occur in the context of drug rash with eosinophilia and systemic symptoms (DRESS).[228,229] BAL eosinophilia may be missing in patients with daptomycin-induced lung disease, despite the presence of peripheral blood eosinophilia.[230]

Eosinophilic lung disease of varying presentation may be due to illicit drugs especially cocaine, crack, heroin, but also cannabis.[62,231] Eosinophilic pneumonia can also be caused by noncigarette smoking products including vaping, waterpipe smoking, and marijuana.[232–234]

Radiation Therapy

A condition similar to ICEP has been reported after radiation therapy for breast cancer in women (similar to the syndrome of radiation-induced organizing pneumonia), with a median delay of 3.5 months and up to 1 year after completion of radiotherapy.[20,235,236] Relapse can occur after withdrawal of corticosteroid therapy.[20]

Idiopathic Hypereosinophilic Obliterative Bronchiolitis

Hypereosinophilic obliterative bronchiolitis[237] is defined by the association of bronchiolitis, peripheral blood and/or alveolar eosinophilia, and persistent airflow obstruction despite high-dose inhaled bronchodilators and corticosteroids. Demonstration of a bronchiolitis may be obtained by lung biopsy[237–241] and/or HRCT showing direct signs of bronchiolitis (eg, centrilobular nodules and branching opacities).[237] Hypereosinophilic obliterative bronchiolitis can be idiopathic, but may also occur in the setting of EGPA, ABPA, drug-induced eosinophilic lung disease (such as minocycline), and possibly in severe asthma.[237]

Patients report cough and exercise dyspnea but generally do not present with intermittent asthma symptoms or wheezes. The blood eosinophil cell count (with a mean value of $2.7 \times 10^9/L$), and the eosinophil differential percentage at BAL are elevated.[237] Airflow obstruction is often severe but reversible with oral corticosteroid therapy;[237,242] however, manifestations often recur when the daily dose of oral prednisone is tapered. Whitish tracheal and bronchial granulations or bronchial ulcerative lesions can be present with prominent tissue eosinophils on bronchial biopsy.[237]

Miscellaneous

ICEP may overlap with, or mimic cryptogenic organizing pneumonia. Eosinophilia may be found in other bronchopulmonary disorders where eosinophilic pneumonia is not prominent,[1] including the eosinophilic phenotype of asthma,[243] hypereosinophilic asthma (ie, with marked blood eosinophilia, >1500/mm³),[244] eosinophilic bronchitis (without asthma),[245] idiopathic eosinophilic systemic vasculitis,[129] bronchocentric granulomatosis,[246] isolated cases of idiopathic interstitial pneumonias (especially desquamative interstitial pneumonia[247]), pulmonary Langerhans cell histiocytosis, sarcoidosis, and in lung transplant recipients.[248]

PRACTICAL APPROACH TO DIAGNOSIS AND TREATMENT

The diagnosis of eosinophilic lung diseases usually relies primarily on characteristic clinical-imaging features and the demonstration of alveolar eosinophilia. BAL is key to confirm the diagnosis, whereas lung biopsy is generally not necessary. Peripheral blood eosinophilia is an excellent diagnostic biomarker but may be absent at presentation, especially in IAEP and in patients who have already received corticosteroid treatment.

Defining the etiology of eosinophilic lung diseases has practical implications for therapeutic intervention, including interruption of a medicinal or illicit drugs, or treatment of infections with parasites or fungi. Laboratory investigations for parasites must take into account the epidemiology of parasites. Biological investigations for ABPA should be prompted by the presence of mucus plugs, peripheral eosinophilia, or very high serum IgE levels in patients with asthma or cystic fibrosis, before proximal bronchiectasis develop. When no cause is found, the eosinophilic lung disease is considered idiopathic. Extrathoracic manifestations are key to the diagnosis of EGPA. The diagnosis of ICEP or IAEP is considered only once all known causes of eosinophilia have been excluded, keeping in mind that the majority of cases of AEP are caused by medications or related to tobacco smoking.

Treatment of eosinophilic lung diseases involves oral corticosteroids in most cases, and withdrawal of the offending agent when appropriate. Immunosuppressive therapy is required in severe cases of EGPA. Therapies that specifically target IL-5/IL-5R have dramatic impact on eosinophils in the lungs, and are increasing used in eosinophilic lung diseases.

CLINICS CARE POINTS

- When doing a bronchoalveolar lavage in the intensive care unit, always perform a differential cell count analysis in addition to microbiology, as acute eosinophilic pneumonia can mimic infectious pneumonia.

- In an asthmatic with poor asthma control, suspect allergic bronchopulmonary aspergillosis in case of peripheral eosinophilia, serum immunoglobulin E levels greater than 1000 ng/mL, or mucous plugs in sputum or at chest imaging.

- When initiating treatment of idiopathic chronic eosinophilic pneumonia, taper the dose of oral corticosteroids over 3 months and inform the patient of the risk of treatment-sensitive relapse.

- When treating a relapse of idiopathic chronic eosinophilic pneumonia, 20 mg per day of oral prednisone is sufficient as a starting dose.

- Therapies that target interleukin 5/interleukin-5 receptor should not be used as first-line therapy in eosinophilic lung diseases

CONFLICTS OF INTEREST

None.

REFERENCES

1. Cordier JF, Cottin V. Eosinophilic pneumonias. In: Schwarz MI, King TE Jr, editors. Interstitial lung disease. 5th ed. Shelton, Connecticut, USA: People's Medical Publishing House-USA; 2011. p. 833–93.
2. Cottin V. Eosinophilic lung diseases. In: Mason RJ, Ernst JD, King TE Jr, et al, editors. Murray and Nadel's textbook of respiratory medicine. 7th ed. Philadelphia: Elsevier; 2022. p. 1322–42.
3. Cottin V. Eosinophilic Lung Diseases. Clin Chest Med 2016;37:535–56.

4. Valent P, Klion AD, Horny HP, et al. Contemporary consensus proposal on criteria and classification of eosinophilic disorders and related syndromes. J Allergy Clin Immunol 2012;130:607–12.

5. Cottin V. Eosinophilic pneumonia. In: Cottin V, Cordier JF, Richeldi L, et al, editors. Orphan lung diseases: a clinical guide to rare lung disease. 2nd edition. London: Springer-Verlag; 2023 (in press).

6. Walsh ER, August A. Eosinophils and allergic airway disease: there is more to the story. Trends Immunol 2010;31:39–44.

7. Hogan SP, Rosenberg HF, Moqbel R, et al. Eosinophils: biological properties and role in health and disease. Clin Exp Allergy 2008;38:709–50.

8. Blanchard C, Rothenberg ME. Biology of the eosinophil. Adv Immunol 2009;101: 81–121.

9. Weller PF, Spencer LA. Functions of tissue-resident eosinophils. Nat Rev Immunol 2017;17:746–60.

10. Wechsler ME, Munitz A, Ackerman SJ, et al. Eosinophils in Health and Disease: A State-of-the-Art Review. Mayo Clin Proc 2021;96:2694–707.

11. Delcros Q, Groh M, Nasser M, et al. Steroid alternatives for managing eosinophilic lung diseases. Expert Opinion on Orphan Drugs 2021;9:205–18.

12. Prin L, Capron M, Gosset P, et al. Eosinophilic lung disease : immunological studies of blood and alveolar eosinophils. Clin Exp Immunol 1986;63:249–57.

13. Janin A, Torpier G, Courtin P, et al. Segregation of eosinophil proteins in alveolar macrophage compartments in chronic eosinophilic pneumonia. Thorax 1993;48: 57–62.

14. Fox B, Seed WA. Chronic eosinophilic pneumonia. Thorax 1980;35:570–80.

15. Akuthota P, Weller PF. Eosinophils and disease pathogenesis. Semin Hematol 2012;49:113–9.

16. Carrington CB, Addington WW, Goff AM, et al. Chronic eosinophilic pneumonia. N Engl J Med 1969;280:787–98.

17. Thomeer MJ, Costabe U, Rizzato G, et al. Comparison of registries of interstitial lung diseases in three European countries. Eur Respir J Suppl 2001;32. 114s-8s.

18. Marchand E, Reynaud-Gaubert M, Lauque D, et al. Idiopathic chronic eosinophilic pneumonia. A clinical and follow-up study of 62 cases. Medicine (Baltim) 1998;77:299–312.

19. Jederlinic PJ, Sicilian L, Gaensler EA. Chronic eosinophilic pneumonia. A report of 19 cases and a review of the literature. Medicine (Baltim) 1988;67:154–62.

20. Cottin V, Frognier R, Monnot H, et al. Chronic eosinophilic pneumonia after radiation therapy for breast cancer. Eur Respir J 2004;23:9–13.

21. Libby DM, Murphy TF, Edwards A, et al. Chronic eosinophilic pneumonia : an unusual cause of acute respiratory failure. Am Rev Respir Dis 1980;122: 497–500.

22. Ivanick MJ, Donohue JF. Chronic eosinophilic pneumonia: a cause of adult respiratory distress syndrome. South Med J 1986;79:686–90.

23. Marchand E, Etienne-Mastroianni B, Chanez P, et al. Idiopathic chronic eosinophilic pneumonia and asthma : how do they influence each other ? The Groupe d'Etudes et de Recherche sur les Maladies "Orphelines" Pulmonaires (GERM"O"P). Eur Respir J 2003;22:8–13.

24. Weynants P, Riou R, Vergnon JM, et al. Pneumopathies chroniques à éosinophiles. Etude de 16 cas. Rev Mal Respir 1985;2:63–8.

25. Johkoh T, Muller NL, Akira M, et al. Eosinophilic lung diseases: diagnostic accuracy of thin-section CT in 111 patients. Radiology 2000;216:773–80.

26. Arakawa H, Kurihara Y, Niimi H, et al. Bronchiolitis obliterans with organizing pneumonia versus chronic eosinophilic pneumonia: high-resolution CT findings in 81 patients. AJR Am J Roentgenol 2001;176:1053–8.

27. Furuiye M, Yoshimura N, Kobayashi A, et al. Churg-Strauss syndrome versus chronic eosinophilic pneumonia on high-resolution computed tomographic findings. J Comput Assist Tomogr 2010;34:19–22.

28. Ebara H, Ikezoe J, Johkoh T, et al. Chronic eosinophilic pneumonia: evolution of chest radiograms and CT features. J Comput Assist Tomogr 1994;18:737–44.

29. Mayo JR, Muller NL, Road J, et al. Chronic eosinophilic pneumonia: CT findings in six cases. AJR Am J Roentgenol 1989;153:727–30.

30. Cottin V, Deviller P, Tardy F, et al. Urinary eosinophil-derived neurotoxin/protein X: a simple method for assessing eosinophil degranulation in vivo. J Allergy Clin Immunol 1998;101:116–23.

31. Shimizudani N, Murata H, Kojo S, et al. Analysis of T cell receptor V(beta) gene expression and clonality in bronchoalveolar fluid lymphocytes from a patient with chronic eosinophilic pneumonitis. Lung 2001;179:31–41.

32. Freymond N, Kahn JE, Legrand F, et al. Clonal expansion of T cells in patients with eosinophilic lung disease. Allergy 2011;66:1506–8.

33. Grantham J, Meadows J, Gleich G. Chronic eosinophilic pneumonia. Evidence for eosinophil degranulation and release of major basic protein. Am J Med 1986; 80:89–94.

34. Durieu J, Wallaert B, Tonnel AB. Long term follow-up of pulmonary function in chronic eosinophilic pneumonia. Eur Respir J 1997;10:286–91.

35. Oyama Y, Fujisawa T, Hashimoto D, et al. Efficacy of short-term prednisolone treatment in patients with chronic eosinophilic pneumonia. Eur Respir J 2015; 45:1624–31.

36. Delcros Q, Taillé C, Vallée A, et al. Targeting interleukin-5/5R for the treatment of idiopathic chronic eosinophilic pneumonia. JACI in Practice 2023 (in press).

37. Badesch DB, King TE, Schwarz MI. Acute eosinophilic pneumonia : a hypersensitivity phenomenon? Am Rev Respir Dis 1989;139:249–52.

38. Allen JD, Pacht ER, Gadek JE, et al. Acute eosinophilic pneumonia as a reversible cause of noninfectious respiratory failure. N Engl J Med 1989;321:569–74.

39. Pope-Harman AL, Davis WB, Allen ED, et al. Acute eosinophilic pneumonia. A summary of 15 cases and a review of the literature. Medicine (Baltim) 1996; 75:334–42.

40. Philit F, Etienne-Mastroianni B, Parrot A, et al. Idiopathic acute eosinophilic pneumonia: a study of 22 patients. Am J Respir Crit Care Med 2002;166: 1235–9.

41. Shorr AF, Scoville SL, Cersovsky SB, et al. Acute eosinophilic pneumonia among US military personnel deployed in or near Iraq. JAMA 2004;292:2997–3005.

42. Rhee CK, Min KH, Yim NY, et al. Clinical characteristics and corticosteroid treatment of acute eosinophilic pneumonia. Eur Respir J 2013;41:402–9.

43. Hayakawa H, Sato A, Toyoshima M, et al. A clinical study of idiopathic eosinophilic pneumonia. Chest 1994;105:1462–6.

44. Cheon JE, Lee KS, Jung GS, et al. Acute eosinophilic pneumonia : radiographic and CT findings in six patients. AJR 1996;167:1195–9.

45. King MA, Pope-Harman AL, Allen JN, et al. Acute eosinophilic pneumonia: radiologic and clinical features. Radiology 1997;203:715–9.

46. Sine CR, Hiles PD, Scoville SL, et al. Acute eosinophilic pneumonia in the deployed military setting. Respir Med 2018;137:123–8.

47. Ajani S, Kennedy CC. Idiopathic acute eosinophilic pneumonia: A retrospective case series and review of the literature. Respir Med Case Rep 2013;10:43–7.

48. Ota K, Sasabuchi Y, Matsui H, et al. Age distribution and seasonality in acute eosinophilic pneumonia: analysis using a national inpatient database. BMC Pulm Med 2019;19:38.

49. Uchiyama H, Suda T, Nakamura Y, et al. Alterations in smoking habits are associated with acute eosinophilic pneumonia. Chest 2008;133:1174–80.

50. Komiya K, Teramoto S, Kawashima M, et al. A case of acute eosinophilic pneumonia following short-term passive smoking: an evidence of very high level of urinary cotinine. Allergol Int 2010;59:421–3.

51. De Giacomi F, Decker PA, Vassallo R, et al. Acute Eosinophilic Pneumonia: Correlation of Clinical Characteristics With Underlying Cause. Chest 2017;152: 379–85.

52. De Giacomi F, Vassallo R, Yi ES, et al. Acute Eosinophilic Pneumonia. Causes, Diagnosis, and Management. Am J Respir Crit Care Med 2018;197:728–36.

53. Tazelaar HD, Linz LJ, Colby TV, et al. Acute eosinophilic pneumonia: histopathologic findings in nine patients. Am J Respir Crit Care Med 1997;155:296–302.

54. Thompson BT, Moss M. A new definition for the acute respiratory distress syndrome. Semin Respir Crit Care Med 2013;34:441–7.

55. Daimon T, Johkoh T, Sumikawa H, et al. Acute eosinophilic pneumonia: Thin-section CT findings in 29 patients. Eur J Radiol 2008;65:462–7.

56. Jhun BW, Kim SJ, Kim K, et al. Clinical implications of initial peripheral eosinophilia in acute eosinophilic pneumonia. Respirology 2014;19:1059–65.

57. Choi JY, Lim JU, Jeong HJ, et al. Association between peripheral blood/bronchoalveolar lavage eosinophilia and significant oxygen requirements in patients with acute eosinophilic pneumonia. BMC Pulm Med 2020;20:22.

58. Taniguchi H, Kadota J, Fujii T, et al. Activation of lymphocytes and increased interleukin-5 levels in bronchoalveolar lavage fluid in acute eosinophilic pneumonia. Eur Respir J 1999;13:217–20.

59. Mochimaru H, Kawamoto M, Fukuda Y, et al. Clinicopathological differences between acute and chronic eosinophilic pneumonia. Respirology 2005;10:76–85.

60. Kawayama T, Fujiki R, Morimitsu Y, et al. Fatal idiopathic acute eosinophilic pneumonia with acute lung injury. Respirology 2002;7:373–5.

61. Jhun BW, Kim SJ, Kim K, et al. Outcomes of rapid corticosteroid tapering in acute eosinophilic pneumonia patients with initial eosinophilia. Respirology 2015;20:1241–7.

62. Sauvaget E, Dellamonica J, Arlaud K, et al. Idiopathic acute eosinophilic pneumonia requiring ECMO in a teenager smoking tobacco and cannabis. Pediatr Pulmonol 2010;45:1246–9.

63. Churg J, Strauss L. Allergic granulomatosis, allergic angiitis, and periarteritis nodosa. Am J Pathol 1951;27:277–301.

64. Jennette JC, Falk RJ, Bacon PA, et al. 2012 Revised International Chapel Hill Consensus Conference Nomenclature of Vasculitides. Arthritis Rheum 2013; 65:1–11.

65. Lanham JG, Elkon KB, Pusey CD, et al. Systemic vasculitis with asthma and eosinophilia: a clinical approach to the Churg-Strauss syndrome. Medicine (Baltim) 1984;63:65–81.

66. Reid AJ, Harrison BD, Watts RA, et al. Churg-Strauss syndrome in a district hospital. Qjm 1998;91:219–29.

67. Chumbley LC, Harrison EG Jr, DeRemee RA. Allergic granulomatosis and angiitis (Churg-Strauss syndrome). Report and analysis of 30 cases. Mayo Clin Proc 1977;52:477–84.

68. Guillevin L, Cohen P, Gayraud M, et al. Churg-Strauss syndrome. Clinical study and long-term follow-up of 96 patients. Medicine (Baltim) 1999;78:26–37.

69. Solans R, Bosch JA, Perez-Bocanegra C, et al. Churg-Strauss syndrome: outcome and long-term follow-up of 32 patients. Rheumatology 2001;40: 763–71.

70. Della Rossa A, Baldini C, Tavoni A, et al. Churg-Strauss syndrome: clinical and serological features of 19 patients from a single Italian centre. Rheumatology 2002;41:1286–94.

71. Keogh KA, Specks U. Churg-Strauss syndrome: clinical presentation, antineutrophil cytoplasmic antibodies, and leukotriene receptor antagonists. Am J Med 2003;115:284–90.

72. Mouthon L, le Toumelin P, Andre MH, et al. Polyarteritis nodosa and Churg-Strauss angiitis: characteristics and outcome in 38 patients over 65 years. Medicine (Baltim) 2002;81:27–40.

73. Sinico RA, Di Toma L, Maggiore U, et al. Prevalence and clinical significance of antineutrophil cytoplasmic antibodies in Churg-Strauss syndrome. Arthritis Rheum 2005;52:2926–35.

74. Sablé-Fourtassou R, Cohen P, Mahr A, et al. Antineutrophil cytoplasmic antibodies and the Churg-Strauss syndrome. Ann Intern Med 2005;143:632–8.

75. Comarmond C, Pagnoux C, Khellaf M, et al. Eosinophilic granulomatosis with polyangiitis (Churg-Strauss): clinical characteristics and long-term followup of the 383 patients enrolled in the French Vasculitis Study Group cohort. Arthritis Rheum 2013;65:270–81.

76. Healy B, Bibby S, Steele R, et al. Antineutrophil cytoplasmic autoantibodies and myeloperoxidase autoantibodies in clinical expression of Churg-Strauss syndrome. J Allergy Clin Immunol 2013;131:571, 576 e1-6.

77. Durel CA, Berthiller J, Caboni S, et al. Long-Term Followup of a Multicenter Cohort of 101 Patients With Eosinophilic Granulomatosis With Polyangiitis (Churg-Strauss). Arthritis Care Res 2016;68:374–87.

78. Cottin V, Bel E, Bottero P, et al. Respiratory manifestations of eosinophilic granulomatosis with polyangiitis (Churg-Strauss). Eur Respir J 2016;48:1429–41.

79. Cottin V, Bel E, Bottero P, et al. Revisiting the systemic vasculitis in eosinophilic granulomatosis with polyangiitis (Churg-Strauss): A study of 157 patients by the Groupe d'Etudes et de Recherche sur les Maladies Orphelines Pulmonaires and the European Respiratory Society Taskforce on eosinophilic granulomatosis with polyangiitis (Churg-Strauss). Autoimmun Rev 2017;16:1–9.

80. Saku A, Furuta S, Hiraguri M, et al. Longterm Outcomes of 188 Japanese Patients with Eosinophilic Granulomatosis with Polyangiitis. J Rheumatol 2018; 45:1159–66.

81. Yoo J, Ahn SS, Jung SM, et al. Could hypereosinophilia at diagnosis estimate the current activity or predict relapse in systemic immunosuppressive drug-naïve patients with eosinophilic granulomatosis with polyangiitis? Rheumatol Int 2019;39:1899–905.

82. Dunogué B, Pagnoux C, Guillevin L. Churg-strauss syndrome: clinical symptoms, complementary investigations, prognosis and outcome, and treatment. Semin Respir Crit Care Med 2011;32:298–309.

83. Vaglio A, Martorana D, Maggiore U, et al. HLA-DRB4 as a genetic risk factor for Churg-Strauss syndrome. Arthritis Rheum 2007;56:3159–66.

84. Bottero P, Bonini M, Vecchio F, et al. The common allergens in the Churg-Strauss syndrome. Allergy 2007;62:1288–94.

85. Wu EY, Hernandez ML, Jennette JC, et al. Eosinophilic Granulomatosis with Polyangiitis: Clinical Pathology Conference and Review. J Allergy Clin Immunol Pract 2018;6:1496–504.

86. Nathani N, Little MA, Kunst H, et al. Churg-Strauss syndrome and leukotriene antagonist use: a respiratory perspective. Thorax 2008;63:883–8.

87. Harrold LR, Patterson MK, Andrade SE, et al. Asthma drug use and the development of Churg-Strauss syndrome (CSS). Pharmacoepidemiol Drug Saf 2007; 16:620–6.

88. Beasley R, Bibby S, Weatherall M. Leukotriene receptor antagonist therapy and Churg-Strauss syndrome: culprit or innocent bystander? Thorax 2008;63:847–9.

89. Hauser T, Mahr A, Metzler C, et al. The leukotriene-receptor antagonist montelukast and the risk of Churg-Strauss syndrome: a case-crossover study. Thorax 2008;63:677–82.

90. Bibby S, Healy B, Steele R, et al. Association between leukotriene receptor antagonist therapy and Churg-Strauss syndrome: an analysis of the FDA AERS database. Thorax 2010;65:132–8.

91. Boita M, Guida G, Circosta P, et al. The molecular and functional characterization of clonally expanded CD8+ TCR BV T cells in eosinophilic granulomatosis with polyangiitis (EGPA). Clin Immunol 2014;152:152–63.

92. Churg A, Brallas M, Cronin SR, et al. Formes frustes of Churg-Strauss syndrome. Chest 1995;108:320–3.

93. Cottin V, Khouatra C, Dubost R, et al. Persistent airflow obstruction in asthma of patients with Churg-Strauss syndrome and long-term follow-up. Allergy 2009; 64:589–95.

94. Szczeklik W, Sokolowska BM, Zuk J, et al. The course of asthma in Churg-Strauss syndrome. J Asthma 2011;48:183–7.

95. Nakamaru Y, Takagi D, Suzuki M, et al. Otologic and Rhinologic Manifestations of Eosinophilic Granulomatosis with Polyangiitis. Audiol Neuro Otol 2016;21: 45–53.

96. Petersen H, Götz P, Both M, et al. Manifestation of eosinophilic granulomatosis with polyangiitis in head and neck. Rhinology 2015;53:277–85.

97. Chen Y, Ding Y, Liu Z, et al. Long-term outcomes in antineutrophil cytoplasmic autoantibody-positive eosinophilic granulomatosis with polyangiitis patients with renal involvement: a retrospective study of 14 Chinese patients. BMC Nephrol 2016;17:101.

98. Vinit J, Bielefeld P, Muller G, et al. Heart involvement in Churg-Strauss syndrome: retrospective study in French Burgundy population in past 10 years. Eur J Intern Med 2010;21:341–6.

99. Neumann T, Manger B, Schmid M, et al. Cardiac involvement in Churg-Strauss syndrome: impact of endomyocarditis. Medicine (Baltim) 2009;88:236–43.

100. Ginsberg F, Parrillo JE. Eosinophilic myocarditis. Heart Fail Clin 2005;1:419–29.

101. Kajihara H, Tachiyama Y, Hirose T, et al. Eosinophilic coronary periarteritis (vasospastic angina and sudden death), a new type of coronary arteritis: report of seven autopsy cases and a review of the literature. Virchows Arch 2013;462: 239–48.

102. Groh M, Masciocco G, Kirchner E, et al. Heart transplantation in patients with eosinophilic granulomatosis with polyangiitis (Churg-Strauss syndrome). J Heart Lung Transplant 2014;33:842–50.

103. Pela G, Tirabassi G, Pattoneri P, et al. Cardiac involvement in the Churg-Strauss syndrome. Am J Cardiol 2006;97:1519–24.
104. Dennert RM, van Paassen P, Schalla S, et al. Cardiac involvement in Churg-Strauss syndrome. Arthritis Rheum 2010;62:627–34.
105. Courand PY, Croisille P, Khouatra C, et al. Churg-Strauss syndrome presenting with acute myocarditis and cardiogenic shock. Heart Lung Circ 2012;21: 178–81.
106. Yune S, Choi DC, Lee BJ, et al. Detecting cardiac involvement with magnetic resonance in patients with active eosinophilic granulomatosis with polyangiitis. Int J Cardiovasc Imaging 2016;32(Suppl 1):155–62.
107. Allenbach Y, Seror R, Pagnoux C, et al. High frequency of venous thromboembolic events in Churg-Strauss syndrome, Wegener's granulomatosis and microscopic polyangiitis but not polyarteritis nodosa: a systematic retrospective study on 1130 patients. Ann Rheum Dis 2009;68:564–7.
108. Szczeklik W, Sokolowska B, Mastalerz L, et al. Pulmonary findings in Churg-Strauss syndrome in chest X-rays and high resolution computed tomography at the time of initial diagnosis. Clin Rheumatol 2010;29:1127–34.
109. Choi YH, Im JG, Han BK, et al. Thoracic manifestation of Churg-Strauss syndrome: radiologic and clinical findings. Chest 2000;117:117–24.
110. Kim YK, Lee KS, Chung MP, et al. Pulmonary involvement in Churg-Strauss syndrome: an analysis of CT, clinical, and pathologic findings. Eur Radiol 2007;17: 3157–65.
111. Chung MP, Yi CA, Lee HY, et al. Imaging of pulmonary vasculitis. Radiology 2010;255:322–41.
112. Worthy SA, Muller NL, Hansell DM, et al. Churg-Strauss syndrome: the spectrum of pulmonary CT findings in 17 patients. AJR Am J Roentgenol 1998;170: 297–300.
113. Wallaert B, Gosset P, Prin L, et al. Bronchoalveolar lavage in allergic granulomatosis and angiitis. Eur Respir J 1993;6:413–7.
114. Cottin V, Tardy F, Gindre D, et al. Urinary eosinophil-derived neurotoxin in Churg-Strauss syndrome. J Allergy Clin Immunol 1995;96:261–4.
115. Vaglio A, Strehl JD, Manger B, et al. IgG4 immune response in Churg-Strauss syndrome. Ann Rheum Dis 2012;71:390–3.
116. Dallos T, Heiland GR, Strehl J, et al. CCL17/thymus and activation-related chemokine in Churg-Strauss syndrome. Arthritis Rheum 2010;62:3496–503.
117. Sokolowska BM, Szczeklik WK, Wludarczyk AA, et al. ANCA-positive and ANCA-negative phenotypes of eosinophilic granulomatosis with polyangiitis (EGPA): outcome and long-term follow-up of 50 patients from a single Polish center. Clin Exp Rheumatol 2014;32:S41–7.
118. Schroeder JW, Folci M, Losappio LM, et al. Anti-Neutrophil Cytoplasmic Antibodies Positivity and Anti-Leukotrienes in Eosinophilic Granulomatosis with Polyangiitis: A Retrospective Monocentric Study on 134 Italian Patients. Int Arch Allergy Immunol 2019;180:64–71.
119. Wieczorek S, Hellmich B, Arning L, et al. Functionally relevant variations of the interleukin-10 gene associated with antineutrophil cytoplasmic antibody-negative Churg-Strauss syndrome, but not with Wegener's granulomatosis. Arthritis Rheum 2008;58:1839–48.
120. Berti A, Cornec D, Casal Moura M, et al. Eosinophilic Granulomatosis With Polyangiitis: Clinical Predictors of Long-term Asthma Severity. Chest 2020;157: 1086–99.

121. Berti A, Volcheck GW, Cornec D, et al. Severe/uncontrolled asthma and overall survival in atopic patients with eosinophilic granulomatosis with polyangiitis. Respir Med 2018;142:66–72.

122. Katzenstein AL. Diagnostic features and differential diagnosis of Churg-Strauss syndrome in the lung. A review. Am J Clin Pathol 2000;114:767–72.

123. Churg A. Recent advances in the diagnosis of Churg-Strauss syndrome. Mod Pathol 2001;14:1284–93.

124. Nasser M, Thivolet-Béjui F, Sève P, et al. Lung-limited or lung-dominant variant of eosinophilic granulomatosis with polyangiitis. J Allergy Clin Immunol Pract 2020; 8:2092–5.

125. Lie JT. Limited forms of Churg-Strauss syndrome. Pathol Annu 1993;28: 199–220.

126. Wechsler ME, Garpestad E, Flier SR, et al. Pulmonary infiltrates, eosinophilia, and cardiomyopathy following corticosteroid withdrawal in patients with asthma receiving zarfirlukast. JAMA 1998;279:455–7.

127. Grayson PC, Ponte C, Suppiah R, et al. American College of Rheumatology/European Alliance of Associations for Rheumatology Classification Criteria for Eosinophilic Granulomatosis with Polyangiitis. Ann Rheum Dis 2022;81:309–14.

128. Wechsler ME, Akuthota P, Jayne D, et al. Mepolizumab or Placebo for Eosinophilic Granulomatosis with Polyangiitis. N Engl J Med 2017;376:1921–32.

129. Lefevre G, Leurs A, Gibier JB, et al. Cereo French National Reference Center for Hypereosinophilic Syndromes. "Idiopathic Eosinophilic Vasculitis": Another Side of Hypereosinophilic Syndrome? A Comprehensive Analysis of 117 Cases in Asthma-Free Patients. J Allergy Clin Immunol Pract 2019;8:1329–40.

130. Nasser M, Thivolet-Béjui F, Cottin V. Idiopathic non-necrotizing eosinophilic vasculitis limited to the lung: Part of a complex spectrum. J Allergy Clin Immunol Pract 2020;8:2454–5.

131. Guillevin L, Lhote F, Gayraud M, et al. Prognostic factors in polyarteritis nodosa and Churg-Strauss syndrome. A prospective study in 342 patients. Medicine (Baltim) 1996;75:17–28.

132. Abu-Shakra M, Smythe H, Lewtas J, et al. Outcome of polyarteritis nodosa and Churg-Strauss syndrome. An analysis of twenty-five patients. Arthritis Rheum 1994;37:1798–803.

133. Cohen P, Pagnoux C, Mahr A, et al. Treatment of Churg-Strauss syndrome (CSS) without poor prognosis factor at baseline with corticosteroids (CS) alone. Preliminary results of a prospective multicenter trial. Arthritis Rheum 2003;48:S209.

134. Guillevin L, Pagnoux C, Seror R, et al. The Five-Factor Score revisited: assessment of prognoses of systemic necrotizing vasculitides based on the French Vasculitis Study Group (FVSG) cohort. Medicine (Baltim) 2011;90:19–27.

135. Moosig F, Richardt G, Gross WL. A fatal attraction: eosinophils and the heart. Rheumatology 2013;52:587–9.

136. Samson M, Puechal X, Devilliers H, et al. Long-term outcomes of 118 patients with eosinophilic granulomatosis with polyangiitis (Churg-Strauss syndrome) enrolled in two prospective trials. J Autoimmun 2013;43:60–9.

137. Groh M, Pagnoux C, Baldini C, et al. Eosinophilic granulomatosis with polyangiitis (Churg-Strauss) (EGPA) Consensus Task Force recommendations for evaluation and management. Eur J Intern Med 2015;26:545–53.

138. Pagnoux C, Quemeneur T, Ninet J, et al. Treatment of systemic necrotizing vasculitides in patients aged sixty-five years or older: results of a multicenter, open-label, randomized controlled trial of corticosteroid and

cyclophosphamide-based induction therapy. Arthritis Rheumatol 2015;67: 1117–27.

139. Chung SA, Langford CA, Maz M, et al. American College of Rheumatology/ Vasculitis Foundation Guideline for the Management of Antineutrophil Cytoplasmic Antibody-Associated Vasculitis. Arthritis Rheumatol 2021;73:1366–83.

140. Bettiol A, Urban ML, Dagna L, et al. Mepolizumab for Eosinophilic Granulomatosis With Polyangiitis: A European Multicenter Observational Study. Arthritis Rheumatol 2022;74:295–306.

141. Cartin-Ceba R, Keogh KA, Specks U, et al. Rituximab for the treatment of Churg-Strauss syndrome with renal involvement. Nephrol Dial Transplant 2011;26: 2865–71.

142. Donvik KK, Omdal R. Churg-Strauss syndrome successfully treated with rituximab. Rheumatol Int 2011;31:89–91.

143. Kaushik VV, Reddy HV, Bucknall RC. Successful use of rituximab in a patient with recalcitrant Churg-Strauss syndrome. Ann Rheum Dis 2006;65:1116–7.

144. Koukoulaki M, Smith KG, Jayne DR. Rituximab in Churg-Strauss syndrome. Ann Rheum Dis 2006;65:557–9.

145. Najem CE, Yadav R, Carlson E. Successful use of Rituximab in a patient with recalcitrant multisystemic eosinophilic granulomatosis with polyangiitis. BMJ Case Rep 2015;2015.

146. Pepper RJ, Fabre MA, Pavesio C, et al. Rituximab is effective in the treatment of refractory Churg-Strauss syndrome and is associated with diminished T-cell interleukin-5 production. Rheumatology 2008;47:1104–5.

147. Saech J, Owczarczyk K, Rosgen S, et al. Successful use of rituximab in a patient with Churg-Strauss syndrome and refractory central nervous system involvement. Ann Rheum Dis 2010;69:1254–5.

148. Thiel J, Hassler F, Salzer U, et al. Rituximab in the treatment of refractory or relapsing eosinophilic granulomatosis with polyangiitis (Churg-Strauss syndrome). Arthritis Res Ther 2013;15:R133.

149. Umezawa N, Kohsaka H, Nanki T, et al. Successful treatment of eosinophilic granulomatosis with polyangiitis (EGPA; formerly Churg-Strauss syndrome) with rituximab in a case refractory to glucocorticoids, cyclophosphamide, and IVIG. Mod Rheumatol 2014;24:685–7.

150. Puechal X, Pagnoux C, Baron G, et al. Non-severe eosinophilic granulomatosis with polyangiitis: long-term outcomes after remission-induction trial. Rheumatology 2019;58:2107–16.

151. Pagnoux C, Mahr A, Hamidou MA, et al. Azathioprine or methotrexate maintenance for ANCA-associated vasculitis. N Engl J Med 2008;359:2790–803.

152. Hiemstra TF, Walsh M, Mahr A, et al. Mycophenolate mofetil vs azathioprine for remission maintenance in antineutrophil cytoplasmic antibody-associated vasculitis: a randomized controlled trial. JAMA 2010;304:2381–8.

153. Tsurikisawa N, Oshikata C, Watanabe M, et al. Clinical Features of Patients with Active Eosinophilic Granulomatosis with Polyangiitis Successfully Treated with Mepolizumab. Int Arch Allergy Immunol 2021;182:744–56.

154. Canzian A, Venhoff N, Urban ML, et al. Use of Biologics to Treat Relapsing and/ or Refractory Eosinophilic Granulomatosis With Polyangiitis: Data From a European Collaborative Study. Arthritis Rheumatol 2021;73:498–503.

155. Manka LA, Guntur VP, Denson JL, et al. Efficacy and safety of reslizumab in the treatment of eosinophilic granulomatosis with polyangiitis. Ann Allergy Asthma Immunol 2021;126:696–701.e1.

156. Guntur VP, Manka LA, Denson JL, et al. Benralizumab as a Steroid-Sparing Treatment Option in Eosinophilic Granulomatosis with Polyangiitis. J Allergy Clin Immunol Pract 2021;9:1186–11893.e1.

157. Celebi Sozener Z, Gorgulu B, Mungan D, et al. Omalizumab in the treatment of eosinophilic granulomatosis with polyangiitis (EGPA): single-center experience in 18 cases. World Allergy Organization journal 2018;11:39.

158. Jachiet M, Samson M, Cottin V, et al. Anti-IgE Monoclonal Antibody (Omalizumab) in Refractory and Relapsing Eosinophilic Granulomatosis With Polyangiitis (Churg-Strauss): Data on Seventeen Patients. Arthritis Rheumatol 2016;68:2274–82.

159. Wechsler ME, Wong DA, Miller MK, et al. Churg-strauss syndrome in patients treated with omalizumab. Chest 2009;136:507–18.

160. Ruppert AM, Averous G, Stanciu D, et al. Development of Churg-Strauss syndrome with controlled asthma during omalizumab treatment. J Allergy Clin Immunol 2008;121:253–4.

161. Winchester DE, Jacob A, Murphy T. Omalizumab for asthma. N Engl J Med 2006;355:1281–2.

162. Puechal X, Rivereau P, Vinchon F. Churg-Strauss syndrome associated with omalizumab. Eur J Intern Med 2008;19:364–6.

163. Bargagli E, Madioni C, Olivieri C, et al. Churg-Strauss vasculitis in a patient treated with omalizumab. J Asthma 2008;45:115–6.

164. Eger K, Pet L, Weersink EJM, et al. Complications of switching from anti-IL-5 or anti-IL-5R to dupilumab in corticosteroid-dependent severe asthma. J Allergy Clin Immunol Pract 2021;9:2913–5.

165. Briegel I, Felicio-Briegel A, Mertsch P, et al. Hypereosinophilia with systemic manifestations under dupilumab and possibility of dual benralizumab and dupilumab therapy in patients with asthma and CRSwNP. J Allergy Clin Immunol Pract 2021;9:4477–9.

166. Ribi C, Cohen P, Pagnoux C, et al. Treatment of Churg-Strauss syndrome without poor-prognosis factors: a multicenter, prospective, randomized, open-label study of seventy-two patients. Arthritis Rheum 2008;58:586–94.

167. Bourgarit A, Le Toumelin P, Pagnoux C, et al. Deaths occurring during the first year after treatment onset for polyarteritis nodosa, microscopic polyangiitis, and Churg-Strauss syndrome: a retrospective analysis of causes and factors predictive of mortality based on 595 patients. Medicine (Baltim) 2005;84:323–30.

168. Geller DE, Kaplowitz H, Light MJ, et al. Allergic bronchopulmonary aspergillosis in cystic fibrosis: reported prevalence, regional distribution, and patient characteristics. Chest 1999;116:639–46.

169. Mastella G, Rainisio M, Harms HK, et al. Allergic bronchopulmonary aspergillosis in cystic fibrosis. A European epidemiological study. Epidemiologic Registry of Cystic Fibrosis. Eur Respir J 2000;16:464–71.

170. Mehta SK, Sandhu RS. Immunological significance of Aspergillus fumigatus in cane-sugar mills. Arch Environ Health 1983;38:41–6.

171. Agarwal R, Muthu V, Sehgal IS, et al. Allergic Bronchopulmonary Aspergillosis. Clin Chest Med 2022;43:99–125.

172. Murdock BJ, Falkowski NR, Shreiner AB, et al. Interleukin-17 drives pulmonary eosinophilia following repeated exposure to Aspergillus fumigatus conidia. Infect Immun 2012;80:1424–36.

173. Ueki S, Tokunaga T, Melo RCN, et al. Charcot-Leyden crystal formation is closely associated with eosinophil extracellular trap cell death. Blood 2018;132:2183–7.

174. Marchand E, Verellen-Dumoulin C, Mairesse M, et al. Frequency of cystic fibrosis transmembrane conductance regulator gene mutations and 5T allele in patients with allergic bronchopulmonary aspergillosis. Chest 2001;119:762–7.

175. Knutsen AP, Kariuki B, Consolino JD, et al. IL-4 alpha chain receptor (IL-4Ralpha) polymorphisms in allergic bronchopulmonary aspergillosis. Clin Mol Allergy 2006;4:3.

176. Brouard J, Knauer N, Boelle PY, et al. Influence of interleukin-10 on Aspergillus fumigatus infection in patients with cystic fibrosis. J Infect Dis 2005;191:1988–91.

177. Saxena S, Madan T, Shah A, et al. Association of polymorphisms in the collagen region of SP-A2 with increased levels of total IgE antibodies and eosinophilia in patients with allergic bronchopulmonary aspergillosis. J Allergy Clin Immunol 2003;111:1001–7.

178. Chauhan B, Santiago L, Kirschmann DA, et al. The association of HLA-DR alleles and T cell activation with allergic bronchopulmonary aspergillosis. J Immunol 1997;159:4072–6.

179. Chauhan B, Santiago L, Hutcheson PS, et al. Evidence for the involvement of two different MHC class II regions in susceptibility or protection in allergic bronchopulmonary aspergillosis. J Allergy Clin Immunol 2000;106:723–9.

180. Chauhan B, Knutsen A, Hutcheson PS, et al. T cell subsets, epitope mapping, and HLA-restriction in patients with allergic bronchopulmonary aspergillosis. J Clin Invest 1996;97:2324–31.

181. Shah A, Khan ZU, Chaturvedi S, et al. Concomitant allergic Aspergillus sinusitis and allergic bronchopulmonary aspergillosis associated with familial occurrence of allergic bronchopulmonary aspergillosis. Ann Allergy 1990;64:507–12.

182. Mussaffi H, Rivlin J, Shalit I, et al. Nontuberculous mycobacteria in cystic fibrosis associated with allergic bronchopulmonary aspergillosis and steroid therapy. Eur Respir J 2005;25:324–8.

183. Dykewicz MS, Rodrigues JM, Slavin RG. Allergic fungal rhinosinusitis. J Allergy Clin Immunol 2018;142:341–51.

184. Agarwal R, Gupta D, Aggarwal AN, et al. Clinical significance of hyperattenuating mucoid impaction in allergic bronchopulmonary aspergillosis: an analysis of 155 patients. Chest 2007;132:1183–90.

185. Logan PM, Muller NL. High-attenuation mucous plugging in allergic bronchopulmonary aspergillosis. Can Assoc Radiol J 1996;47:374–7.

186. Martinez S, Heyneman LE, McAdams HP, et al. Mucoid impactions: finger-in-glove sign and other CT and radiographic features. Radiographics 2008;28:1369–82.

187. Refait J, Macey J, Bui S, et al. CT evaluation of hyperattenuating mucus to diagnose allergic bronchopulmonary aspergillosis in the special condition of cystic fibrosis. J Cyst Fibros 2019;18:e31–6.

188. Agarwal R, Gupta D, Aggarwal AN, et al. Allergic bronchopulmonary aspergillosis: lessons from 126 patients attending a chest clinic in north India. Chest 2006;130:442–8.

189. Ward S, Heyneman L, Lee MJ, et al. Accuracy of CT in the diagnosis of allergic bronchopulmonary aspergillosis in asthmatic patients. AJR Am J Roentgenol 1999;173:937–42.

190. Rosenberg M, Patterson R, Roberts M, et al. The assessment of immunologic and clinical changes occurring during corticosteroid therapy for allergic bronchopulmonary aspergillosis. Am J Med 1978;64:599–606.

191. Alghamdi NS, Barton R, Wilcox M, et al. Serum IgE and IgG reactivity to Aspergillus recombinant antigens in patients with cystic fibrosis. J Med Microbiol 2019;68:924–9.

192. Muthu V, Singh P, Choudhary H, et al. Diagnostic Cutoffs and Clinical Utility of Recombinant Aspergillus fumigatus Antigens in the Diagnosis of Allergic Bronchopulmonary Aspergillosis. J Allergy Clin Immunol Pract 2020;8:579–87.

193. Agarwal R, Maskey D, Aggarwal AN, et al. Diagnostic performance of various tests and criteria employed in allergic bronchopulmonary aspergillosis: a latent class analysis. PLoS One 2013;8. e61105.

194. Sehgal IS, Agarwal R. Specific IgE is better than skin testing for detecting Aspergillus sensitization and allergic bronchopulmonary aspergillosis in asthma. Chest 2015;147:e194.

195. Chakrabarti A, Sethi S, Raman DS, et al. Eight-year study of allergic bronchopulmonary aspergillosis in an Indian teaching hospital. Mycoses 2002;45:295–9.

196. Pashley CH, Fairs A, Morley JP, et al. Routine processing procedures for isolating filamentous fungi from respiratory sputum samples may underestimate fungal prevalence. Medical mycology 2012;50:433–8.

197. Agarwal R, Chakrabarti A, Shah A, et al. Allergic bronchopulmonary aspergillosis: review of literature and proposal of new diagnostic and classification criteria. Clin Exp Allergy 2013;43:850–73.

198. Bosken C, Myers J, Greenberger P, et al. Pathologic features of allergic bronchopulmonary aspergillosis. Am J Surg Pathol 1988;12:216–22.

199. Saxena P, Choudhary H, Muthu V, et al. Which Are the Optimal Criteria for the Diagnosis of Allergic Bronchopulmonary Aspergillosis? A Latent Class Analysis. J Allergy Clin Immunol Pract 2021;9:328–35.e1.

200. Asano K, Hebisawa A, Ishiguro T, et al. New clinical diagnostic criteria for allergic bronchopulmonary aspergillosis/mycosis and its validation. J Allergy Clin Immunol 2021;147:1261–8.e5.

201. Chowdhary A, Agarwal K, Kathuria S, et al. Allergic bronchopulmonary mycosis due to fungi other than Aspergillus: a global overview. Crit Rev Microbiol 2014; 40:30–48.

202. Agarwal R, Aggarwal AN, Dhooria S, et al. A randomised trial of glucocorticoids in acute-stage allergic bronchopulmonary aspergillosis complicating asthma. Eur Respir J 2016;47:385–7.

203. Greenberger PA. Allergic bronchopulmonary aspergillosis. J Allergy Clin Immunol 2002;110:685–92.

204. Singh Sehgal I, Agarwal R. Pulse methylprednisolone in allergic bronchopulmonary aspergillosis exacerbations. Eur Respir Rev 2014;23:149–52.

205. Patterson R, Greenberger PA, Lee TM, et al. Prolonged evaluation of patients with corticosteroid-dependent asthma stage of allergic bronchopulmonary aspergillosis. J Allergy Clin Immunol 1987;80:663–8.

206. Salez F, Brichet A, Desurmont S, et al. Effects of itraconazole therapy in allergic bronchopulmonary aspergillosis. Chest 1999;116:1665–8.

207. Wark P. Pathogenesis of allergic bronchopulmonary aspergillosis and an evidence-based review of azoles in treatment. Respir Med 2004;98:915–23.

208. Agarwal R, Dhooria S, Singh Sehgal I, et al. A Randomized Trial of Itraconazole vs Prednisolone in Acute-Stage Allergic Bronchopulmonary Aspergillosis Complicating Asthma. Chest 2018;153:656–64.

209. Godet C, Meurice JC, Roblot F, et al. Efficacy of nebulised liposomal amphotericin B in the attack and maintenance treatment of ABPA. Eur Respir J 2012;39:1261–3.

210. van der Ent CK, Hoekstra H, Rijkers GT. Successful treatment of allergic bronchopulmonary aspergillosis with recombinant anti-IgE antibody. Thorax 2007; 62:276–7.
211. Zirbes JM, Milla CE. Steroid-sparing effect of omalizumab for allergic bronchopulmonary aspergillosis and cystic fibrosis. Pediatr Pulmonol 2008;43:607–10.
212. Kanu A, Patel K. Treatment of allergic bronchopulmonary aspergillosis (ABPA) in CF with anti-IgE antibody (omalizumab). Pediatr Pulmonol 2008;43:1249–51.
213. Tillie-Leblond I, Germaud P, Leroyer C, et al. Allergic bronchopulmonary aspergillosis and omalizumab. Allergy 2011;66:1254–6.
214. Perez-de-Llano LA, Vennera MC, Parra A, et al. Effects of omalizumab in Aspergillus-associated airway disease. Thorax 2011;66:539–40.
215. Fauci AS, Harley JB, Roberts WC, et al. The idiopathic hypereosinophilic syndrome : clinical, pathophysiologic and therapeutic considerations. Ann Intern Med 1982;97:78–92.
216. Dulohery MM, Patel RR, Schneider F, et al. Lung involvement in hypereosinophilic syndromes. Respir Med 2011;105:114–21.
217. Kang EY, Shim JJ, Kim JS, et al. Pulmonary involvement of idiopathic hypereosinophilic syndrome: CT findings in five patients. J Comput Assist Tom 1997;21: 612–5.
218. Chung KF, Hew M, Score J, et al. Cough and hypereosinophilia due to FIP1L1-PDGFRA fusion gene with tyrosine kinase activity. Eur Respir J 2006;27:230–2.
219. Roufosse F, Heimann P, Lambert F, et al. Severe Prolonged Cough as Presenting Manifestation of FIP1L1-PDGFRA+ Chronic Eosinophilic Leukaemia: A Widely Ignored Association. Respiration 2016;91:374–9.
220. Xie J, Zhang J, Zhang X, et al. Cough in hypereosinophilic syndrome: case report and literature review. BMC Pulm Med 2020;20:90.
221. Kunst H, Mack D, Kon OM, et al. Parasitic infections of the lung: a guide for the respiratory physician. Thorax 2011;66:528–36.
222. Vijayan VK. How to diagnose and manage common parasitic pneumonias. Curr Opin Pulm Med 2007;13:218–24.
223. Fiorentini LF, Bergo P, Meirelles GSP, et al. Pictorial Review of Thoracic Parasitic Diseases: A Radiologic Guide. Chest 2020;157:1100–13.
224. Ming DK, Armstrong M, Lowe P, et al. Clinical and Diagnostic Features of 413 Patients Treated for Imported Strongyloidiasis at the Hospital for Tropical Diseases, London. Am J Trop Med Hyg 2019;101:428–31.
225. Spagnolo P, Bonniaud P, Rossi G, et al. Drug-induced interstitial lung disease. Eur Respir J 2022;60.
226. Sitbon O, Bidel N, Dussopt C, et al. Minocycline pneumonitis and eosinophilia. A report on eight patients. Arch Intern Med 1994;154:1633–40.
227. Sovijarvi AR, Lemola M, Stenius B, et al. Nitrofurantoin-induced acute, subacute and chronic pulmonary reactions. Scand J Respir Dis 1977;58:41–50.
228. Husain Z, Reddy BY, Schwartz RA. DRESS syndrome: Part II. Management and therapeutics. J Am Acad Dermatol 2013;68. 709 e1-9; quiz; 18-20.
229. Husain Z, Reddy BY, Schwartz RA. DRESS syndrome: Part I. Clinical perspectives. J Am Acad Dermatol 2013;68. 693.e1-14; quiz; 706-8.
230. Pham TT, Garreau R, Craighero F, et al. Seventeen Cases of Daptomycin-Induced Eosinophilic Pneumonia in a Cohort of Patients Treated for Bone and Joint Infections: Proposal for a New Algorithm. Open Forum Infect Dis 2022;9: ofac577.
231. Brander PE, Tukiainen P. Acute eosinophilic pneumonia in a heroin smoker. Eur Respir J 1993;6:750–2.

232. Chaaban T. Acute eosinophilic pneumonia associated with non-cigarette smoking products: a systematic review. Advances in respiratory medicine 2020;88:142–6.
233. Puebla Neira D, Tambra S, Bhasin V, et al. Discordant bilateral bronchoalveolar lavage findings in a patient with acute eosinophilic pneumonia associated with counterfeit tetrahydrocannabinol oil vaping. Respir Med Case Rep 2020;29:101015.
234. Mull ES, Erdem G, Nicol K, et al. Eosinophilic Pneumonia and Lymphadenopathy Associated With Vaping and Tetrahydrocannabinol Use. Pediatrics 2020;145.
235. Miranowski AC, Ditto AM. Eosinophilic pneumonia in a patient with breast cancer: idiopathic or not. Ann Allergy Asthma Immunol 2006;97:557–8.
236. Cottin V, Cordier JF. Eosinophilic pneumonia in a patient with breast cancer: idiopathic or not? Ann Allergy Asthma Immunol 2006;97:557–8.
237. Cordier JF, Cottin V, Khouatra C, et al. Hypereosinophilic obliterative bronchiolitis: a distinct, unrecognised syndrome. Eur Respir J 2013;41:1126–34.
238. Takayanagi N, Kanazawa M, Kawabata Y, et al. Chronic bronchiolitis with associated eosinophilic lung disease (eosinophilic bronchiolitis). Respiration 2001;68:319–22.
239. Fukushima Y, Kamiya K, Tatewaki M, et al. A patient with bronchial asthma in whom eosinophilic bronchitis and bronchiolitis developed during treatment. Allergol Int 2010;59:87–91.
240. Kobayashi T, Inoue H, Mio T. Hypereosinophilic obliterative bronchiolitis clinically mimicking diffuse panbronchiolitis: four-year follow-up. Intern Med 2015;54:1091–4.
241. Tang TT, Cheng HH, Zhang H, et al. Hypereosinophilic obliterative bronchiolitis with an elevated level of serum CEA: a case report and a review of the literature. Eur Rev Med Pharmacol Sci 2015;19:2634–40.
242. Wang LH, Tsai YS, Yan JJ, et al. Reversing rapidly deteriorating lung function in eosinophilic bronchiolitis by pulse steroid and anti-IgE therapy. J Formos Med Assoc 2014;113:326–7.
243. Carr TF, Zeki AA, Kraft M. Eosinophilic and Noneosinophilic Asthma. Am J Respir Crit Care Med 2018;197:22–37.
244. Cordier JF. Asthmes hyperéosinophiliques. Rev Fr Allergol Immunol Clin 2004;44:92–5.
245. Gibson PG, Fujimura M, Niimi A. Eosinophilic bronchitis: clinical manifestations and implications for treatment. Thorax 2002;57:178–82.
246. Ward S, Heyneman LE, Flint JD, et al. Bronchocentric granulomatosis: computed tomographic findings in five patients. Clin Radiol 2000;55:296–300.
247. Ishiguro T, Takayanagi N, Kurashima K, et al. Desquamative interstitial pneumonia with a remarkable increase in the number of BAL eosinophils. Intern Med 2008;47:779–84.
248. Verleden SE, Ruttens D, Vandermeulen E, et al. Elevated bronchoalveolar lavage eosinophilia correlates with poor outcome after lung transplantation. Transplantation 2014;97:83–9.

Occupational Interstitial Lung Diseases

Hayley Barnes, PhD, MPH, MBBS[a,b,c,*], Ian Glaspole, PhD, MBBS[a,c]

KEYWORDS

- Occupational lung disease • Interstitial lung disease • Asbestosis • Silicosis
- Hypersensitivity pneumonitis

KEY POINTS

- Silicosis, asbestosis, and coal worker's pneumoconiosis are commonly encountered in pulmonary clinics, and are related to dust and asbestos exposure.
- Wood dust, gases, vapors and fumes, silica, and agricultural dusts, are associated with idiopathic pulmonary fibrosis.
- Silica, welding fumes, solvents, heavy metals, and particulate matter, are associated with connective tissue disease-associated ILD.
- Bird, mold, and agricultural exposures are associated with hypersensitivity pneumonitis.
- There are limited treatment options; reduction of exposure is essential to reduce disease progression.

INTRODUCTION

Interstitial lung diseases (ILDs) are a heterogeneous group of parenchymal lung diseases, some of which arise as a result of genetic susceptibility, as well as external noxious stimuli, of which occupational and environmental exposures contribute. Such exposures may by directly causal, such as in the case of dust-related pneumoconioses, or partly contributory, such as in the case of idiopathic pulmonary fibrosis (IPF) and connective tissue disease associated interstitial lung diseases (CTD-ILDs) (**Table 1**). This review will outline our current understanding of the occupational burden of common ILDs, highlight limitations of our current knowledge, and propose future research directions.

OCCUPATIONAL INTERSTITIAL LUNG DISEASES
Pneumoconioses

The pneumoconioses are parenchymal lung diseases that arise from the inhalation of inorganic dust particles. It comprises a heterogenous group of parenchymal lung

[a] Department of Respiratory Medicine, Alfred Hospital, 34 Commercial Road, Melbourne 3004, Australia; [b] Monash Centre for Occupational and Environmental Health, Monash University, Melbourne, Australia; [c] Central Clinical School, Monash University, Melbourne, Australia
* Corresponding author. Department of Respiratory Medicine, Alfred Hospital, 34 Commercial Road, Melbourne 3004, Australia.
E-mail address: Hayley.Barnes@monash.edu

Immunol Allergy Clin N Am 43 (2023) 323–339
https://doi.org/10.1016/j.iac.2023.01.006
0889-8561/23/© 2023 Elsevier Inc. All rights reserved.
immunology.theclinics.com

Table 1
Common interstitial lung diseases and associated occupational exposures

ILD	Relevant Occupations
Silicosis	Miners, artificial stone benchtop fabrication, sandblasting, and jewelry polishing
Asbestosis	Miner, asbestos production, insulation, lagging, cement production, boilermaker, shipyard and railway workers, car mechanics, demolition, and WTC first responders
Coal worker's pneumoconiosis	Coal miners and coal production
Chronic beryllium disease	Aerospace and defense industries, alloy and automotive industries
IPF	Silica-related industries, vapors, gases, dusts, fumes, wood dusts, and agricultural dusts
CTD-ILD	Silica-related industries, petrochemical industries, motor vehicle production, dry cleaning, particulate matter, welding fumes, and heavy metals
Sarcoidosis	Agriculture, bakers, food production workers, silica-associated industries, firefighters, WTC first responders, dental technicians, machine operators, and aerospace industry
Hypersensitivity pneumonitis	Farming, food production workers, bird breeding, and poor ventilation/contaminated water systems

Abbreviations: CTD-ILD, connective tissue disease-associated interstitial lung disease; ILD, interstitial lung disease; IPF, idiopathic pulmonary fibrosis; WTC, World Trade Center.

diseases, whose pathogenicity and disease sequelae vary depending on the dust composition, the degree of exposure, and associated comorbidities.

Silicosis

Prevalence

Silicosis is a fibrotic lung disease resulting from the inhalation and deposition of respirable crystalline silicon dioxide. Recognition of silicosis emerged in in the 1st century with Pliny the Elder, again in 1716 by Bernadino Ramazzini, and in the early 1900s in South Africa and elsewhere.[1] Historically, those at most risk of silicosis were workers who encountered silica in its natural environment, including miners, tunnel, and quarry workers. Although a greater understanding of the risks of silica and the development of dust control measures had resulted in a decline in silicosis morbidity and mortality, rates remain unacceptably high and are increasing in some areas. More recently, there has been an increase in pneumoconiosis attributable to silica exposure in Central Appalachian coal miners.[2] This highlights that constant dust control vigilance is required. Rates have also increased in newer industries including artificial stone benchtop fabrication, denim jean production (sandblasting),[3] and jewelry polishing,[4] where silica has been introduced without recognition or control of its hazards. Artificial stone is formed from finely crushed rocks (predominantly quartz), with added constituents including colored glass, shells, metals, and adhesives, all of which are bound by a polymer resin, molded into shape, and heat-cured.[5] Artificial stone contains up to 95% crystalline silica, far higher than any other commonly used stone.[6] Stone slabs are most commonly cut and shaped for benchtop fabrication using high powered hand tools that generate extremely high levels of respirable crystalline silica dust. The current permissible crystalline silica exposure limit in the United States is 0.05 mg/m^3 over an 8-h work period.[7]

By way of example, dry cutting artificial stone generates silica dust levels of 44 mg/m^3 over 30 minutes; over 300 times the permissible limit.[8] More than 500 workers with silicosis have been identified from the artificial stone benchtop industry in Australia,[9] and cases are rapidly emerging in North America,[10] Spain,[11] and elsewhere. In Israel where much of the artificial stone is produced, at least 82 workers with silicosis were identified, and at least 18 workers having undergone lung transplantation for this condition, representing a 15-fold increase in the expected rate of transplantation.[12]

Pathogenesis

The development of silicosis is related to factors specific to silica exposure including the concentration of silica dust, fibrogenicity of silica particles, additional constituents of the silica-containing products, as well as other contributory factors such as smoking, infections, and genetic and autoimmune susceptibilities.

Silica mediates interstitial damage both directly and indirectly through the upregulation of inflammatory and fibrotic pathways. When silica particles are inhaled in the lungs, they are engulfed by alveolar macrophages, which stimulate pro-inflammatory and pro-fibrotic pathways. Dust-laden macrophages enter the interstitium both directly and via the hilar lymph nodes, and a perpetual cycle of inflammation and fibrosis ensues. Silica particles also enter the interstitium directly, and freshly fractured silica, which is generated through newer industries, is more likely to directly penetrate the epithelium. These silica particles are more likely to generate free radicals, leading to oxidative stress and stimulation of cytokine transcription factors, which further stimulates a pro-inflammatory and pro-fibrotic response[13,14] (**Fig. 1**).

Persistent silica uptake and its associated immunologic effects leads to the formation of parenchymal silicotic nodules, tending to occur around respiratory bronchioles in the subpleural and paraseptal areas. Over time, these nodules conglomerate and obliterate the surrounding small airways and pulmonary vessels, and results in progressive massive fibrosis (PMF).[11,12]

Diagnosis

Diagnosis of silicosis requires a history of silica exposure, concordant radiological findings, and exclusion of other diseases that mimic silicosis. Additional investigations including bronchoalveolar lavage (BAL), and lymph node or lung biopsy may be required (**Table 2**).

Plain chest x-ray (CXR) using the International Labour Classification (ILO) has traditionally been used in screening and diagnosis of silica-affected workers. However, the higher resolution of computed tomography (CT) makes it superior to CXR in the detection and characterization of disease and has supplanted the use of CXR for diagnosis in high-resourced countries. Simple silicosis tends to be characterized on CT by diffuse centrilobular nodules (up to 1 cm in size), usually in an upper lobe predominant distribution. As silicosis progresses, nodules coalesce to form conglomerate masses (>1 cm in size) with central cavitation. Distortion of the surrounding lung parenchyma and peribronchial vessels occurs and is often associated with pleural thickening. Lymphadenopathy with or without calcification may be seen (**Fig. 2**). Rarely, in silicoproteinosis, crazy paving with septal thickening and airspace consolidation may be identified.[15,16]

Additional tests include BAL fluid analysis, where a predominance of macrophages may be seen in the cell count differential (though nonspecific), and birefringent silica particles may be visualized and quantified. Histopathology shows well-demarcated fibrotic nodules containing birefringent silica particles, histiocytes, and interstitial fibrosis.[11,12]

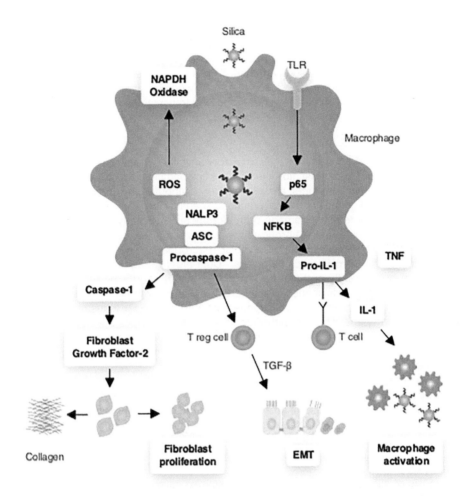

Fig. 1. Biological pathways in silicosis. NALP3 (NACHT, LLR, and PYD domains containing protein 3), ASC (apoptosis-associated speckle-like protein containing a CARD), and procaspase-1 form the inflammasome. EMT, epithelial mesenchymal transition; IL, interleukin; NADPH, nicotinamide adenine dinucleotide phosphate; NF-κB, nuclear factor kappa-light-chain-enhancer of activated B cells; ROS, reactive oxygen species; TGF-β, transforming growth factor beta; TLR, toll-like receptor; TNF, tumor necrosis factor. (*From* Barnes H, Goh NSL, Leong TL, Hoy R. Silica-associated lung disease: An old-world exposure in modern industries. *Respirology*. 2019;24(12):1165-1175.)

Disease Behavior and Treatment

Outcomes range from subclinical pathologic changes on imaging, to lung damage, reduced ventilatory capacity, diminished quality of life and reduced life expectancy.

The mainstay of management of silicosis is reduction or elimination of the exposure, according to the hierarchy of controls (**Fig. 3**), as persistent exposure is associated with disease progression. However, it is also important to note that some will continue to progress even after exposure cessation.[3] Workplace reporting and compensation programs vary between states and countries, and clinicians should make themselves and their patients aware of the options for workplace remediation and ongoing support.

Table 2
Common interstitial lung diseases and associated imaging and histopathological findings

ILD	Imaging Findings	Additional Tests
Silicosis	Simple silicosis—diffuse centrilobular nodules in an upper zone distribution Complicated silicosis—conglomerate masses with cavitation and distortion of the surrounding parenchyma Mediastinal and hilar lymphadenopathy	BAL—macrophage predominant, birefringent silica crystals Histopathology– well demarcated fibrotic nodules containing silica crystals, interstitial fibrosis
Asbestosis	Bilateral lower zone fibrosis, parenchymal bands, traction bronchiectasis, honeycombing, subpleural dot-like opacities, pleural plaques, diffuse pleural thickening, pleural effusions	Histopathology—peribronchiolar and subpleural fibrosis, asbestos bodies
Coal worker's pneumoconiosis	Small round reticular nodular opacities, upper zone predominant. Progressive massive fibrosis with conglomerate masses and parenchymal distortion Mediastinal and hilar lymphadenopathy	Histopathology—nodules containing dust-filed macrophages, with adjacent fibrosis and collagen, and surrounded by a halo of emphysema

Abbreviations: BAL, bronchoalveolar lavage; CTD-ILD, connective tissue disease-associated interstitial lung disease; ILD, interstitial lung disease; IPF, idiopathic pulmonary fibrosis.

Whole lung lavage is an experimental therapy considered in carefully selected patients. Although there are no clearly established criteria, radiological presence of diffuse ground glass nodules with minimal evidence of PMF is likely to confer the greatest benefit. Given that some patients improve after exposure cessation, whole lung lavage is generally reserved for those who continue to progress despite cessation. There is limited evidence of reduction in radiological and physiologic progression in the short term,[17,18] though the long-term effects are still unknown. Anti-fibrotic therapy in those who display a progressive-fibrosing phenotype may be indicated, though not specifically studied in this population.[19] Lung transplantation may be indicated for end-stage disease in otherwise suitable patients. In addition to specific therapies, smoking cessation and treatment of coexisting infections including mycobacterial infections are important.

Asbestosis

Asbestosis is an ILD caused specifically by exposure to asbestos fibers. Other respiratory effects of asbestos include benign pleural plaques, diffuse pleural thickening, mesothelioma, and lung cancer.

Asbestos is a naturally occurring mineral, and is used to strengthen, insulate, and fireproof materials. Asbestos is still used in the United States, and although its use is now banned in many other countries, its lag time in developing disease makes it a still relevant occupational risk factor. Asbestosis may develop 20 to 40 years after exposure, and risk of disease is dose dependent.[20] Those most at risk include

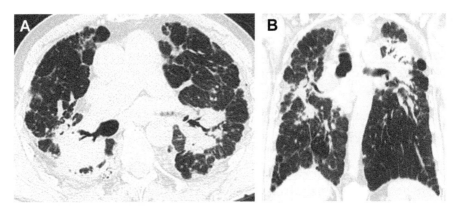

Fig. 2. Axial (*A*) and coronal (*B*) HRCT images of silicosis with progressive massive fibrosis. Numerous perilymphatic nodules are present, and coalesce in the upper lobes with marked upper volume loss and masslike fibrosis.

miners of asbestos, boilermakers, those working with insulation and cement, shipyard and railway workers and those involved in demolition. In addition, first responders of the World Trade Center had significant asbestos exposure (see **Table 1**).[21]

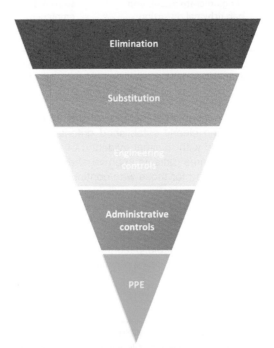

Fig. 3. Hierarchy of workplace controls. Elimination (including physical removal of the hazard) and substitution (including replacing the hazardous material) are the most effective hazard reduction measures, though then tend to be the most difficult to implement. Administrative controls include changing the way people work and engineering controls which includes isolating people from the hazard. Personal protective equipment (PPE) includes respirators, masks, gloves, ear plugs, and other equipment which the employee wears to reduce the risk of exposure. PPE tends to reduce but not eliminate risk.

Pathogenesis

Asbestosis results from inflammation and fibrosis that occurs both directly from asbestosis fibers and indirectly from the activation of the innate immune system. When asbestos fibers are inhaled into the lung, they are engulfed by alveolar macrophages, which subsequently lyse, releasing cytokines that attract further macrophages, CD4+ T lymphocytes, and mast cells, perpetuating an inflammatory response. Ingestion of asbestos fibers by alveolar macrophages also stimulates the NLRP3 (NACHT, LRR and PYD domains-containing protein 3) inflammasome to produce interleukin-1 (IL-1) and recruit fibroblasts. Persistent inflammation and stimulation of pro-fibrotic cytokines increases fibrogenesis. Hypertrophy and hyperplasia of type II epithelial cells promote fibrogenesis, and the upregulation of proto-oncogenes, leading not only to fibrosis but an increase in the risk of lung cancer[22,23] (**Fig. 4**).

Diagnosis

A detailed occupational history is essential to confirm sufficient exposure to asbestos. Common sources include brake pads, insulation products, and mined material. In addition, patients may be indirectly exposed through regular household contacts in the relevant industries.[24]

Imaging. High-resolution computed tomography (HRCT) chest findings include bilateral fibrosis, predominantly lower zone and subpleural in distribution, with parenchymal bands, traction bronchiectasis, and honeycombing (**Fig. 5**). Features which differentiate asbestosis from IPF can be subtle or absent and includes the presence of subpleural dot-like or branching centrilobular opacities and associated pleural disease (see **Table 2**).[25]

Histopathology. Lung biopsy specimens show an initially peribroncholar and subpleural fibrotic pattern, which advances beyond the pleural in the later stages. Asbestosis may share similar histopathological properties to usual interstitial pattern (UIP), though asbestosis tends to lack significant inflammation, and is collagenous rather than fibroblastic.[26] Asbestos bodies may be detected through light microscopy or electron microscopy.[26] Two or more asbestos bodies per 1 cm^2 of a 5 mm thick lung section, plus associated findings of pulmonary fibrosis, are required to confirm diagnosis.[26]

Disease Behavior and Treatment

Asbestosis tends to be less rapidly progressive than untreated IPF, although cases of progressive asbestosis do occur.[27] There are no specific treatments for asbestosis. Avoidance of ongoing exposure is essential to reduce further progression. Monitoring for pleural disease including mesothelioma and lung cancer is important. Patients who meet criteria for progressive-fibrosing ILD may be candidates for anti-fibrotic therapy.[19] A small single-arm exploratory study examining the use of pirfenidone in those with asbestosis found no significant safety signals.[28] There was a stability in FVC in the 24 weeks of treatment, but the study was not powered to detect differences in efficacy. Supportive treatments including oxygen supplementation, pulmonary rehabilitation, and palliative care referral should be used where indicated.

Coal Worker's Pneumoconiosis

Coal worker's pneumoconiosis (CWP), also known as 'black lung', is an irreversible ILD resulting from chronic inhalation of coal dust. In addition to CWP, coal dust can also cause silicosis, chronic obstructive pulmonary disease (COPD), and chronic

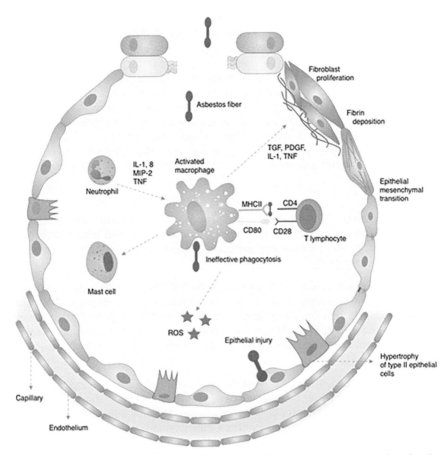

Fig. 4. Immunopathogenesis of asbestosis. Asbestos fibers are inhaled into the alveolar space. Macrophages are activated and stimulate production of neutrophils, mast cells, and T lymphocytes. Activated macrophages produce cytokines to stimulate fibroblast production. Ineffective phagocytosis of asbestos fibers results in release of reactive oxygen species (ROS). Direct epithelial injury leads to hypertrophy and hyperplasia of type II epithelial cells. Repeated epithelial injury and cytokine production leads to epithelial mesenchymal transition, fibrin deposition, and fibroblast proliferation.

bronchitis. Coal dust contributed to 25,000 deaths worldwide in 2013.[29] There has been a resurgence in the prevalence of CWP in the United States in the last few decades (1970s—6.5%, 1990s—2.1%, and 2000s—3.2%), specifically contributed by cases in Central Appalachia, and in this population there has also been an increase in the rate of PMF.[30] The factors for this increase are multifactorial, and may be explained by increased exposure to silica due to change in rock composition and more powerful mechanization, longer work hours, and reduced vigilance in dust control measures.

Diagnosis
Many countries have implemented screening programs for at-risk workers. Patients therefore may present with a wide spectrum of disease, from asymptomatic to advanced illness. Common signs and symptoms include cough productive of black

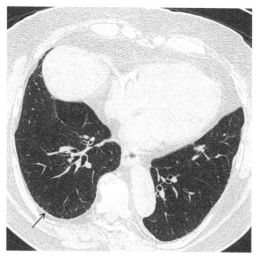

Fig. 5. Axial HRCT image of asbestosis, with a calcified pleural plaque in the left posterior thorax (*arrow*). Septal thickening is noted.

sputum, dyspnea, and air flow obstruction. Development of PMF may lead to respiratory failure and death.

Imaging. CXR is commonly used in screening programs to identify presence of disease. HRCT is more commonly used for diagnosis and to characterize disease progression. Imaging typically depicts small round reticular nodular opacities, in a diffuse perilymphatic upper zone predominant distribution. PMF with coalescence of nodules, surrounding parenchymal distortion, and mediastinal and hilar lymphadenopathy may also be present (see **Table 2**; **Fig. 6**).[31]

Histopathology. Lung biopsy is rarely required. If performed, the histopathology typically displays nodules containing dust-filled macrophages around a terminal bronchovascular bundle, with fibrosis and collagen surrounding it. A halo of emphysema surrounding the nodule may also be present. Evidence of PMF with coalescence of fibrotic masses, distortion of the surrounding parenchyma, and presence of other dust diseases such as silicosis may also be noted.[31,32]

Disease Behavior and Treatment
There are no specific therapies for CWP. Avoidance of further dust exposure may reduce progression. Although not specifically studied in these patients, those with PMF who meet criteria for progressive fibrosing-ILD (PF-ILD) could consider antifibrotic therapy. Disease progression is dependent on the level of exposure, profusion of nodules, presence of PMF, and concomitant risk factors including advancing age, smoking, and tuberculosis.[33]

Granulomatous Lung Diseases

Inhalation of metals can cause granulomatous lung disease, the most common of which is chronic beryllium disease. Occupations with heavy beryllium exposure include aerospace and defense industries, alloy, and automotive industries.

Patients with chronic beryllium disease may present with cough, fever, night sweats, and fatigue. Diagnosis is made on confirmatory occupational history, a positive serum

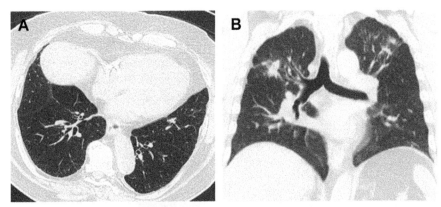

Fig. 6. Axial and coronal HRCT images of coal worker's pneumoconiosis, with upper lobe predominant peribronchovascular nodules and conglomerate masses.

or BAL beryllium lymphocyte proliferation test, and evidence of granulomatous inflammation on lung biopsy (either via transbronchial or VATS or open biopsy).[34] Chronic beryllium disease may have a similar radiological and histopathological appearance to sarcoidosis, although chronic beryllium disease may display less prominent lymphadenopathy, and lack extra-pulmonary features showed in sarcoidosis (**Fig. 7**). Differentiation between sarcoidosis and chronic beryllium disease is not only important to reduce ongoing exposure from occupational sources, but may also alter treatment regimens; chronic beryllium disease commonly requires ongoing immunosuppression whereas in a proportion of sarcoidosis patients, immunosuppression is not needed or required for a short term to induce remission.[35–37] Avoidance of exposure is important once the diagnosis of chronic beryllium disease is made. Treatment includes immunosuppression using corticosteroids and steroid sparing agents, though this is based on limited retrospective evidence.[38]

Hard Metal Lung Disease

Hard metal lung disease is derived from exposure to cobalt, tungsten, titanium, nickel, and chromium. These metals themselves are not "hard," rather their combination results in a strong and heat resistant composite material used in drilling, cutting, and mining.[39] These cases are rare, and limited to small case series.[40] Histopathology shows presence of "cannibalistic" giant cells (giant cell interstitial pneumonitis) with or without fibrosis. The altered appearance of these giant cells differentiates hard metal lung disease from other granulomatous diseases such as chronic beryllium disease, sarcoidosis, and hypersensitivity pneumonitis (HP).[39,40]

OCCUPATIONAL BURDEN OF OTHER INTERSTITIAL LUNG DISEASES

Although some ILDs are directly attributable to occupational and environmental exposures, there is a growing body of evidence to support the contributory pathogenic role of exposures in other ILDs. A large meta-analysis found that occupational exposures contributed to at least 26% of IPF, 19% of HP, and 30% of sarcoidosis cases.[41]

Idiopathic Pulmonary Fibrosis

IPF, the most common and prototypical ILD, is caused by a combination of intrinsic genetic factors in addition to external noxious stimuli and other contributory factors.

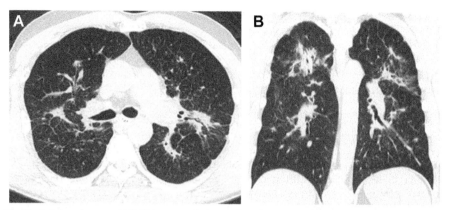

Fig. 7. Axial and coronal HRCT images of chronic beryllium disease, with upper lung predominant fine nodularity with septal thickening and peribronchovascular coalescent nodules.

Repeated microinjury of the alveolar epithelium is considered the initiating factor, leading to aberrant repair processes and ultimately the development of fibrosis.[42] Occupational exposures that are associated with IPF include vapors, gases, dusts, and fumes, wood dusts, agricultural dusts, and silica. In addition, smoking, microbial agents, and particulate matter from air pollution may play a role in the pathogenesis of IPF.[43,44]

Connective Tissue Disease-Associated Interstitial Lung Diseases

The link between occupational and environmental exposure and a subgroup of CTD-ILD cases has long been described.[45] Although complete mechanisms are yet to be fully elucidated, it is thought that ingestion of silica particles by alveolar macrophages stimulates pro-inflammatory cytokine production, activation of the adaptive immune system, loss of tolerance, and the production of autoantibodies.[46,47] Autoantibodies, in turn, exert direct effects on the epithelial endothelium, or form antigen-antibody complexes, which initiate further inflammation and fibrosis.[48]

Silica-associated scleroderma is more common in men, and associated with greater risk of ILD, as well as a diffuse phenotype, digital ulcers, cardiac dysfunction, and cancer, in addition to greater mortality. Positive anti-topoisomerase I antibodies are detected with greater frequency in silica-exposed patients. Cases of rheumatoid arthritis, systemic lupus erythematosus, dermatomyositis, polymyositis, and ANCA-vasculitis in association with silica have been described.[49]

Other exposures associated with CTD-ILDs include organic solvents, typically aromatic compounds, trichloroethylene, and ketones, derived from petrochemical industries, motor vehicle production, and dry cleaning. Particulate matter from air pollution, welding fumes, pesticides, and heavy metals may also increase risk.[49]

Sarcoidosis

Sarcoidosis is a granulomatous disease that predominantly affects the lungs, but can also show extrapulmonary manifestations including cardiac, renal, dermatologic, and neurologic manifestations. Sarcoidosis is typically considered a diagnosis of exclusion, that is, attributable no other cause. However, occupational and environmental exposures as well as other noxious stimuli can play a role in initiation and perpetuation of inflammation and fibrosis. Clinical signs, symptoms, imaging, pathology, and exposure may overlap with other parenchymal lung diseases including silicosis, HP, and rarer granulomatous diseases.

Commonly implicated exposures associated with sarcoidosis included organic dusts (agriculture, bakers, food makers), inorganic dusts (silica including miners, fire-fighting, World Trade Center first responders, and dental technicians), and solvents (machine operators, aerospace industry).[50]

Hypersensitivity Pneumonitis

HP is an immune-mediated ILD that arises as a result of occupational and environmental exposures to inhaled antigens, in susceptible individuals. The first cases of HP were described in farmers, attributable to moldy hay (*Saccharomyces spp.*).[51,52] Reports of HP associated with maple bark and sugar cane processing,[53] mushroom cultivation,[54] and cleaning pigeon excreta[55] soon followed. Prevalence of exposure varies with geography and seasonality, but common occupational sources include farming and manufacturing industries, bird breeding, and poor ventilation or contaminated water systems.[56] Additional risk factors including occupational exposure to pesticides,[57] and previous viral infections,[58] also increase risk. Unlike other workplaces exposures such as asbestosis and silicosis where the exposure is obvious, the exposures associated with the development of HP can be difficult to elicit. Furthermore, multiple exposures may be present, derived from the workplace or home. A detailed clinical history, serum precipitins testing, and in select cases specific inhalational challenge may aid in elicitation and differentiation of relevant exposures.[59] Workplace visits may be useful to identify exposures for the individual, and risk for others such as in the case of metal-working fluid contamination or swimming pool outbreaks. Similar to other ILDs, identification and remediation of the exposure significantly reduces the risk of progression of HP.[60]

LIMITATIONS OF THE EVIDENCE AND FUTURE RESEARCH DIRECTIONS

Occupational exposures remain an under-recognized risk factor in the development of ILDs. Drawing associations between occupation and the development of disease requires clinicians to take a detailed clinical history (**Box 1**) and requires systematic incorporation of such details into ILD registries. An occupational exposure history should include not only presence or absence of exposure, but also the nature of the tasks undertaken, frequency, duration, what type of reduction of exposure and personal protective equipment was used, and additional relevant risk factors. These details will allow us to better understand the pathologic link between exposure and disease, and the steps required to reduce disease occurrence.

The current literature reflects that there are few treatment options for many occupationally derived diseases. Although the pathogenesis of many occupational-related ILDs is predicated on the up-regulation of inflammatory pathways, the effect of immunosuppression has been disappointing. Availability of antifibrotic treatment for those who display a progressive-fibrosing phenotype may add possible options to the treatment arsenal but is unlikely to be a panacea. Further research into more effective treatment options is required in these ILDs.

In addition to addressing mortality and prevention of disease progression in these patients, focus should also be on assessment and improvement of quality of life. Work is good for our health, and in many cases our occupation forms part of our identity. Advising patients that work may have contributed to their disease, and advising work cessation, has considerable effects on quality of life, and this should also be considered in the overall care of the patients.

Box 1
Taking an occupational history

Respiratory Symptoms
What are the relevant symptoms and signs? (eg, cough, wheeze, dyspnea, chest tightness, and reduced exercise tolerance)
Do symptoms worsen when at work and improve when away from work?
Are other workers experiencing similar symptoms?

Occupational details
What is your current job?
What industry is that in?
What tasks do you do?
What materials do you work with?
Are there exposure protections in place? (eg, dust suppression, wet cutting, extraction, ventilation, personal protective equipment)
How long have you been in this job?
What job did you do before this? (for each previous job, ask about the industry, tasks, exposure protections, etc.).

Other environmental exposures
Do you have frequent and prolonged exposure to birds, mold, wood dust, metals, gases, vapors, or fumes?
Are there any hobbies or environmental exposures from which you experience respiratory symptoms?
Is there anyone in the household who has prolonged exposure to occupational exposures of concern?

Relevant medical history
Do you have a history of smoking, previous respiratory infections, symptoms, and signs of autoimmune disease?
Do you have any medical conditions?
Is there a family history of respiratory or autoimmune disease?

SUMMARY

Occupational exposures contribute to a significant burden of ILDs. Exposure may be partly or wholly contributory. A detailed clinical history paired with radiological and additional biological tests are required to confirm a diagnosis. Management includes reduction and avoidance of ongoing exposure; beyond that, treatment options are often limited. Further research into the systematic inclusion of occupational details in ILD registries, therapeutic options for these patients, and a focus on quality of life, is needed.

CLINICS CARE POINTS

- Clinicians should consider occupation as a potential contributing factor to those with interstitial lung diseases (ILDs).

- A detailed occupational history includes job details, tasks involved, and whether symptoms are associated with work.

- Diagnosis requires a detailed occupational history, compatible high-resolution computed tomography findings, and histopathology where indicated.

- Clinicians should assist patients in reduction or cessation of workplace exposures if causative of their ILD.

DISCLOSURES

H. Barnes and I. Glaspole do not have any disclosures relevant to this article.

AUTHOR CONTRIBUTIONS

H. Barnes and I. Glaspole conceived, drafted, and edited the article, and both approved the final version.

ACKNOWLEDGMENTS

The authors thank Professor David Lynch, National Jewish Health, for providing the radiological images.

REFERENCES

1. Rosen G. The history of miners' diseases: a medical and social interpretation. Schuman's; 1943.
2. Antao VC, Petsonk EL, Sokolow LZ, et al. Rapidly progressive coal workers' pneumoconiosis in the United States: geographic clustering and other factors. Occup Environ Med 2005;62(10):670–4.
3. Akgun M, Araz O, Ucar EY, et al. Silicosis Appears Inevitable Among Former Denim Sandblasters: A 4-Year Follow-up Study. Chest 2015;148(3):647–54.
4. Jiang CQ, Xiao LW, Lam TH, et al. Accelerated silicosis in workers exposed to agate dust in Guangzhou, China. Am J Ind Med 2001;40(1):87–91.
5. Caesarstone. The facts about quartz. Available at: http://www.caesarstone.com.au/AboutUs/TheFactsAboutQuartz/. Accessed 7 January 2019.
6. Caesarstone. Safety Data Sheet. 2016.WorkCover, Queensland.
7. OSHA. OSHA's Respirable Crystalline Silica Standard for General Industry and Maritime. Available at: https://www.osha.gov/sites/default/files/publications/OSHA3682.pdf2022.
8. American Conference of Governmental Industrial Hygienists. TLVs and BEIs: threshold limit values for chemical substances and physical agents and biological exposure indices. Cincinnati, OH: American Conference of Governmental Industrial Hygienists; 2008.
9. Almberg KS GL, Yates DH, Waite TD, Cohen RA. Silicosis Return to Work review: Return to Work and Vocational Rehabilitation Support for Workers Suffering from Silicosis, 2020.
10. Rose C, Heinzerling A, Patel K, et al. Severe Silicosis in Engineered Stone Fabrication Workers - California, Colorado, Texas, and Washington, 2017-2019. MMWR Morb Mortal Wkly Rep, 2019. http://europepmc.org/abstract/MED/31557149. https://doi.org/10.15585/mmwr.mm6838a1. https://europepmc.org/articles/PMC6762184. https://europepmc.org/articles/PMC6762184?pdf=render (accessed 2019/09//).
11. Perez-Alonso A, Cordoba-Dona JA, Millares-Lorenzo JL, et al. Outbreak of silicosis in Spanish quartz conglomerate workers. Int J Occup Environ Health 2014;20(1):26–32.
12. Kramer MR, Blanc PD, Fireman E, et al. Artificial stone silicosis [corrected]: disease resurgence among artificial stone workers. Chest 2012;142(2):419–24.
13. Greenberg MI, Waksman J, Curtis J. Silicosis: a review. Dis Mon 2007;53(8):394–416.
14. Leung CC, Yu IT, Chen W. Silicosis. Lancet 2012;379(9830):2008–18.

15. Ozmen CA, Nazaroglu H, Yildiz T, et al. MDCT findings of denim-sandblasting-induced silicosis: A cross-sectional study. Environ Health: A Global Access Science Source 2010;9(1) (no pagination)(17).

16. Marchiori E, Ferreira A, Saez F, et al. Conglomerated masses of silicosis in sandblasters: high-resolution CT findings. Eur J Radiol 2006;59(1):56–9.

17. Chambers DC, Apte SH, Deller D, et al. Radiological outcomes of whole lung lavage for artificial stone-associated silicosis. Respirology 2021;26(5):501–3.

18. Zhang Y, Zhang H, Wang W, et al. Long-term therapeutic effects of whole lung lavage in the management of silicosis. [Chinese]. Zhonghua lao dong wei sheng zhi ye bing za zhi = Zhonghua laodong weisheng zhiyebing zazhi = Chinese journal of industrial hygiene and occupational diseases 2012;30(9):690–3.

19. Flaherty KR, Wells AU, Cottin V, et al. Nintedanib in Progressive Fibrosing Interstitial Lung Diseases. N Engl J Med 2019;381(18):1718–27.

20. Paris C, Thierry S, Brochard P, et al. Pleural plaques and asbestosis: dose- and time-response relationships based on HRCT data. Eur Respir J 2009;34(1):72–9.

21. Bartrip PW. History of asbestos related disease. Postgrad Med J 2004; 80(940):72–6.

22. Mossman BT, Churg A. Mechanisms in the pathogenesis of asbestosis and silicosis. Am J Respir Crit Care Med 1998;157(5 Pt 1):1666–80.

23. Matsuzaki H, Maeda M, Lee S, et al. Asbestos-induced cellular and molecular alteration of immunocompetent cells and their relationship with chronic inflammation and carcinogenesis. J Biomed Biotechnol 2012;2012:492608.

24. Soeberg M, Vallance DA, Keena V, et al. Australia's Ongoing Legacy of Asbestos: Significant Challenges Remain Even after the Complete Banning of Asbestos Almost Fifteen Years Ago. Int J Environ Res Public Health 2018;15(2).

25. Akira M, Yamamoto S, Inoue Y, et al. High-resolution CT of asbestosis and idiopathic pulmonary fibrosis. AJR Am J Roentgenol 2003;181(1):163–9.

26. Roggli VL, Gibbs AR, Attanoos R, et al. Pathology of asbestosis- An update of the diagnostic criteria: Report of the asbestosis committee of the college of american pathologists and pulmonary pathology society. Arch Pathol Lab Med 2010; 134(3):462–80.

27. Keskitalo E, Salonen J, Vahanikkila H, et al. Survival of patients with asbestosis can be assessed by risk-predicting models. Occup Environ Med 2021;78(7):516.

28. Miedema JR, Moor CC, Veltkamp M, et al. Safety and tolerability of pirfenidone in asbestosis: a prospective multicenter study. Respir Res 2022;23(1):139.

29. Mortality GBD. Causes of Death C. Global, regional, and national age-sex specific all-cause and cause-specific mortality for 240 causes of death, 1990-2013: a systematic analysis for the Global Burden of Disease Study 2013. Lancet 2015;385(9963):117–71.

30. Laney AS, Attfield MD. Coal workers' pneumoconiosis and progressive massive fibrosis are increasingly more prevalent among workers in small underground coal mines in the United States. Occup Environ Med 2010;67(6):428–31.

31. Chong S, Lee KS, Chung MJ, et al. Pneumoconiosis: comparison of imaging and pathologic findings. Radiographics 2006;26(1):59–77.

32. Cohen RA, Rose CS, Go LHT, et al. Pathology and Mineralogy Demonstrate Respirable Crystalline Silica Is a Major Cause of Severe Pneumoconiosis in U.S. Coal Miners. Ann Am Thorac Soc 2022;19(9):1469–78.

33. Go LHT, Cohen RA. Coal Workers' Pneumoconiosis and Other Mining-Related Lung Disease: New Manifestations of Illness in an Age-Old Occupation. Clin Chest Med 2020;41(4):687–96.

34. MacMurdo MG, Mroz MM, Culver DA, et al. Chronic Beryllium Disease: Update on a Moving Target. Chest 2020;158(6):2458–66.
35. Baughman RP, Valeyre D, Korsten P, et al. ERS clinical practice guidelines on treatment of sarcoidosis. Eur Respir J 2021;58(6):2004079.
36. Culver DA. Beryllium disease and sarcoidosis: still besties after all these years? Eur Respir J 2016;47(6):1625–8.
37. Culver DA, Dweik RA. Chronic Beryllium Disease. Clin Pulm Med 2003;10(2).
38. Sood A. Current treatment of chronic beryllium disease. J Occup Environ Hyg 2009;6(12):762–5.
39. Nemery B, Abraham JL. Hard metal lung disease: still hard to understand. Am J Respir Crit Care Med 2007;176(1):2–3.
40. Tanaka J, Moriyama H, Terada M, et al. An observational study of giant cell interstitial pneumonia and lung fibrosis in hard metal lung disease. BMJ Open 2014; 4(3):e004407.
41. Blanc PD, Annesi-Maesano I, Balmes JR, et al. The Occupational Burden of Nonmalignant Respiratory Diseases. An Official American Thoracic Society and European Respiratory Society Statement. Am J Respir Crit Care Med 2019; 199(11):1312–34.
42. Wijsenbeek M, Cottin V. Spectrum of Fibrotic Lung Diseases. N Engl J Med 2020; 383(10):958–68.
43. Abramson MJ, Murambadoro T, Alif SM, et al. Occupational and environmental risk factors for idiopathic pulmonary fibrosis in Australia: case-control study. Thorax 2020;75(10):864–9.
44. Park Y, Ahn C, Kim TH. Occupational and environmental risk factors of idiopathic pulmonary fibrosis: a systematic review and meta-analyses. Sci Rep 2021;11(1): 4318.
45. Caplan A. Certain unusual radiological appearances in the chest of coal-miners suffering from rheumatoid arthritis. Thorax 1953;8(1):29–37.
46. Pollard KM. Silica, Silicosis, and Autoimmunity. Front Immunol 2016;7:97.
47. Yates DH, Miles SE. Silica and Connective Tissue Disorders: The Important Role of the Dermatologist. Journal of Dermatology and Skin Science 2022;4(2):10–9.
48. Chung L, Utz PJ. Antibodies in scleroderma: direct pathogenicity and phenotypic associations. Curr Rheumatol Rep 2004;6(2):156–63.
49. Ouchene L, Muntyanu A, Lavoue J, et al. Toward Understanding of Environmental Risk Factors in Systemic Sclerosis [Formula: see text]. J Cutan Med Surg 2021; 25(2):188–204.
50. Newman KL, Newman LS. Occupational causes of sarcoidosis. Curr Opin Allergy Clin Immunol 2012;12(2):145–50.
51. Campbell JM. Acute Symptoms Following Work with Hay. BMJ 1932;2:1143–4.
52. Fawcitt R. Fungoid Conditions of the Lung—Part I. Brit J Radiol 1936;9(99): 172–95.
53. Towey JW, Sweany HC, Huron WH. Severe bronchial asthma apparently due to fungus spores found in maple bark. JAMA 1932;99(6):453–9.
54. Bringhurst LS, Byrne RN, Gershon-Cohen J. Respiratory disease of mushroom workers; farmer's lung. J Am Med Assoc 1959;171:15–8.
55. Feldman HA, Sabin AB. Pneumonitis of unknown aetiology in a group of men exposed to pigeon excreta. J Clin Invest 1948;27:533.
56. Barnes H, Lu J, Glaspole I, et al. Exposures and associations with clinical phenotypes in hypersensitivity pneumonitis: A scoping review. Respir Med 2021;184: 106444.

57. Hoppin JA, Umbach DM, Kullman GJ, et al. Pesticides and other agricultural factors associated with self-reported farmer's lung among farm residents in the Agricultural Health Study. Occup Environ Med 2007;64(5):334–41.
58. Wuyts WA, Agostini C, Antoniou KM, et al. The pathogenesis of pulmonary fibrosis: a moving target. Eur Respir J 2013;41(5):1207–18.
59. Johannson KA, Barnes H, Bellanger AP, et al. Exposure Assessment Tools for Hypersensitivity Pneumonitis. An Official American Thoracic Society Workshop Report. Ann Am Thorac Soc 2020;17(12):1501–9.
60. Gimenez A, Storrer K, Kuranishi L, et al. Change in FVC and survival in chronic fibrotic hypersensitivity pneumonitis. Thorax 2018;73(4):391–2.

Drug-Induced Interstitial Lung Diseases

Nicole Ng, MD, PharmD[a],*, Maria L. Padilla, MD[a], Philippe Camus, MD[b]

KEYWORDS

- Drug-induced interstitial lung disease • Interstitial lung disease
- Infiltrative lung disease • Lung toxicity • Pulmonary toxicity • Pneumonitis
- Iatrogenic • Chest imaging • Respiratory system

KEY POINTS

- Drug-induced (interstitial) lung disease is a potentially severe and life-threatening adverse reaction to drugs.
- A high index of suspicion and systematic approach is necessary to properly identify the culprit drug and secure the diagnosis.
- Drug withdrawal is the cornerstone of management (underlying illness permitting) and other drugs in severe cases glucocorticoids may be administered.

INTRODUCTION

Iatrogenic respiratory disease is defined as damage to the lung or intrathoracic organs due to therapy with medications or interventions.[1] Drug-induced respiratory disease can involve the airways, parenchyma, pulmonary vasculature, mediastinum, pleura, and/or neuromuscular system. Drug-induced interstitial lung disease (DI-ILD) is the most prevalent form of iatrogenic respiratory disease and is the focus of this article. Of note, drug-induced cardiac toxicity should be distinguished as it may also cause pulmonary infiltrates, pulmonary edema, and/or pleural effusion.

DI-ILD occurs from exposure to treatments that results in injury to the lung parenchyma manifesting by varying patterns of edema, inflammation, and fibrosis. It is a subtype of diffuse parenchymal lung disease (DPLD) according to the American Thoracic Society (ATS) and European Respiratory Society (ERS); DI-ILD accounts for 2.5% to 5% of all DPLDs (**Fig. 1**).[2–6] There are over 1654 causes of iatrogenic respiratory disease and over 380 drugs/substances implicated in DI-ILD on the growing list compiled on the Drug-Induced Respiratory Disease free website,

[a] Division of Pulmonary, Critical Care, and Sleep Medicine, Icahn School of Medicine at Mount Sinai, 1 Gustave L Levy Place, PO Box 1232, New York, NY 10029, USA; [b] Pulmonary and Intensive Care at Universite de Bourgogne, 1 Rue Marion, F21079, Dijon, France
* Corresponding author.
E-mail address: nicole.ng2@mountsinai.org

Immunol Allergy Clin N Am 43 (2023) 341–357
https://doi.org/10.1016/j.iac.2023.01.009
0889-8561/23/© 2023 Elsevier Inc. All rights reserved.

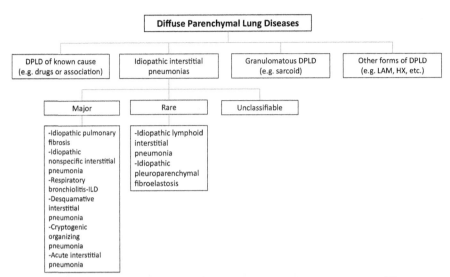

Fig. 1. Classification of DPLD, adapted from ATS/ERS classifications 2002, 2013.[2,3] Drugs can cause several of these patterns as an adverse reaction.[8] DPLD, diffuse parenchymal lung disease; HX, histiocytosis X; ILD, interstitial lung disease; LAM, lymphangioleiomyomatosis. (*Adapted from* American Thoracic Society/European Respiratory Society International Multidisciplinary Consensus Classification of the Idiopathic Interstitial Pneumonias. *Am J Respir Crit Care Med.* 2002/01/15 2002;165(2):277-304.)

www.pneumotox.com.[7] Of these, 15 have been implicated in more than 200 cases, 10 in 100 to 200 cases, 13 in 50 to 100 cases, 45 in 10 to 50 cases, and 299 in less than 10 cases.

EPIDEMIOLOGY

The epidemiology of DI-ILD is difficult to determine as the availability of drugs may change with time. For example, pneumonitis secondary to use of penicillamine and gold has declined (as their use has fallen out of favor); on the contrary, methotrexate, and biologics have supplanted their use in the treatment of rheumatoid arthritis.[1,9] Nonetheless, cases of DI-ILD have increased almost exponentially likely reflecting increased awareness and a true increase as more drugs are available. The incidence of DI-ILD varies widely depending on drugs, doses, and accuracy of reporting. In a PRISMA (Preferred Reporting Items for Systematic Reviews and Meta-Analysis)-compliant systematic review by Skeoch and colleagues,[6] over 6000 cases of DI-ILD were included; however, the papers were of such low quality that a meta-analysis could not be performed. The literature suffered from poor quality, high risk of biases, and lack of standardized case definition for DI-ILD (eg, physician or patient-reported diagnosis, radiologic diagnosis, lack of workup to exclude alternative causes). In this now-turned descriptive review, the incidence of DI-ILD for individual drugs ranged from less than 1% to nearly 60%, the incidence of DI-ILD at a population level ranged from 4.1 to 12.4 cases/million/year, and the prevalence of DI-ILD within ILD populations ranged from 2.6% to 5%. Incidence rates in Japan were found to be several-fold higher compared with the rest of the world; whether this reflects distinct susceptibility or reporting bias is unknown.

PATHOGENESIS AND RISK FACTORS

The pathogenesis of DI-ILD is not well understood and is thought to involve drug kinetics and metabolism in the lung via cytotoxic, immune-mediated mechanisms and/or immune dysregulation in the initiation and propagation of injury.[10,11] Cytotoxic pulmonary injury occurs through direct damage to alveolar epithelial or capillary endothelial cells, with subsequent edema and inflammation. Toxicity is usually idiosyncratic or rarely dose-dependent, and is a result of injury from inflammatory mediators (eg, cytokines, leukotrienes, or proteases from neutrophils, macrophages, or eosinophils) and/or reactive oxygen species.[12] This can be seen in cytotoxic drugs—from classes of drugs such as alkylating agents (eg, cyclophosphamide) to individual drugs such as bleomycin and methotrexate, and in non-cytotoxic drugs such as nitrofurantoin and amiodarone.[7,13]

Immune-mediated mechanisms are dose-independent and may rely on prior sensitization to the offending agent.[10] Subsequent interaction of the drug with humoral antibodies or sensitized lymphocytes causes injury by several types of hypersensitivity reactions. Type IV (cell-mediated) hypersensitivity is a delayed non-antibody-dependent reaction produced by sensitized T lymphocytes.[14] It is the most commonly implicated hypersensitivity reaction in DI-ILD and includes drugs such as minocycline, methotrexate, and amiodarone to name a few.[10,15]

Immune dysregulation is a newer mechanism of DI-ILD recognized since the introduction of biologics and immune checkpoint inhibitors (ICIs).[11] ICIs re-activate T cells to kill cancer cells by blocking the inhibitory programmed death receptor 1/ligand 1 (PD-1/PDL-1) and cytotoxic T lymphocyte-associated antigen 4 (CTLA-4) pathways. As such, checkpoint inhibitor pneumonitis is thought to occur from heightened T cell responses to cross-antigens against not only tumors but also self normal tissues. Increased levels of preexisting autoantibodies and elevated levels of inflammatory cytokines are also thought to play a role in these immune-related adverse events. In this regard, many organs other than the lung can also develop severe adverse effects from ICIs.[16]

Despite proposed mechanisms, it remains unclear why in a large population of treated individuals; only some develop DI-ILD. Although limiting doses have been identified in a few drugs (eg, bleomycin, nitrosoureas, amiodarone), DI-ILD mostly occurs at therapeutic doses and as such, its occurrence is largely idiosyncratic and unpredictable. Retrospective studies have identified several potential host risk factors for DI-ILD including advanced age, current smoking, renal impairment, preexisting interstitial lung disease, abnormal baseline pulmonary function tests (PFTs), prior pneumonectomy, radiation exposure, high fractional oxygen concentration, genetic predispositions (eg, HLA), and underlying disease for which the drug is being given; identifying the real culprit can be very challenging.[1,6,9,17] Whether these factors make the lung more susceptible to injury or reduce the threshold for symptom manifestation is unclear. Additionally, polypharmacy and use of multiple pneumotoxic drugs may increase the risk of toxicity through interactions within metabolic/detoxification pathways in specific cell types and synergistic pneumotoxicity, respectively.

CLINICAL PRESENTATION

The presentation of a DI-ILD is highly variable among drugs and even with the same drug; it can occur hours, days, years after exposure, or rarely even after termination of treatment. Acute pneumonitis manifests with fevers, shortness of breath, cough, and hypoxemia. Subacute or chronic DI-ILD presents with worsening dyspnea or decreased exercise tolerance and persistent cough. Physical examination may reveal

"Velcro-like" crackles. PFTs may show restriction and/or impaired diffusing capacity for carbon monoxide (DLCO). Overall, these findings are nonspecific for the diagnosis of DI-ILD, but the temporal relationship with exposure to the drug is key.

There are few laboratory biomarkers, radiographic patterns, or histologic features that are truly diagnostic or pathognomonic for DI-ILD (except for foreign body reactions in the lung, eg, kayexalate aspiration).[7] The evaluation is particularly difficult when a potentially pneumotoxic drug is used to treat a condition with associated ILD manifestations (eg, rheumatologic diseases, left ventricular failure, solid organ or hematologic malignancies (lymphangitic carcinomatosis)), in a patient on multiple pneumotoxic drugs. The differential diagnosis in these cases can be wide and include underlying lung disease, infection, or DI-ILD from several possible culprit medications. Additionally, medications, and in particular antineoplastic agents can cause pneumotoxicity and cardiotoxicity which can present similarly.[18] Cardiotoxic complications include cardiomyopathy, myocarditis, arrhythmias, and pericardial disease.[19] A similar database of cardiotoxic drugs can be found on the Drug-Induced Cardiovascular Disease App, Cardiotox.[20]

Naranjo and colleagues published the Adverse Drug Reaction Probability Scale in 1981 which can still be applied to suspected DI-ILD (**Table 1**).[21] A caveat to this scale

Table 1
Adverse drug reaction probability scale (Naranjo)

		Yes	No	Don't Know	Score
1	Are there previous conclusive reports on this reaction?	+1	0	0	
2	Did the adverse event appear after the suspected drug was administered?	+2	−1	0	
3	Did the adverse reaction improve when the drug was discontinued, or a specific antagonist was administered?	+1	0	0	
4	Did the adverse reaction reappear when the drug was readministered?	+2	−1	0	
5	Are there alternative causes (other than the drug) that could on their own have caused the reaction?	−1	+2	0	
6	Did the reaction reappear when a placebo was given?	−1	+1	0	
7	Was the drug detected in the blood (or other fluids) in concentrations known to be toxic?	+1	0	0	
8	Was the reaction more severe when the dose was increased, or less severe when the dose was decreased?	+1	0	0	
9	Did the patient have a similar reaction to the same or similar drugs in any previous exposure?	+1	0	0	
10	Was the adverse event confirmed by any objective evidence?	+1	0	0	
				Total Score	

Total scores range from −4 to +13. An ADR is classified as definite (score ≥9), probable (score 5 to 8), possible (score 1 to 4), or doubtful (score ≤ 0).

From Naranjo CA, Busto U, Sellers EM, et al. A method for estimating the probability of adverse drug reactions. *Clin Pharmacol Ther.* 1981;30(2):239-245.

is the inclusion of (toxic) drug levels which is flawed in the setting of idiosyncratic drug reactions and is rarely performed nowadays, except in evaluating respiratory disease in presumed drug abusers.

DIAGNOSIS

The diagnosis of DI-ILD requires several elements: (1) clinical suspicion with the exposure history of potentially pneumotoxic drug, (2) appropriate temporal relationship between drug and symptoms, (3) clinical, physiologic, and radiographic findings consistent with ILD from the given medication, (4) exclusion of another cause such as infection, pulmonary edema, underlying or incidental lung disease, (5) improvement upon removal of drug, and rarely feasible (6) recurrence with rechallenge. Despite the systematic approach, the diagnosis of DI-ILD and the assessment of causality is fraught with challenges.

Diagnosis of DI-ILD is exclusionary against the backdrop of a wide differential diagnosis including primary lung diseases with progression or exacerbation, classic and opportunistic infections, cardiovascular etiologies, radiation pneumonitis, and malignancy.[22] This assessment can be complicated, for example, in patients with cancer who are at baseline immunosuppressed, potentially taking multi-agent regimens with additive immunosuppressive and/or pneumotoxic effects, and as such prone to infections including *Pneumocystis jiroveci* pneumonia. Other differential diagnostic considerations include ILD from radiation or stem cell transplantation, both of which are independently associated with increased risk of DI-ILD, as well as immune reconstitution inflammatory syndrome and engraftment syndrome.

The importance of a DI-ILD diagnosis is the potential improvement and/or reversal of lung injury after early drug cessation, thereby eliminating exposure to unnecessary treatments and/or interventions. The challenge with confirmation of DI-ILD is manifold. First, the onset can occur any time after exposure—within hours (eg, transfusion-related acute lung injury), days to weeks (eg, nitrofurantoin), weeks to months (eg, chemotherapy, amiodarone), or even years (eg, amiodarone). Next, drugs can produce any pattern of ILD, both radiographically and histopathologically.[8] These presentations are the same as those from classically known and idiopathic ILDs (eg, connective-tissue disease ILD, idiopathic pulmonary fibrosis [IPF]). Furthermore, the severity can range from asymptomatic and incidentally detected radiographic abnormalities to life-threatening acute respiratory failure or end-stage lung fibrosis or death. The National Cancer Institute proposed the Common Terminology Criteria for Adverse Events (CTCAE), including for respiratory failure that was initially used in clinical trials (**Table 2**).[23]

Laboratory findings are nonspecific. Less commonly, eosinophilia may be seen to suggest eosinophilic pneumonia (EP); however, it is neither sensitive nor specific. Research is ongoing to identify serum biomarkers for DI-ILD. Krebs von den Lungen-6 and serum surfactant proteins A and D have been reported to be elevated in patients with DI-ILD.[24,25] However, these markers are more extensively studied in exacerbations in IPF and coronavirus disease-2019 pneumonia, and are more likely indicative of any acute lung injury rather than for specific subtypes of ILD, including DI-ILD.[26,27]

Bronchoscopy may support clinical/pathologic patterns of lung involvement, but its main role is in the exclusion of alternative causes of respiratory failure, especially infection and malignancy.[28] This is particularly relevant when the causal drug is immunosuppressive or the patient is immunocompromised. On bronchoalveolar lavage (BAL), several types of alveolitis (eg, lymphocytic, neutrophilic, eosinophilic, mixed,

Table 2
Common terminology criteria for adverse events

Grade 1	Mild	Asymptomatic; clinical or diagnostic observations only; intervention not indicated
Grade 2	Moderate	Symptomatic; medical intervention indication; limiting instrumental ADL
Grade 3	Severe	Severe symptoms; limiting self-care ADL; oxygen indicated
Grade 4	Life-threatening	Life-threatening respiratory compromise; urgent intervention indication (eg, intubation)
Grade 5	Fatal	

Abbreviation: ADL, activities of daily living.

Data from Common terminology criteria for adverse events (CTCAE), version 5.0. U.S. Department of Health and Human Services. 2017. Available at: https://ctep.cancer.gov/protocoldevelopment/electronic_applications/docs/CTCAE_v5_Quick_Reference_8.5x11.pdf. Accessed on October 31, 2022.

or foamy or lipid-laden macrophages) or diffuse alveolar hemorrhage (DAH) may be seen with DI-ILD.[29,30] A classic finding is a CD8+ predominant lymphocytic alveolitis; however, a CD4+ increase has been reported with ampicillin/sulbactam, methotrexate, nitrofurantoin, and sirolimus.[7,31–34]

Histopathology, by transbronchial, cryo, or surgical biopsy, is not routinely indicated in the evaluation of DI-ILD. The findings are mostly nonspecific as discussed above, nearly all histologic ILD subtypes can be seen with DI-ILD and they range from patterns of acute lung injury: acute interstitial pneumonia (AIP), diffuse alveolar damage (DAD), DAH, organizing pneumonia (OP), and EP, to more subacute and chronic patterns: nonspecific interstitial pneumonia (NSIP), lymphoid interstitial pneumonia (LIP), granulomatous interstitial pneumonia (GIP), sarcoid-like reactions, pulmonary alveolar proteinosis (PAP), hypersensitivity pneumonitis (HP), and usual interstitial pneumonia (UIP), as well as lung nodules and lymphadenopathy.[7,35–37] Some drugs are known to induce stereotypical reactions in the lung (eg, minocycline with EP), whereas others induce an array of different histopathologic patterns (eg, amiodarone with DAD, OP, NSIP, and UIP).[38,39]

Thin section high-resolution computed tomography (HRCT) of the chest remains the cornerstone for the diagnosis of ILD and DI-ILD by describing the extent and distribution of lung injury. The radiographic criteria for DI-ILD as defined by the Fleischner Society are: (1) new pulmonary parenchymal opacities, (2) temporal association with therapeutic agent, and (3) exclusion of alternative causes.[40] Similar to histopathologic patterns, almost all radiographic patterns of ILD can be associated with DI-ILD (**Fig. 2**). Although radiographic patterns are often used to predict histologic patterns of disease, correlation is poor.[35,41] Nonetheless, HRCT is the preferred noninvasive method to assess for the presence of ILD as well as for monitoring its appearance, progression, and resolution.[42]

IMPLICATED DRUGS

There are various ways to categorize DI-ILDs—from individual agents or classes of medications to mechanisms of lung injury, or radiographic/histologic and BAL patterns. A comprehensive search by individual drugs or patterns can be performed on Pneumotox with referenced articles.[7] In this article, classes of the most implicated drugs are discussed. Recent additions include lung damage from ICIs and e-cigarettes.[7]

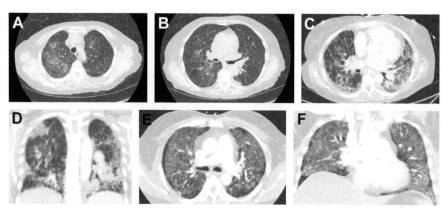

Fig. 2. CT images of the chest of confirmed DI-ILD cases. (*A, B*) Amiodarone pulmonary toxicity—axial CT images with patchy ground glass opacities and interlobular septal thickening with a nonspecific radiographic pattern; liver or lung density may be increased. (*C, D*) Infliximab toxicity—axial and coronal CT images with patchy dense, consolidative ground glass opacities consistent with OP and/or NSIP patterns. (*E, F*) Melphalan toxicity—axial and coronal CT images with extensive, diffuse ground glass opacities associated with subpleural sparing consistent with a DAD pattern.

In the largest descriptive review by Skeoch and corroborated on Pneumotox, the most common pneumotoxic drugs identified in unselected DI-ILD cohorts were chemotherapeutic agents accounting for 23% to 51% of cases, followed by disease-modifying antirheumatic drugs (DMARDS, 6% to 72%) and antibiotics (6% to 26%), which will be discussed along with cardiovascular drugs and others.[6,7]

Traditional Antineoplastic Agents

Pulmonary toxicity has been reported to occur in 6% to 20% of patients who receive chemotherapeutic agents, although incidence varies depending on specific medication or dose.[6,43–45] The risk of injury increases with multiagent chemotherapy regimen or (prior or current) radiation therapy, high fractional oxygen concentration, and in patients with subclinical ILD or in those treated for lung cancer.[46]

The clinical presentation generally occurs weeks to a few months after initiation of therapy; rarely delayed fibrosis can be observed with nitrosoureas and bleomycin, and delayed pleuroparenchymal fibroelastosis (PPFE) observed with alkylating agents, which can occur more than 10 years after exposure.[47–49] The types of DI-ILD can vary along the continuum from benign transient infiltrates and pulmonary edema, to DAD and ARDS; as well as recognized patterns of EP, OP, GIP, lung nodules, and fibrotic lung disease.[1,7]

Bleomycin is the most prevalent and well-defined chemotherapeutic-induced lung disease. It is an antineoplastic antibiotic used for curative intent in germ cell tumors and Hodgkin's lymphoma, which commonly affects young individuals. The reported risk for lung toxicity ranges from 6.8% to 32%, with mortality up to 25%.[50–54] Risk factors for bleomycin pulmonary toxicity include older age, underlying lung disease, prior radiation to the chest (radiation recall), renal failure, cumulative dose, and rapid intravenous infusion rates.[55] The presentation of lung injury can range from subclinical ILD to acute fatal ARDS; however, most commonly causes interstitial pulmonary fibrosis ("fibrosing alveolitis").[1,7] The respective merit of systematic chest auscultation, PFT (DLCO decreasing by more than 40%), and chest imaging during exposure is debated; watchful waiting, avoiding rapid infusion, monitoring renal function, and minimizing oxygen therapy as able should be borne in mind. Of note, bleomycin-induced pneumonitis is a well-recognized research tool to induce lung fibrosis in mice, although this model differs from the disease in humans.[56]

Alkylating agents act directly on DNA to cause crosslinking and strand breaks. The agents most implicated in DI-ILD are busulfan and cyclophosphamide, but also include nitrosoureas (eg, carmustine, melphalan) and chlorambucil. Busulfan was the first cytotoxic drug associated with lung toxicity.[57] The pattern of injury is most commonly pulmonary fibrosis, but DAD, OP, and PAP have also been reported.[57–60] Cyclophosphamide is associated with two distinct clinical patterns: early-onset pneumonitis or ILD (onset one to 6 months, with favorable prognosis) and late-onset pneumonitis/fibrosis, sometimes mimicking PPFE (onset months to years, with progressive respiratory failure).[61]

Taxanes stabilize microtubules to prevent disassembly thereby inhibiting cell replication. Implicated taxanes are paclitaxel and docetaxel, which cause AIP, OP, pulmonary opacities with peripheral eosinophilia, and pulmonary fibrosis.[1,62–65] Of note, paclitaxel has additional anti-proliferative properties to reduce the risk of in-stent restenosis and its use even in drug-eluting stents (DES) have been reported to cause fatal AIPs.[66]

Molecularly Targeted Antineoplastic Agents

ICIs are immunomodulatory antibodies that enhance the immune system by targeting PD-1 (eg, nivolumab, pembrolizumab), PDL-1 (eg, atezolizumab, avelumab, durvalumab), and CTLA (eg, ipilimumab).[67] Pneumonitis is described with every class of ICIs, but highest in PD-1 inhibitors and combination ICIs with incidence rates up to 3.6% and mortality 9.4% with a median onset of 2.3 months, ranging from 0.2 to 27.4 months.[68,69] The radiographic patterns of injury were most frequently reported to be consistent with OP and NSIP, followed by AIP and HP-like patterns; autopsies and biopsies have revealed histopathologic patterns of DAD, interstitial fibrosis, and sarcoid-like reactions/GIP.[70] The differential diagnosis of ICI pneumonitis should also include tumor progression or pseudo-progression.[71] Owing to the incidence and severity of ICI pneumonitis, guidelines exist on their grading and management, which will be discussed in the next section.

Other molecularly targeted therapies associated with DI-ILD include anti-epidermal growth factor receptor (EGFR) agents (eg, erlotinib, gefitinib, osimertinib), anaplastic lymphoma kinase (ALK) inhibitors (eg, crizotinib), Bcr-Abl TKIs (eg, dasatinib), poly ADP-ribose polymerase (PARP) inhibitors (eg, olaparib), and mammalian target of rapamycin (mTOR) inhibitors (eg, sirolimus, temsirolimus, everolimus).[72–76] Similar to paclitaxel, everolimus is also used in DES and has been implicated in case reports of OP.[77,78] The possible positive effect of mTOR and ICI-induced (respiratory) adverse effects on outcome of the basic disease is a current area of intense investigation.

Lastly, monoclonal antibodies, particularly, fam-trastuzumab deruxtecan (T-DXd), has been an increasingly recognized cause of DI-ILD. Trastuzumab is a monoclonal antibody against the human epidermal growth factor receptor 2, which was first available as conventional trastuzumab, followed by ado-trastuzumab emtansine (T-DM1, antibody-drug conjugate incorporated with a microtubule inhibitor), and most recently T-DXd (antibody-drug conjugate incorporated with a topoisomerase I inhibitor).[79,80] These progressive modifications render the drugs more stable, selective, and specific for cancer cells, and more cytotoxic, with favorable clinical trial results to support this. Yet with these enhancements, increasing frequency of acute pneumonitis has been seen with T-DM1 with an incidence of 0.5% to 4.0%.[81] Moreover, incidence with

T-DXd ranged from 5.4% to 26.4%; a systemic review found 10.7% to be grade 3 or 4% and 10.7% to be fatal.[81,82]

Disease-Modifying Antirheumatic Drugs

DMARDs are commonly classified as conventional (eg, methotrexate), or biologic (eg, tumor necrosis factor (TNF)-α inhibitors). Methotrexate is a mainstay agent in rheumatology and used in some malignancies. Acute/subacute lung toxicity tends to occur after weeks to months on low dose oral therapy but can occur earlier with higher dose parenteral administration.[83–85] Chronic pneumonitis and fibrosis associated with methotrexate has not been well established and remains controversial,[86] though recent studies suggest no association, delayed presentation, or slower progression of rheumatoid arthritis associated ILD in patients on MTX3351506732646919.[87,88]

TNF-α inhibitors (eg, etanercept, infliximab) are an increasingly recognized cause of DI-ILD. The most common histopathologic patterns are UIP, NSIP, and OP; however, sarcoid-like reactions, DAD, DAH, LIP, and OP have also been described.[89,90] TNF-α inhibitors also increase the risk of developing pulmonary or extrapulmonary tuberculosis. Careful pretherapy investigation using interferon-gamma release assays before treatment initiation is warranted in all cases.

Antibiotics

Nitrofurantoin is frequently used for the treatment and prophylaxis of urinary tract infections. Acute pneumonitis accounts for over 80% of nitrofurantion-induced ILD cases and occurs within 1 to 2 weeks of exposure, or sooner (eg, hours) with prior exposure; whereas chronic pneumonitis/fibrosis develops months to years after extended prophylactic therapy.[91,92] Radiographic patterns of chronic pneumonitis include ground-glass, masses, or remodeling (eg, bronchiectasis) with varying degrees of associated fibrosis.[93]

Cardiovascular Drugs

Amiodarone is one of the most common causes of DI-ILD. The incidence of amiodarone pulmonary toxicity is estimated to range from 1.2% to 8.8% (depending on dose) with mortality rates of 3% to 37%.[6] Onset of symptoms generally occurs within 6 to 12 months but can range from under 2 months to several years into treatment.[1] Pulmonary toxicity can manifests as EP, OP, DAD, DAH, or shaggy/necrotic lung nodules.[17] Of note, the presence of foamy macrophages (accumulation of phospholipids) on BAL cells can be seen but is not entirely pathognomonic for pulmonary toxicity, although its absence suggests amiodarone lung toxicity is unlikely.

Other Considerations

Radiation-induced lung injury (RILI) can present in two forms: acute radiation pneumonitis or chronic radiation fibrosis, generally from thoracic irradiation for the treatment of lung, breast, or hematologic malignancies.[94] Risk factors for RILI include method of irradiation, volume of irradiated lung, and dosage and frequency of irradiation. Imaging is key in the evaluation of RILI in which lung involvement may not conform to anatomic units but rather to the confines of the radiation port; less commonly additional patterns of acute diffuse pneumonitis and migratory areas of OP can also be seen.[95] Yttrium-90 radioembolization induced ILD is distinctive.

MANAGEMENT, TREATMENT, AND PROGNOSIS

Discontinuation of the offending agent is the cornerstone of treatment, underlying illness permitting. In patients with mild presentations of acute pneumonitis, early withdrawal generally leads to complete reversal. However, in patients with disabling or progressive disease, or in those not responding to drug discontinuation, glucocorticoids (GCs) are considered despite the lack of robust data. The efficacy of GCs is difficult to assess due to overall low-quality data, with variability in GC agents, doses, and duration used for different forms of DI-ILD, as well as lack of analysis of dechallenge alone.[6] However, many case reports point to efficacy in non-fibrotic DI-ILD. High doses (boluses) are of uncertain efficacy. Treatment response is highly variable from no improvement in DAD, to 46% improvement in NSIP and 75% improvement in OP. More guidance is in place for the management of pneumonitis in ICIs based on the CTCAE grading criteria with management guidelines from the American Society of Clinical Oncology (ASCO)—where grade 1 (G1) is managed with holding the ICI, G2 with addition of prednisone 1 to 2 mg/kg/d, G3-4 with higher dose intravenous methylprednisolone 1 to 2 mg/kg/d, and if no response, potential addition of further immunosuppressive agents.[23,96] This may serve to be a useful framework for the management of DI-ILDs as a whole and to provide standardization of care; thereby allowing for improvements in outcomes and more robust evidence based data in the future.[40] Of note, the decision to initiate GCs long-term may be challenging given patients' susceptibility to infections even at low dosages. Bronchoscopic evaluation and BAL to rule out infection is recommended, if feasible. Otherwise, there is a low threshold to initiate concurrent empiric antibiotics.

In patients with chronic pneumonitis and evidence of fibrosis (eg, radiographic UIP pattern or features of honeycombing and PFTs with restriction and low DLCO) which can occur months to years after drug exposure with progression of disease and poor response to steroids, antifibrotic therapy has been considered.[17,40]

Risk factors predicting mortality include acute severe presentation, particularly, with need for mechanical ventilation or extracorporeal membrane oxygenation (ECMO), as well as radiologic patterns suggesting DAD or honeycombing with chronic interstitial pneumonitis.[6] In patients who continue to progress to end-stage respiratory failure, referral should be made to lung transplant. ECMO can be considered for bridge to recovery or lung transplantation and should follow the Extracorporeal Life Support Organization (ELSO) guidelines for candidacy.[97]

In patients who fully recover from DI-ILD, rechallenge is generally not recommended as fatal cases have been recorded. However, in cases where therapeutic alternatives are limited, rechallenge using stepwise dosages may be considered on a case-by-case basis in a multidisciplinary setting. The severity must be limited to CTCAE grade 1 or 2 with consideration for concomitant GC (eg, methylprednisolone 1 mg/kg) administration.[68]

DISCUSSION

DI-ILD affects many patients globally with a significant impact on morbidity and mortality that is underrecognized. The burden of DI-ILD will probably continue to grow as new medications are brought into the market. In particular, molecularly targeted agents have been shown to be one of the biggest culprits of DI-ILD and will continue to pose concerns as the field of personalized medicine evolves.

The start to understanding DI-ILD is to recognize the entity and be aware of the potential pneumotoxicity of drugs (and at least aware of the resources to find this information). In a study by Speirs and colleagues, 125 prescribers of long-term nitrofurantoin (82.4% general practitioners, 12% urologists) were given a question-naire to understand prescribing and monitoring practices: 28% were unaware of lung complications, 52.8% never monitored for lung issues, and 46.7% of urologists did not believe they were responsible for drug monitoring (eg, is the general practi-tioner's responsibility).[93] This highlights not only gaps in common knowledge as nitrofurantoin-ILD has been frequently reported since 1962, but also gaps in moni-toring, care, and responsibility.[98] At the same time, it is important to distinguish minor lung shadows (eg, "interstitial lung abnormalities") on CT that do not necessary equate to ILD or DI-ILD. Careful evaluation is needed at all times, short of that, withdrawal of a vital drug may bear dire consequences.

Despite the preponderance of literature on DI-ILD, the majority is of heterogeneous, suboptimal quality and difficult to synthesize.[6] This is hindered by the inherent difficulty and unreliability in the diagnosis and management of DI-ILD leading to heterogeneity of data. From the variable and nonspecific clinical manifesta-tions of DI-ILD, to the common lack of specific physiologic, radiographic, or histopath-ologic findings, the diagnosis remains one of thoughtful exclusion. Beyond this, there remains a dearth of evidence for the management of DI-ILDs. Consideration can be made for standardizing treatment approach by adopting the guidelines used in ICI pneumonitis for other DI-ILDs, but this would require consensus.[23,96]

Overall more research is needed across this spectrum. Useful sources for practi-tioners include Pneumotox which is continuously updated and can serve as a quick and trusted diagnostic aid in drug-induced respiratory diseases.[7]

SUMMARY

The DI-ILDs are a heterogenous group of conditions caused by a list of medications that is ever growing. The clinical, radiologic, and histopathologic findings may be sug-gestive of DI-ILD, but confirmatory diagnosis requires a high index of suspicion with careful history taking and low threshold for deeper investigation into potential causality while excluding typical etiologies. Withdrawal of the culprit drug usually leads to res-olution; however, more severe presentations may warrant administration of GCs. Rechallenge is generally not recommended but can be considered on a case-by-case basis in mild presentations with lack of therapeutic alternative. Not to be forgotten, aside from ILD, drugs can occasion other pulmonary manifestations from large and small airways to serosal surfaces, pulmonary circulation, mediastinum, and neuromuscular system that drives ventilation and oxygenation.

CLINICS CARE POINTS

- Drug-induced respiratory disease can involve the airways, pulmonary vasculature, mediastinum, pleura, and/or neuromuscular system, but parenchymal involvement with interstitial lung disease (ILD) is the most prevalent.

- The incidence and prevalence of drug-induced interstitial lung disease (DI-ILD) vary widely but is estimated to range from 4.1 to 12.4 cases/million/year and 3% to 5% of ILD cases, respectively.

- Presentation is highly variable among drugs and even with the same drug; it can occur hours, days, or even years after exposure with a wide range of severity.

- There are no specific tests diagnostic of DI-ILD; diagnosis requires clinical suspicion with relevant exposure history and appropriate temporal relationship, as well as clinical, physiologic, and radiographic findings suggestive of ILD and exclusion of alternative causes.

- Discontinuation of the offending agent (underlying illness permitting) is the mainstay of treatment, but in severe cases administration of glucocorticoids should be considered. Rechallenge is generally not recommended.

DISCLOSURE

The authors have no commercial or financial conflicts of interest that affect the writing or publication of this article.

ACKNOWLEDGMENTS

The authors would like to thank Dr Adam Bernheim for contributing the radiographs included in this article.

REFERENCES

1. Schwarz MI, King TE. Interstitial lung disease. Shelton, CT: People's Medical Publishing House; 2011.
2. Travis WD, Costabel U, Hansell DM, et al. An official American Thoracic Society/European Respiratory Society statement: Update of the international multidisciplinary classification of the idiopathic interstitial pneumonias. Am J Respir Crit Care Med 2013;188(6):733–48.
3. American Thoracic Society/European Respiratory Society International Multidisciplinary Consensus Classification of the Idiopathic Interstitial Pneumonias. Am J Respir Crit Care Med 2002;165(2):277–304.
4. Coultas DB, Zumwalt RE, Black WC, et al. The epidemiology of interstitial lung diseases. Am J Respir Crit Care Med 1994;150(4):967–72.
5. Thomeer MJ, Costabe U, Rizzato G, et al. Comparison of registries of interstitial lung diseases in three European countries. Eur Respir J Suppl 2001;32:114s–8s.
6. Skeoch S, Weatherley N, Swift AJ, et al. Drug-Induced Interstitial Lung Disease: A Systematic Review. J Clin Med 2018;7(10). https://doi.org/10.3390/jcm7100356.
7. Camus P. The Drug-induced respiratory disease website. Pneumotox 2022. Available at: https://www.pneumotox.com. Accessed February 17, 2023.
8. Roden AC, Camus P. Iatrogenic pulmonary lesions. Semin Diagn Pathol 2018;35(4):260–71.
9. Camus P, Foucher P, Bonniaud P, et al. Drug-induced infiltrative lung disease. Eur Respir J 2001;18(32 suppl):93s.
10. Matsuno O. Drug-induced interstitial lung disease: mechanisms and best diagnostic approaches. Respir Res 2012;13(1):39.
11. Zhai X, Zhang J, Tian Y, et al. The mechanism and risk factors for immune checkpoint inhibitor pneumonitis in non-small cell lung cancer patients. Cancer Biol Med 2020;17(3):599–611.
12. Pietra GG. Pathologic mechanisms of drug-induced lung disorders. J Thorac Imaging 1991;6(1):1–7.
13. Erasmus JJ, McAdams HP, Rossi SE. High-resolution CT of drug-induced lung disease. Radiol Clin North Am 2002;40(1):61–72.
14. Marwa K, Kondamudi NP. Type IV Hypersensitivity Reaction. In: StatPearls [Internet]. Treasure Island (FL): StatPearls Publishing; 2022. Available at: https://www.ncbi.nlm.nih.gov/books/NBK562228/. Accessed October 31, 2022.
15. Guillon JM, Joly P, Autran B, et al. Minocycline-induced cell-mediated hypersensitivity pneumonitis. Ann Intern Med 1992;117(6):476–81.

16. Ramos-Casals M, Brahmer JR, Callahan MK, et al. Immune-related adverse events of checkpoint inhibitors. Nat Rev Dis Primers 2020;6(1):38.

17. Spagnolo P, Bonniaud P, Rossi G, et al. Drug-induced interstitial lung disease. Eur Respir J 2022;2102776. https://doi.org/10.1183/13993003.02776-2021.

18. Hradska K, Hajek R, Jelinek T. Toxicity of Immune-Checkpoint Inhibitors in Hematological Malignancies. Review. Front Pharmacol 2021. https://doi.org/10.3389/fphar.2021.733890.

19. Stone JR, Kanneganti R, Abbasi M, et al. Monitoring for Chemotherapy-Related Cardiotoxicity in the Form of Left Ventricular Systolic Dysfunction: A Review of Current Recommendations. JCO Oncol Pract 2021;17(5):228–36.

20. Cardiotox: the drug-induced cardiovascular disease app. Version 1.0. Cactus Mobile. Updated August 23, 2022.

21. Naranjo CA, Busto U, Sellers EM, et al. A method for estimating the probability of adverse drug reactions. Clin Pharmacol Ther 1981;30(2):239–45.

22. Müller NL, White DA, Jiang H, et al. Diagnosis and management of drug-associated interstitial lung disease. Br J Cancer 2004;91(2):S24–30.

23. Common terminology criteria for adverse events (CTCAE), version 5.0. U.S. Department of Health and Human Services. Available at: https://ctep.cancer.gov/protocoldevelopment/electronic_applications/docs/CTCAE_v5_Quick_Reference_8.5x11.pdf. Accessed on October 31, 2022.

24. Inomata S, Takahashi H, Nagata M, et al. Acute lung injury as an adverse event of gefitinib. Anti Cancer Drugs 2004;15(5):461–7.

25. Ohnishi H, Yokoyama A, Yasuhara Y, et al. Circulating KL-6 levels in patients with drug induced pneumonitis. Thorax 2003;58(10):872–5.

26. Wang K, Ju Q, Cao J, et al. Impact of serum SP-A and SP-D levels on comparison and prognosis of idiopathic pulmonary fibrosis: A systematic review and meta-analysis. Med (Baltimore) 2017;96(23):e7083.

27. Tong M, Xiong Y, Zhu C, et al. Serum surfactant protein D in COVID-19 is elevated and correlated with disease severity. BMC Infect Dis 2021;21(1):737.

28. Meyer KC, Raghu G, Baughman RP, et al. An Official American Thoracic Society Clinical Practice Guideline: The Clinical Utility of Bronchoalveolar Lavage Cellular Analysis in Interstitial Lung Disease. Am J Respir Crit Care Med 2012;185(9):1004–14.

29. Costabel U, Uzaslan E, Guzman J. Bronchoalveolar lavage in drug-induced lung disease. Clin Chest Med 2004;25(1):25–35.

30. Costabel U, Guzman J, Bonella F, et al. Bronchoalveolar lavage in other interstitial lung diseases. Semin Respir Crit Care Med 2007;28(5):514–24.

31. Miyashita N, Nakajima M, Kuroki M, et al. [Sulbactam/ampicillin-induced pneumonitis]. Nihon Kokyuki Gakkai Zasshi 1998;36(8):684–9.

32. Brutinel WM, Martin WJ. Chronic Nitrofurantoin Reaction Associated with T-Lymphocyte Alveolitis. Chest 1986;89(1):150–2.

33. Morelon E, Stern M, Israël-Biet D, et al. Characteristics of sirolimus-associated interstitial pneumonitis in renal transplant patients. Transplantation 2001;72(5):787–90.

34. Schnabel A, Richter C, Bauerfeind S, et al. Bronchoalveolar lavage cell profile in methotrexate induced pneumonitis. Thorax 1997;52(4):377–9.

35. Cleverley JR, Screaton NJ, Hiorns MP, et al. Drug-induced lung disease: high-resolution CT and histological findings. Clin Radiol 2002;57(4):292–9.

36. Flieder DB, Travis WD. Pathologic characteristics of drug-induced lung disease. Clin Chest Med 2004;25(1):37–45.

37. Camus P, Fanton A, Bonniaud P, et al. Interstitial Lung Disease Induced by Drugs and Radiation. Respiration 2004;71(4):301–26.
38. Sitbon O, Bidel N, Dussopt C, et al. Minocycline Pneumonitis and Eosinophilia: A Report on Eight Patients. Arch Intern Med 1994;154(14):1633–40.
39. Wolkove N, Baltzan M. Amiodarone pulmonary toxicity. Can Respir J 2009; 16(2):43–8.
40. Johkoh T, Lee KS, Nishino M, et al. Chest CT Diagnosis and Clinical Management of Drug-related Pneumonitis in Patients Receiving Molecular Targeting Agents and Immune Checkpoint Inhibitors: A Position Paper from the Fleischner Society. Radiol 2021;298(3):550–66.
41. Myers JL, Limper AH, Swensen SJ. Drug-induced lung disease: a pragmatic classification incorporating HRCT appearances. Semin Respir Crit Care Med 2003;24(4):445–54.
42. Silva CI, Müller NL. Drug-induced lung diseases: most common reaction patterns and corresponding high-resolution CT manifestations. Semin Ultrasound CT MR 2006;27(2):111–6.
43. Limper AH. Chemotherapy-induced lung disease. Clin Chest Med 2004;25(1): 53–64.
44. Dimopoulou I, Bamias A, Lyberopoulos P, et al. Pulmonary toxicity from novel anti-neoplastic agents. Ann Oncol 2006;17(3):372–9.
45. Fujimoto D, Kato R, Morimoto T, et al. Characteristics and Prognostic Impact of Pneumonitis during Systemic Anti-Cancer Therapy in Patients with Advanced Non-Small-Cell Lung Cancer. PLoS One 2016;11(12):e0168465.
46. Li F, Liu H, Wu H, et al. Risk factors for radiation pneumonitis in lung cancer patients with subclinical interstitial lung disease after thoracic radiation therapy. Radiat Oncol 2021;16(1):70.
47. Vahid B, Marik PE. Pulmonary Complications of Novel Antineoplastic Agents for Solid Tumors. Chest 2008;133(2):528–38.
48. O'Driscoll BRMDM, Hasleton PSMDF, Taylor PMMF, et al. Active Lung Fibrosis Up to 17 Years after Chemotherapy with Carmustine (BCNU) in Childhood. N Engl J Med 1990;323(6):378–82.
49. Beynat-Mouterde C, Beltramo G, Lezmi G, et al. Pleuroparenchymal fibroelastosis as a late complication of chemotherapy agents. Eur Respir J 2014;44(2):523.
50. O'Sullivan JM, Huddart RA, Norman AR, et al. Predicting the risk of bleomycin lung toxicity in patients with germ-cell tumours. Ann Oncol 2003;14(1):91–6.
51. Delanoy N, Pécuchet N, Fabre E, et al. Bleomycin-Induced Pneumonitis in the Treatment of Ovarian Sex Cord–Stromal Tumors: A Systematic Review and Meta-analysis. Int J Gynecol Cancer 2015;25(9):1593.
52. Ngeow J, Tan IB, Kanesvaran R, et al. Prognostic impact of bleomycin-induced pneumonitis on the outcome of Hodgkin's lymphoma. Ann Hematol 2011;90(1): 67–72.
53. Stamatoullas A, Brice P, Bouabdallah R, et al. Outcome of patients older than 60 years with classical Hodgkin lymphoma treated with front line ABVD chemotherapy: frequent pulmonary events suggest limiting the use of bleomycin in the elderly. Br J Haematol 2015;170(2):179–84.
54. Evens AM, Helenowski I, Ramsdale E, et al. A retrospective multicenter analysis of elderly Hodgkin lymphoma: outcomes and prognostic factors in the modern era. Blood 2012;119(3):692–5.
55. Broaddus VC, Ernst JD, King TE, et al. Murray & Nadel's Textbook of Respiratory Medicine E-Book. Elsevier Health Sciences 2021.

56. Ruscitti F, Ravanetti F, Bertani V, et al. Quantification of Lung Fibrosis in IPF-Like Mouse Model and Pharmacological Response to Treatment by Micro-Computed Tomography. Original Research. Front Pharmacol 2020. https://doi.org/10.3389/fphar.2020.01117.

57. Oliner H, Schwartz R, Rubio F, et al. Interstitial pulmonary fibrosis following busulfan therapy. Am J Med 1961;31(1):134–9.

58. About I, Lauque D, Levenes H, et al. [Alveolar opacities and busulfan pneumonia]. Rev Mal Respir 1993;10(1):39–41. Opacités alvéolaires et pneumopathie au busulfan.

59. Kedia RK, Sullivan A, Stephens M, et al. A breathless female. Eur Respir J 1999; 13(1):207–9.

60. Heard BE, Cooke RA. Busulphan lung. Thorax 1968;23(2):187–93.

61. Malik SW, Myers JL, DeRemee RA, et al. Lung toxicity associated with cyclophosphamide use. Two distinct patterns. Am J Respir Crit Care Med 1996;154(6 Pt 1): 1851–6.

62. Anoop TM, Joseph R, Unnikrishnan P, et al. Taxane-induced acute interstitial pneumonitis in patients with breast cancer and outcome of taxane rechallenge. Lung India 2022;39(2):158–68.

63. Bielopolski D, Evron E, Moreh-Rahav O, et al. Paclitaxel-induced pneumonitis in patients with breast cancer: case series and review of the literature. J Chemother 2017;29(2):113–7.

64. Ostoros G, Pretz A, Fillinger J, et al. Fatal pulmonary fibrosis induced by paclitaxel: a case report and review of the literature. Int J Gynecol Cancer 2006; 16(Suppl 1):391–3.

65. Ardolino L, Lau B, Wilson I, et al. Case Report: Paclitaxel-Induced Pneumonitis in Early Breast Cancer: A Single Institution Experience and Review. Front Oncol 2021;11:701424. https://doi.org/10.3389/fonc.2021.701424.

66. Fujimaki T, Kato K, Fukuda S, et al. Acute interstitial pneumonitis after implantation of paclitaxel-eluting stents: a report of two fatal cases. Int J Cardiol 2011; 148(2):e21–4.

67. Bukamur H, Alkrekshi A, Katz H, et al. Immune Checkpoint Inhibitor-Related Pulmonary Toxicity: A Comprehensive Review, Part II. South Med J 2021;114(9): 614–9.

68. Delaunay M, Cadranel J, Lusque A, et al. Immune-checkpoint inhibitors associated with interstitial lung disease in cancer patients. Eur Respir J 2017;50(2): 1700050.

69. Khunger M, Rakshit S, Pasupuleti V, et al. Incidence of Pneumonitis With Use of Programmed Death 1 and Programmed Death-Ligand 1 Inhibitors in Non-Small Cell Lung Cancer: A Systematic Review and Meta-Analysis of Trials. Chest 2017;152(2):271–81.

70. Chuzi S, Tavora F, Cruz M, et al. Clinical features, diagnostic challenges, and management strategies in checkpoint inhibitor-related pneumonitis. Cancer Manag Res 2017;9:207–13.

71. Wang H, Guo X, Zhou J, et al. Clinical diagnosis and treatment of immune checkpoint inhibitor-associated pneumonitis. Thorac Cancer 2020;11(1):191–7.

72. Shi L, Tang J, Tong L, et al. Risk of interstitial lung disease with gefitinib and erlotinib in advanced non-small cell lung cancer: a systematic review and meta-analysis of clinical trials. Lung Cancer 2014;83(2):231–9.

73. Yoneda KY, Scranton JR, Cadogan MA, et al. Interstitial Lung Disease Associated With Crizotinib in Patients With Advanced Non-Small Cell Lung Cancer: Independent Review of Four PROFILE Trials. Clin Lung Cancer 2017;18(5):472–9.

74. Bergeron A, Réa D, Levy V, et al. Lung abnormalities after dasatinib treatment for chronic myeloid leukemia: a case series. Am J Respir Crit Care Med 2007;176(8): 814–8.

75. Ma Z, Sun X, Zhao Z, et al. Risk of pneumonitis in cancer patients treated with PARP inhibitors: A meta-analysis of randomized controlled trials and a pharmaco-vigilance study of the FAERS database. Gynecol Oncol 2021;162(2):496–505.

76. Willemsen AECAB, Grutters JC, Gerritsen WR, et al. mTOR inhibitor-induced interstitial lung disease in cancer patients: Comprehensive review and a practical management algorithm. Int J Cancer 2016;138(10):2312–21.

77. Sakamoto S, Kikuchi N, Ichikawa A, et al. Everolimus-induced pneumonitis after drug-eluting stent implantation: a case report. Cardiovasc Intervent Radiol 2013; 36(4):1151–4.

78. Kobayashi H. Everolimus-Eluting Stent-induced Pneumonitis. Am J Respir Crit Care Med 2022;205(6):12–3.

79. Cortés J, Kim S-B, Chung W-P, et al. Trastuzumab Deruxtecan versus Trastuzu-mab Emtansine for Breast Cancer. N Engl J Med 2022;386(12):1143–54.

80. Verma S, Miles D, Gianni L, et al. Trastuzumab Emtansine for HER2-Positive Advanced Breast Cancer. N Engl J Med 2012;367(19):1783–91.

81. Tarantino P, Modi S, Tolaney SM, et al. Interstitial Lung Disease Induced by Anti-ERBB2 Antibody-Drug Conjugates: A Review. JAMA Oncol 2021;7(12):1873–81.

82. Abuhelwa Z, Alloghbi A, Alqahtani A, et al. Trastuzumab Deruxtecan-Induced Interstitial Lung Disease/Pneumonitis in ERBB2-Positive Advanced Solid Malig-nancies: A Systematic Review. Drugs 2022;82(9):979–87.

83. Kremer JM, Alarcón GS, Weinblatt ME, et al. Clinical, laboratory, radiographic, and histopathologic features of methotrexate-associated lung injury in patients with rheumatoid arthritis: a multicenter study with literature review. Arthritis Rheum 1997;40(10):1829–37.

84. Imokawa S, Colby TV, Leslie KO, et al. Methotrexate pneumonitis: review of the literature and histopathological findings in nine patients. Eur Respir J 2000; 15(2):373.

85. Le Guillou F, Dominique S, Dubruille V, et al. [Acute respiratory distress syndrome due to pneumonitis following intrathecal methotrexate administration]. Rev Mal Respir 2003;20(2 Pt 1):273–7. Insuffisance respiratoire aiguë avec pneumopathie après administration intrathécale de méthotrexate.

86. Conway R, Low C, Coughlan RJ, et al. Methotrexate use and risk of lung disease in psoriasis, psoriatic arthritis, and inflammatory bowel disease: systematic liter-ature review and meta-analysis of randomised controlled trials. Br Med J 2015; 13(350):h1269.

87. Dawson JK, Quah E, Earnshaw B, et al. Does methotrexate cause progressive fibrotic interstitial lung disease? A systematic review, Rheumatol Int, 41(6), 2021, 1055-1064.

88. Juge PA, Lee JS, Lau J, et al. Methotrexate and rheumatoid arthritis associated interstitial lung disease, Eur Respir J, 57(2), 2000337, 2021.

89. Perez-Alvarez R, Perez-de-Lis M, Diaz-Lagares C, et al. Interstitial lung disease induced or exacerbated by TNF-targeted therapies: analysis of 122 cases. Semin Arthritis Rheum 2011;41(2):256–64.

90. Theunssens X, Bricman L, Dierckx S, et al. Anti-TNF Induced Sarcoidosis-Like Disease in Rheumatoid Arthritis Patients: Review Cases from the RA UCLouvain Brussels Cohort. Rheumatol Ther 2022;9(2):763–70.

91. Holmberg L, Boman G. Pulmonary reactions to nitrofurantoin. 447 cases reported to the Swedish Adverse Drug Reaction Committee 1966-1976. Eur J Respir Dis 1981;62(3):180–9.

92. Sovijärvi AR, Lemola M, Stenius B, et al. Nitrofurantoin-induced acute, subacute and chronic pulmonary reactions. Scand J Respir Dis 1977;58(1):41–50.

93. Speirs TP, Tuffin N, Mundy-Baird F, et al. Long-term nitrofurantoin: an analysis of complication awareness, monitoring, and pulmonary injury cases. BJGP Open 2021;5(6).

94. Hanania AN, Mainwaring W, Ghebre YT, et al. Radiation-Induced Lung Injury: Assessment and Management. Chest 2019;156(1):150–62.

95. Davis SD, Yankelevitz DF, Henschke CI. Radiation effects on the lung: clinical features, pathology, and imaging findings. AJR Am J Roentgenol 1992;159(6): 1157–64.

96. Schneider BJ, Naidoo J, Santomasso BD, et al. Management of Immune-Related Adverse Events in Patients Treated With Immune Checkpoint Inhibitor Therapy: ASCO Guideline Update. J Clin Oncol 2021;39(36):4073–126.

97. Extracorporal Membrane Oxygenation (ECMO). Available at: https://elso.org/ ecmo-resources/elso-ecmo-guidelines.aspx. Accessed October 31, 2022.

98. Israel HL, Diamond P. Recurrent Pulmonary Infiltration and Pleural Effusion Due to Nitrofurantoin Sensitivity. N Engl J Med 1962;266(20):1024–6.

Lymphangioleiomyomatosis and Other Cystic Lung Diseases

Matthew Koslow, MD[a,b],*, David A. Lynch, MB[c],
Carlyne D. Cool, MD[d,e], Steve D. Groshong, MD[b],
Gregory P. Downey, MD, FRCPC[b,f,g]

KEYWORDS

- Cystic lung disease • Lymphangioleiomyomatosis (LAM)
- Birt-Hogg-Dubé syndrome (BHD) • Lymphoid interstitial pneumonia
- Pulmonary Langerhans cell histiocytosis (LCH) • Amyloidosis
- Light chain deposition disease

KEY POINTS

- Distinguish cysts from cavities and define anatomic distribution as focal versus diffuse.
- Identify tempo of disease progression and the clinical context.
- Review of high-resolution computed tomography (HRCT) scan with expert radiologists will help identify key features and refine diagnostic possibilities.
- Blood biomarkers and genetic testing may be required to establish diagnosis.
- Some conditions (ie, LAM and BHD) require surveillance of extrapulmonary manifestations such as renal and other abdominal tumors.

INTRODUCTION

Pulmonary cysts and cavities are commonly encountered on chest imaging. The differential diagnosis is broad because both congenital and acquired processes can cause such findings. This article reviews common diffuse cystic lung diseases and a systematic approach to diagnosis.

[a] Division of Pulmonary, Critical Care, and Sleep Medicine, National Jewish Health, 1400 Jackson St, Denver, CO 80206, USA; [b] Department of Medicine, National Jewish Health, 1400 Jackson St, Denver, CO 80206, USA; [c] Department of Radiology, National Jewish Health, 1400 Jackson St, Denver, CO 80206, USA; [d] Department of Pathology, University of Colorado School of Medicine Anschutz Medical Campus, 13001 E 17th Pl, Aurora, CO 80045, USA; [e] Division of Pathology, Department of Medicine, National Jewish Health, Denver, CO, USA; [f] Department of Pediatrics, National Jewish Health; [g] Department of Immunology and Genomic Medicine, National Jewish Health
* Corresponding author.
E-mail address: koslowm@njhealth.org

Immunol Allergy Clin N Am 43 (2023) 359–377
https://doi.org/10.1016/j.iac.2023.01.003
0889-8561/23/© 2023 Elsevier Inc. All rights reserved.
immunology.theclinics.com

DEFINITION

Cysts and cavities are foci of decreased lung density with discernible walls as assessed by high-resolution computed tomography (HRCT). In contrast, emphysematous airspaces typically lack a perceptible wall. A cyst is typically surrounded by a thin wall (≤2 mm) of uniform thickness, whereas a lung cavity is a gas-filled space with a relatively thick wall (>4 mm), and may be surrounded by consolidation or mass.[1] A cavity often develops from drainage of a necrotic lesion via the bronchial tree and may contain a fluid level. This distinction is useful because "cysts" are rarely malignant, but a cavitary lesion raises concern for malignancy, infection, or vasculitis, especially in a high-risk patient.[2]

The distribution of cysts is classified as focal or multifocal versus diffuse (involving all lobes). The presence of lung cysts in a diffuse distribution limits the differential diagnosis to certain disorders and is the focus of this article.

LYMPHANGIOLEIOMYOMATOSIS
Background

Lymphangioleiomyomatosis (LAM) is a rare, slowly progressive neoplastic and metastasizing disorder characterized by progressive cystic destruction of the lung with marked female predominance. Clinical manifestations include exertional dyspnea, recurrent pneumothoraces, chylous effusions in the chest and abdomen, and abdominal tumors such as renal angiomyolipomas (AMLs).

LAM can be associated with the tuberous sclerosis complex (TSC-LAM) or sporadic (S-LAM), in which patients do not have TSC gene mutations or its clinical manifestations. TSC is an autosomal dominant genetic disorder that in its most severe form is associated with seizures and cognitive impairment, and central nervous system (CNS), cutaneous, and systemic lesions. TSC-LAM has been reported in 10% of men and 30% of women, although studies indicate that symptomatic TSC-LAM is nearly completely limited to women.[3] In S-LAM, lymphangiomas, AMLs, and sclerotic bone lesions may accompany the cystic lung changes but CNS and skin lesions are lacking.[4]

Variable phenotypes in S-LAM in the face of negative TSC1/TSC2 genetic testing of peripheral blood leukocytes may be explained by genetic mosaicism, the occurrence of somatic cells in a single organism with different genetic compositions, which occurs from random errors in DNA replication after fertilization and during embryogenesis. For example, Han and colleagues[5] report the case of an otherwise normal man who presented with apparent S-LAM and mosaicism for a TSC2 mutation yet no other TSC manifestations including a normal brain magnetic resonance imaging (MRI). Ogorek and colleagues[6] report a similar case of LAM with mosaicism for a pathogenic TSC2 mutation among 61 female patients with apparent sporadic LAM. The investigators hypothesize whether bilateral AMLs and sclerotic bone lesions (present in their index case yet rare among the cohort) could predict mosaicism for TSC2 mutations in sporadic LAM.[6]

Pathogenesis

LAM is caused by mutations in either of the 2 known TSC genetic loci: TSC1 on chromosome 9q34 or TSC2 on chromosome 16p13.[7,8] Dysregulation of the PI3/Akt signaling pathway enables activation of mechanistic target of rapamycin (mTOR) that promotes abnormal LAM cell proliferation and survival.[9,10] Disease progression is aided by abnormal lymphangiogenesis, immune evasion mechanisms, and antiapoptotic effects of sex steroids such as estrogen.

A model for LAM suggests that LAM cells metastasize to the lung from a remote source hypothesized to be the lymphatic system,[11] the uterus,[12] or AMLs.[9] Recently, single-cell transcriptomic analysis identified a unique population of LAM cells (LAM^{core} cells) with similar gene expression profiles in both pulmonary and uterine LAM^{core} cells providing support for the concept of a uterine source for pulmonary LAM cells.[13] The novel LAM^{core} cell discovery may serve to develop biomarkers and future therapeutic targets.

Nearly one-third of patients with LAM have abdominal or thoracic lymph node enlargement, usually due to lymphangiomyomatous tissue (**Fig. 1**).[14,15] Clusters of LAM cells enter the venous circulation at the thoracic duct, disseminate through the pulmonary capillary bed, and can be found in chylous pleural fluid.[11] Expression of lymphatic endothelial markers such as vascular endothelial growth factor receptors is critical to the process. Elevated levels of vascular endothelial growth factor D ([VEGF-D] > 800 pg/mL) can be useful to distinguish LAM from other cystic lung diseases[16] and predict response to therapy.[17]

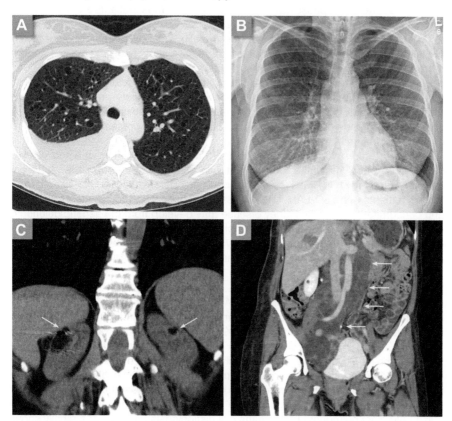

Fig. 1. Typical CT findings of LAM. (*A*) Axial CT image shows a moderate right chylous effusion and thin-walled cysts of variable sizes evenly distributed throughout the lungs. (*B*) Chest radiograph shows a resolved effusion following 4 months of medical therapy. (*C*) Coronal CT image in a different patient shows bilateral fat-containing renal angiomyolipomas (*arrows*). Metal artifact in the right kidney is from arterial embolization coils. (*D*) Coronal CT in a different patient shows a large tubular and lobulated fluid-attenuating structure in the retroperitoneum (*arrows*) compatible with retroperitoneal lymphangeioleiomyoma, which resolved with prolonged therapy (not shown). A large right chylous effusion is also present.

Estrogen may play a critical role in LAM cell survival, proliferation, and destructive potential. Estrogen regulates gene transcription and may modulate signaling to activate mTOR. Animal studies have shown that estrogen may promote metastases and the survival of TSC-2-deficient cells,[18] whereas estrogen suppression (by ovariectomy or aromatase inhibition) decreases mTOR activity and inhibits myometrial proliferation.[19,20] Targeting the estrogen-ERK pathway, along with the mTOR pathway, could be a potential therapeutic approach for LAM.

The pathogenesis of LAM has many similarities to the mechanisms of other human cancers, such as immune evasion strategies and tissue destruction. For example, targeted monoclonal antibodies (eg, anti-PD-L1) reduced tumor burden and prolonged survival in an animal model of TSC-LAM[21,22] and suggests immunotherapy as a potential treatment strategy for human LAM.

Clinical and Radiologic Manifestations

LAM typically presents during the reproductive years, although examples of LAM presenting well after menopause have been reported.[23,24] Most patients are nonsmokers, and LAM does not seem to be smoking related.

The most common clinical presentations are exertional dyspnea from disease progression, spontaneous pneumothorax, or incidental discovery of lung cysts. Pneumothorax is common (up to two-thirds of patients) with a high recurrence rate (70%),[24–26] and may precede the diagnosis of LAM in most patients. The accumulation of chyle in pleural and extrathoracic locations, such as the airway (chyloptysis) and genitourinary tract (chyluria), may occur. Fistulous communication with the gut can result in chyle in stool, and retrograde chylous parenchymal congestion can present with ground-glass or reticular change in the lung.[27]

AMLs are tumors composed of fat, smooth muscle, and abnormal blood vessels, which most often affect the kidneys but can present anywhere in the chest and abdomen (see **Fig. 1C**). AMLs are seen in one-third of patients with S-LAM and nearly 90% of patients with TSC-LAM.[4] Renal cysts have been reported in patients with LAM, and concomitant polycystic kidney disease may develop from the genetic deletion of PKD1, which is adjacent to TSC2.[28] Lymphangioleiomyomas are masses of LAM cell clusters within lymphatic vessels and lymph nodes that can mimic lymphomas, ovarian or renal cancers, or other malignant tumors (see **Fig. 1D**).[29]

Radiologic-Pathologic Correlation

On the chest radiograph, early signs of LAM include fine nodular, reticular, or reticulonodular opacities. Over time, the reticular pattern may progress into a more irregular pattern, lung volumes may increase (50% of cases), and pulmonary cysts become visible.[30] CT will invariably show diffuse cysts of varying size and profusion (see **Fig. 1**).[31] The lung cysts in LAM are typically round, thin walled (1–2 mm), and diffusely distributed throughout the otherwise normal lung. The number of cysts is typically greater among those with symptomatic pulmonary impairment than in asymptomatic patients.[30] The involvement of pulmonary cysts in the costophrenic sulci can distinguish LAM from pulmonary Langerhans cell histiocytosis (pLCH) that typically shows upper lung predominance with sparing of the sulci.[32]

The pulmonary cysts may develop from air trapping by smooth muscle proliferation in the small airways.[33] The LAM muscle cells stain with a monoclonal antibody, HMB-45 (human melanoma black-45), specific for LAM in this context (**Fig. 2**).[34] There is profound lymphatic duct and lymph node involvement and obstruction, which accounts for the chylous accumulation in the pleura and peritoneum among patients with LAM, yet unusual among those with TSC-LAM.[35] Other lung findings described

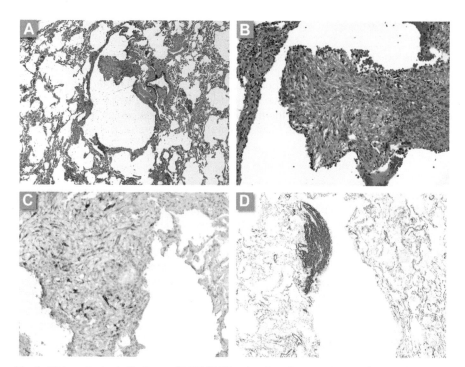

Fig. 2. Histopathologic findings of LAM (H&E-stained section at 5X magnification.) (*A*) H&E-stained section at low power shows a cystic structure with a nodule of LAM cells protruding into the cyst space in a polypoid manner (H&E stain). (*B*) High-power image of the LAM nodule demonstrating clusters of spindle-shaped cells growing in a haphazard manner (H&E stain). (*C*) HMB45 immunohistochemical stain of LAM cells shows patchy cytoplasmic staining (HMB45 stain). (*D*) SMA (smooth muscle active) immunohistochemistry stain highlights the nodules of smooth muscle cells within the wall of a cyst in LAM (SMA stain). (*Courtesy of* Carlyne D. Cool, MD, and Steve D. Groshong, MD, Denver, CO.)

include septal thickening, presumed to be consequent to lymphatic obstruction[36]; centrilobular nodules that may reflect pneumocyte hyperplasia; and ground-glass opacities or focal consolidations that may reflect hemosiderosis or hemorrhage.[37]

Renal AMLs are common (30%–50% of patients) (see **Fig. 1**). Other intra-abdominal findings include hepatic AMLs, lymphangiomyomas, retroperitoneal lymph nodes, and chylous peritoneum. The presence of characteristic lung cysts associated with either hepatic or renal AMLs and/or chylothorax supports a confident diagnosis of LAM.[26]

Management and Clinical Trails

Based on the landmark MILES trial (Multicenter International LAM Efficacy of Sirolimus),[38] inhibition of mTOR is indicated for patients with abnormal lung function (forced expiratory volume in the first second of expiration < 70% predicted), progressive lung disease, or clinically significant chylous effusions. mTOR inhibitors are also effective for other presentations such as AMLs and lymphangiomyomas and may decrease the frequency of pneumothoraces.[39,40] The MILED (Multicenter Interventional LAM Early Disease) trial is investigating the safety and efficacy of low-dose treatment to preserve lung function in earlier stages of disease (NCT03150914). Several other clinical trials are investigating novel therapies involving mTOR inhibitors and other investigational treatments, which can be found at The LAM Foundation Web site.[41]

BIRT-HOGG-DUBÉ
Background

The Birt-Hogg-Dubé (BHD) syndrome (BHDS) was first described in a case report of 2 siblings with unique skin lesions and a strong family history of similar skin lesions; one of the siblings later developed colon cancer.[42] In 1977, Birt and colleagues[43] described the autosomal dominance of the disorder among a large kindred with hereditary medullary carcinoma of the thyroid and skin lesions, which they diagnosed histologically as fibrofolliculomas. Most patients (~80%) currently present with diffuse pulmonary cysts.[44]

Pathogenesis

Numerous studies have defined the genetics and pathogenesis of BHDS. In 2001, the BHD gene locus was mapped to chromosome 17p[45] and later narrowed to a 700-kb region on chromosome 17p11.2.[46] In 2005, Schmidt and colleagues[47] reported germline mutations in 84% of affected families, and more than 150 unique mutations in the folliculin (FLCN) gene have since been reported. Most result in loss-of-function mutations and support the role of FLCN as a tumor suppressor gene. The loss of FLCN leads to BHD-associated tumors such as kidney tumors, the most serious manifestation, occurring in up to 34% of patients by age 50 years.[48] BHDS has been associated with other neoplasms such as colorectal cancer,[49] melanoma,[50] and thyroid and parathyroid tumors,[51] although data are limited to case reports and small series and the risk is uncertain.

Clinical and Radiologic Manifestations

The phenotypic expression of BHDS is highly variable even among families sharing the same FLCN mutation. Patients may present with any combination of skin, pulmonary, and renal findings. However, the absence of skin and renal manifestations does not exclude the diagnosis. Many patients with BHDS presenting with a pneumothorax are misdiagnosed as primary spontaneous pneumothorax or emphysema given the rarity of the syndrome.[52]

Skin manifestations include fibrofolliculomas and acrochordons, which are difficult to distinguish and may be spectrums of the same lesion.[43] These manifestations are characterized by round, grayish white papules 2 to 4 mm in size and most often distributed along the face, trunk, and neck, including the posterior ear (**Fig. 3**).[53] Although fibrofolliculomas are the most prevalent lesion, they may be subtle and patients may not seek medical care.

Pulmonary cysts are the most common systemic manifestation and typically appear after the fourth and fifth decades but can appear during teenage years. Pulmonary cysts are elliptical or "floppy," thin walled, and typically distributed along the basilar medial region of the lungs (see **Fig. 3**). Studies suggest that the number and size of the cysts typically remain stable.[30] Cysts do not typically impact pulmonary function until the development of a pneumothorax. Histopathologic examination of cysts in patients with BHDS with recurrent pneumothorax reveals inner surfaces lined with type II pneumocytelike cells suggesting slow-growing, hamartomatous cysts that may rupture.[54]

Escalon and colleagues[55] studied 47 subjects with isolated cystic lung disease in which thoracic radiologists were blinded to the final diagnoses, limited to BHD, lymphocytic interstitial pneumonia (LIP), or LAM. Lower lung-predominant cysts were significantly more likely among BHD or LIP compared with LAM, in which cysts were diffusely distributed. Furthermore, patients with BHDS were more likely to

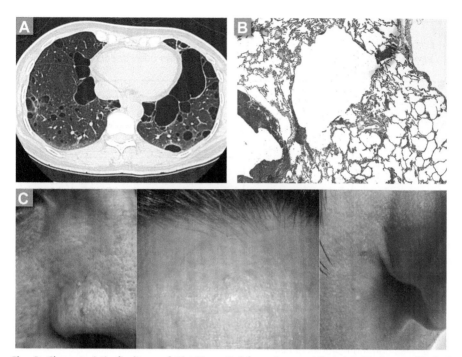

Fig. 3. Characteristic findings of Birt-Hogg-Dubé syndrome. (*A*) Axial CT shows elliptical thin-walled pulmonary cysts predominating in the paracardiac regions of the lower lungs. (*B*) Subpleural cystic structure lined by bland alveolar cells without atypical morphology (2X magnification, H&E stain). (*C*) White/gray papules on midface, forehead, and postauricular region of a patient with Birt-Hogg-Dubé syndrome characteristic of fibrofolliculomas or similar lesions (eg, acrochordons). ([*A*] *Courtesy of* Carlyne D. Cool, MD, and Steve D. Groshong, MD, Denver, CO.)

have elliptical, paramediastinal cysts. The investigators propose an algorithm to reliably differentiate BHDS from other cystic lung diseases (**Fig. 4**).[55]

Management

Similar to LAM, pulmonary cysts predispose patients to develop pneumothoraces. Although the risk for initial pneumothorax is relatively low (~24%), the risk for recurrence is high (75%).[56] For this reason, pleurodesis has been suggested with the first event to avoid the morbidity associated with repeat events.[57] Certain activities, such as scuba diving, increase the risk of pneumothorax due to potential expansion of cysts from transthoracic pressure changes. Although air travel is considered safe among patients with diffuse cystic lung disease,[58] subtle symptoms of pneumothorax may go unrecognized by patients.[58] For this reason, patients with extensive cystic disease, prior pneumothoraces, or new symptoms of chest pain should seek evaluation before air travel. Tobacco smoking and of other substances is discouraged despite limited data that such exposure increased the risk of pneumothorax.[56]

Screening for renal tumors should begin at age 20 years (per expert opinion)[59] or at the time of diagnosis preferably with MRI, which is more sensitive and specific than ultrasonography, and avoids the cumulative radiation exposure with CT. Surveillance should continue at least every 36 months until a mass is identified, which will determine management.[60] Most tumors have an indolent behavior. The risk of metastases

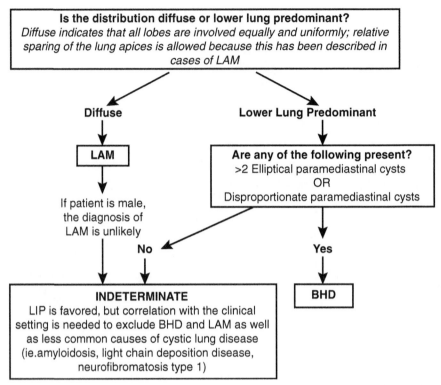

Fig. 4. Algorithm to differentiate BHDS, LIP, and LAM in patients with isolated cystic lung disease. (*From* Escalon JG, Richards JC, Koelsch T, Downey GP, Lynch DA. Isolated Cystic Lung Disease: An Algorithmic Approach to Distinguishing Birt-Hogg-Dubé Syndrome, Lymphangioleiomyomatosis, and Lymphocytic Interstitial Pneumonia. AJR Am J Roentgenol. 2019;1-5. Copyright © 2022 American Journal of Roentgenology.)

increases with tumor size, and kidney-sparing resection is recommended for tumors larger than 3 cm in diameter, along with resection of all additional tumors detected during surgery.[60]

Genetic testing may detect germline mutations in the folliculin (FLCN) gene, which confirms the diagnosis. Some patients (~5%) may be FLCN mutation-negative by DNA sequencing yet carry intragenic deletions/duplications detectable by more advanced molecular diagnostic methods.[61] The penetrance of FLCN mutations is high among affected families, and genetic counseling should be encouraged for first-degree relatives of patients. Carriers of FLCN mutations should undergo regular (every 3 years) imaging surveillance for kidney tumors.[60]

LYMPHOID INTERSTITIAL PNEUMONIA
Background

LIP is characterized by infiltration of the pulmonary interstitium by dense lymphoid tissue.[62] The radiographic LIP pattern is most commonly seen as a pulmonary manifestation of systemic collagen vascular diseases.[63] Other disease associations with LIP include dysproteinemias, infections (eg, Epstein-Barr virus, human T lymphotropic virus 1, or human immunodeficiency virus [HIV]), and rarely drug reactions (eg, phenytoin).[64] The dense accrual of lymphoid tissue implies risk for lymphoproliferative disease, particularly small B-cell lymphomas of extranodal marginal zone type, as well as polyclonal lymphoproliferative conditions associated with viral infections.[63] Idiopathic LIP is rare and must be distinguished from systemic and lymphoproliferative conditions.

Pathogenesis

The histopathologic pattern involves a dense layer of lymphocytes, plasma cells, and histiocytes with alveolar septal infiltration and along the bronchi and vasculature. (**Fig. 5**C) Granulomatous and lymphocytic interstitial lung disease (GLILD) is considered a variant of LIP associated with common variable immunodeficiency (CVID), but cysts are rarely seen in GLILD.[65] Germinal centers may become prominent along the airways and lymphatic channels, in which case lymphoproliferative conditions should be considered (**Fig. 5**D). In the idiopathic form of LIP, immunophenotyping would show absence of clonality.[66] When the nodular lymphoid hyperplasia is prominent along the bronchioles then Sjögren syndrome should be strongly considered[67] and coexisting amyloidosis may also be seen in this context[68] (**Fig. 5**B).

Clinical and Radiologic Manifestations

The cystic airspaces associated with LIP range from 1 to 30 mm, are typically peribronchovascular in distribution, and seem to represent dilated small bronchi and bronchioles from partial obstruction by lymphocytic infiltration (**Fig. 5**A).[69,70] Ground-glass opacities, poorly defined centrolobular nodules, and bronchovascular and septal thickening may also be seen (**Fig. 5**E,F).[71] The ground-glass opacities may improve with treatment, but new cysts may develop in areas of centrilobular nodules and consolidations may evolve into honeycombing.[72] Larger nodules (11–30 mm in diameter), consolidations, and pleural effusions are more common among LIP associated with lymphoma.[67,73]

Management Considerations

The natural history of LIP varies according to the underlying disease process. When LIP is associated with autoimmune disease (eg, Sjögren syndrome), management is based on the severity of pulmonary impairment and evidence of progression. Treatment is directed at the underlying condition, and some regimens may treat both systemic and pulmonary manifestations.[63,74] It is important to exclude secondary conditions such as GLILD among patients with CVID, HIV, and secondary infections from immune deficiency syndromes or secondary to immunosuppression. Lymphoma may develop in approximately 5% of patients with LIP with an increased risk in those with Sjögren syndrome.[63] Malignant transformation may be suggested by larger nodules or those increasing in size, pleural effusions, and alveolar consolidations[67,73]; polyclonality is key to differentiate LIP from lymphoma.[75]

AMYLOIDOSIS AND LIGHT CHAIN DEPOSITION
Background and Pathogenesis

Amyloidosis is the abnormal deposition of low-molecular-weight proteins into highly structured fibrils, which, in their native state, would otherwise circulate in plasma. The deposition of "amyloid deposits" results in a broad range of clinical manifestations depending on their type and location. The major types of systemic amyloidosis include the primary types (light chain [AL] and transthyretin [ATTR]), which account for most systemic amyloid.[76] Secondary amyloidosis (AA) is a rare systemic complication of chronic disease resulting in sustained production of serum amyloid A, an acute phase reactant, and most often affects the kidney leading to proteinuria.[77] Light chain

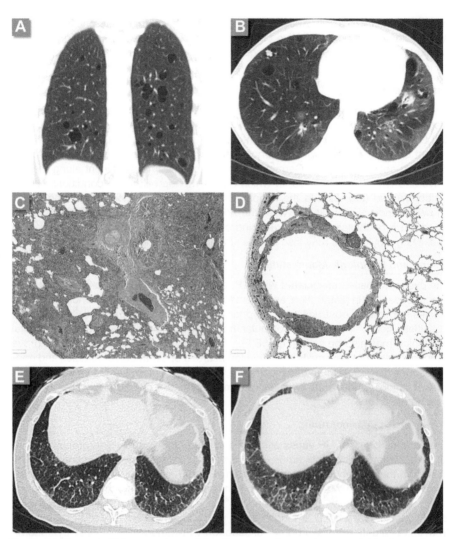

Fig. 5. (*A*) Coronal CT in a patient with Sjögren syndrome shows multiple lower lung-predominant thin-walled cysts with peribronchovascular predominance, compatible with LIP. (*B*) Axial CT through the lower lungs in a patient with biopsy-proven LIP and amyloidosis in Sjögren syndrome shows a combination of irregular nodules, cysts, and ground-glass opacities. (*C*) Low-power image demonstrating diffuse interstitial infiltrate by mature lymphocytes and plasma cells. Cysts are seen adjacent to airways (2X magnification, H&E stain). (*D*) Lymphoid follicles with germinal centers in a patient with Sjögren syndrome and cystic lung disease (2X magnification, H&E stain). (*E, F*) CT scans 2 years apart in a patient with LIP and Sjögren syndrome show increased ground-glass abnormality and septal thickening indicating progression of lymphocytic infiltrates. Bronchoalveolar lavage demonstrated 60% lymphocytic predominance without monoclonality or infection. ([*C, D*] *Courtesy of* Carlyne D. Cool, MD, and Steve D. Groshong, MD, Denver, CO.)

deposition disease (LCDD) reflects the presence of monoclonal deposits composed of light chains only and is typically associated with lymphoproliferative diseases with prominent kidney involvement.[78]

Clinical and Radiologic Manifestations

Pulmonary amyloidosis typically presents with multiple lung nodules. Cystic pulmonary amyloidosis is rare and may be associated with Sjögren syndrome or mucosa-associated lymphoid tissue lymphoma (**Fig. 6**).[79,80] The lung cysts are thought to arise from obstruction of distal airways from amyloid deposits.[79] Pulmonary lung function tests may be normal, obstructive, or have an isolated reduction in diffusing capacity.[79]

Management

The diagnosis of pulmonary amyloidosis requires lung biopsy to demonstrate amyloid deposits, which stain with Congo red dye or exhibit apple-green birefringence under polarized light. Biopsy is usually considered for growth of a nodule to exclude other processes (eg, lung cancer or lymphoma). LCDD can be progressive and lead to

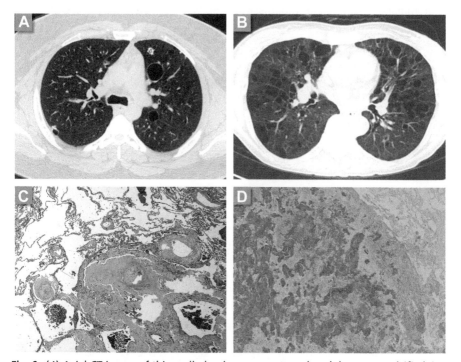

Fig. 6. (A) Axial CT image of thin-walled pulmonary cysts and nodules, some calcified, in a patient with biopsy-proven LIP and amyloidosis. (B) Axial CT image of diffuse lung cysts in the mid and upper lung zones in a patient with advanced LCDD of the kidney secondary to multiple myeloma. (C) Nodular amyloidosis characterized by intra-alveolar and interstitial deposits of amorphous eosinophilic material (2X magnification, H&E stain). (D) Congo red stain highlights the amyloid material (2X magnification, congo red stain). ([C] *Courtesy of* Carlyne D. Cool, MD, Denver, CO; and [D] *From* Achchar RD, Groshong SD and Cool CD. Differential Diagnoses in Surgical Pathology: Pulmonary Pathology. Wolters Kluwer; 2016.)

respiratory failure. Treatment is directed at the underlying lymphoproliferative disease, if present.[81]

PULMONARY LANGERHANS CELL HISTIOCYTOSIS
Background

pLCH, previously called pulmonary eosinophilic granuloma or histiocytosis X, is a smoking-related lung disease predominantly seen in young adults.[82] By contrast, systemic Langerhans cell histiocytosis (LCH) is a rare histiocytic disorder characterized by single or multiple osteolytic lesions, although histocytes can infiltrate any organ, particularly bones (although sparing the heart and kidneys). Systemic LCH may be diagnosed at any age but is more common in children (especially younger children) and has no apparent association with cigarette smoking.[83] The 2 conditions seem to be unrelated yet are indistinguishable histologically when the systemic eosinophilic granuloma of LCH involves the lung.[84]

Pathogenesis

pLCH has 2 distinct histopathologic manifestations: a cellular phase and a fibrotic phase. The natural history of pLCH includes the early cellular form with abundance of Langerhans cells and tissue eosinophilia.[85] As the lesions age, Langerhans and other immune cells become progressively depleted and overshadowed by fibrosis.

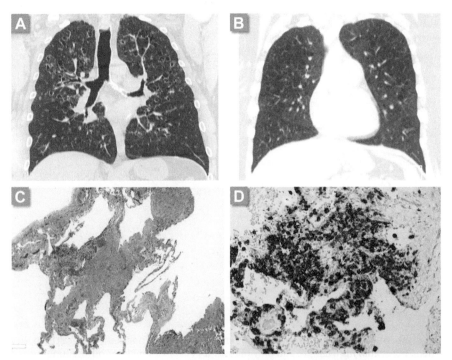

Fig. 7. (*A, B*) Coronal CT images in a patient with pLCH show characteristic irregular cysts with mid to upper zone predominance, relative sparing of the costophrenic sulci, and scattered small nodules [(A, 5X magnification, H&E stain) (B, 10X magnification, CD1a stain)]. (*C*). Bronchiolocentric stellate (*starlike*) scars develop with aging of the lesions and depletion of the Langerhans cells. (*D*) Immunohistochemical stain for CD1a highlights the Langerhans cells. ([*C, D*] Courtesy of Steve D. Groshong, MD, Denver, CO.)

In some patients, only the residual stellate scar may be left with pulmonary function significantly compromised.[86,87] In such cases, imaging may demonstrate diffuse disease, yet biopsied tissue may exhibit only stellate fibrotic lesions centered on the terminal airways without any identifiable interstitial inflammatory disease (**Fig. 7**).

Clinical and Radiologic Manifestations

pLCH typically presents in young adults (ages 20–40 years) who are cigarette smokers, with nonspecific pulmonary symptoms (cough, dyspnea, chest pain), pneumothorax, or may be incidentally diagnosed on imaging. Some may present with systemic symptoms (fatigue, weight, fever). Pulmonary cysts are seen in almost all cases; these may be thin or thick walled, often irregular in outline, and usually predominate in the mid and upper parts of lungs (see **Fig. 7**). Nodules are seen in many cases, and the combination of cysts and nodules in a cigarette smoker should always suggest pLCH. Extrapulmonary manifestations may involve the pituitary, bone, skin, and lymph nodes, and patients may present with bone pain or pathologic fractures, signs of diabetes insipidus, or atypical skin lesions. Longitudinal study suggests that 5% of patients with pulmonary involvement alone at diagnosis may subsequently develop extrapulmonary manifestations.[88]

Management Considerations

Evaluation should exclude other causes of cystic lung disease, including testing for alpha-1 antitrypsin deficiency particularly if there is airflow obstruction, and identify

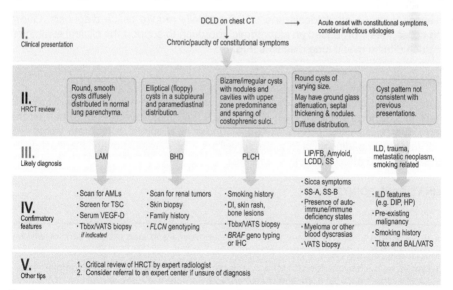

Fig. 8. An algorithmic approach to the diagnosis of diffuse cystic lung disease. BAL, bronchoalveolar lavage; BRAF, v-Raf murine sarcoma viral oncogene homolog; DCLD, diffuse cystic lung disease; DI, diabetes insipidus; DIP, desquamative interstitial pneumonia; FB, follicular bronchiolitis; FLCN, folliculin; HP, hypersensitivity pneumonitis; IHC, immunohistochemistry; ILD, interstitial lung disease; SS, Sjögren syndrome; Tbbx, transbronchial biopsy; VATS, video-assisted thoracoscopic surgery. (Modified with permission of the American Thoracic Society. Copyright © 2022 American Thoracic Society. All rights reserved. Gupta et al. 2015, Diffuse Cystic Lung Disease Part II, AJRCCM, Vol 192 p17-29. The American Journal of Respiratory and Critical Care Medicine is an official journal of the American Thoracic Society.)

symptoms suggesting extrapulmonary involvement. Lung function impairment, especially airflow obstruction, is predictive of adverse outcomes,[85] and early diagnosis with lung function testing may facilitate early intervention. Once the diagnosis is confirmed, management includes (1) smoking cessation and avoidance of all second-hand smoking exposure, (2) consideration for pharmacotherapy (eg, bronchodilators and chemotherapy), and (3) assessment for pulmonary-related complications such as hypoxemic respiratory failure, pneumothoraces, and secondary pulmonary hypertension.[89]

For systemic LCH and other histiocytic disorders, somatic mutations in the MAPK pathway, such as BRAF V600 E, seem to correlate with more severe disease,[90] and treatment with vemurafenib, an inhibitor of BRAF V600 kinase, may decrease risk for disease progression.[91] The role of targeted therapy for MAPK pathway mutations remains unclear, particularly for pLCH; however, testing at the time of diagnosis should be considered whenever possible (ie, surgical lung biopsy) given the future potential for treatment in refractory cases.

Diagnostic Approach to Diffuse Cystic Lung Diseases

A systematic approach can narrow the differential diagnosis of diffuse cystic lung disease and starts with a detailed history and physical examination. For example, sicca symptoms may suggest autoimmune-related LIP, and smoking exposure is a requisite for pLCH. A family history of recurrent pneumothoraces, skin lesions, or kidney cancer may suggest BHDS, and physical examination may reveal BHD skin lesions or clues to TSC-LAM. Additional testing may provide diagnostic confirmation such as elevated serum VEGF-D level for LAM or pathogenic FLCN gene mutation for BHD. Other diseases such as amyloidosis and LCDD typically require tissue diagnosis. Gupta and colleagues[59] proposed an algorithmic approach to support the clinical evaluation for such diffuse cystic lung diseases (**Fig. 8**).

SUMMARY

Lung cysts are commonly encountered with chest imaging and can be a diagnostic challenge. Expert review of chest HRCT is still the most valuable tool to narrow the diagnostic possibilities.[92] An accurate diagnosis is required to facilitate treatment, and, in some conditions, adequate surveillance of extrapulmonary manifestations for patients and affected family members.

CLINICS CARE POINTS

- It is essential to distinguish lung cysts from emphysema and lung cavities, each of which convey different diagnostic considerations.

- Lymphangioleiomyomatosis (LAM) occurs in patients with tuberous sclerosis complex (TSC-LAM) or the "sporadic" form and characterized by progressive cystic destruction of the lung, recurrent pneumothoraces, chylous effusions and renal angiomyolipomas. Elevated levels of vascular endothelial growth factor (VEGF-D) > 800 pg/ml can distinguish LAM from other cystic lung diseases. Inhibition of mTOR is indicated for patients with impaired lung function (FEV1 < 70% predicted), progressive lung disease, or clinically significant chylous effusions.

- Birt-Hogg-Dube syndrome is an autosomal dominant disorder attributed to mutations in the folliculin (FLCN) gene which confirms the diagnosis. Clinical features include fibrofolliculomas (along the face, trunk and neck), pneumothoraces, and paramediastinal lung cysts. Surveillance for renal tumors should begin at age 20 years, preferably with MRI, every 36 months.

- Lymphoid interstitial pneumonia (LIP) is characterized by lung cysts with peribronchovascular distribution and most often associated with autoimmune disease. It is important to exclude secondary conditions such as immune dysregulation (e.g. CVID) and infections. Lymphoma may develop in 5% of cases suggested by lung nodules, pleural effusions and alveolar consolidations; polyclonality is key to distinguish LIP from lymphoma.

- Pulmonary Langerhans Cell Histiocytosis (pLCH) is a smoking-related lung disease characterized by the combination of lung nodules and irregular lung cysts which predominate in the mid and upper lung. Evaluation should exclude alpha-1 antitrypsin deficiency and extrapulmonary involvement. Smoking cessation and avoidance of all second-hand smoking exposure is essential.

DISCLOSURE

The authors have no disclosures related to the content of this work.

REFERENCES

1. Hansell DM, Bankier AA, MacMahon H, et al. Fleischner Society: glossary of terms for thoracic imaging. Radiology 2008;246(3):697–722.
2. Woodring JH, Fried AM. Significance of wall thickness in solitary cavities of the lung: a follow-up study. AJR Am J Roentgenol 1983;140(3):473–4.
3. Moss J, Avila NA, Barnes PM, et al. Prevalence and clinical characteristics of lymphangioleiomyomatosis (LAM) in patients with tuberous sclerosis complex. Am J Respir Crit Care Med 2001;164(4):669–71.
4. Ryu JH, Moss J, Beck GJ, et al. The NHLBI lymphangioleiomyomatosis registry: characteristics of 230 patients at enrollment. Am J Respir Crit Care Med 2006; 173(1):105–11.
5. Han MK, Tyburczy ME, Darling TN, et al. Apparent Sporadic Lymphangioleiomyomatosis in a Man as a Result of Extreme Mosaicism for a TSC2 Mutation. Ann Am Thorac Soc 2017;14(7):1227–9.
6. Ogorek B, Hamieh L, Lasseter K, et al. Generalised mosaicism for TSC2 mutation in isolated lymphangioleiomyomatosis. Eur Respir J 2019;54(4). https://doi.org/ 10.1183/13993003.00938-2019.
7. European Chromosome 16 Tuberous Sclerosis C. Identification and characterization of the tuberous sclerosis gene on chromosome 16. Cell 1993;75(7):1305–15.
8. van Slegtenhorst M, de Hoogt R, Hermans C, et al. Identification of the tuberous sclerosis gene TSC1 on chromosome 9q34. Science 1997;277(5327):805–8.
9. Henske EP, McCormack FX. Lymphangioleiomyomatosis - a wolf in sheep's clothing. J Clin Invest 2012;122(11):3807–16.
10. Krymskaya VP, McCormack FX. Lymphangioleiomyomatosis: A Monogenic Model of Malignancy. Annu Rev Med 2017;68:69–83.
11. Kumasaka T, Seyama K, Mitani K, et al. Lymphangiogenesis-mediated shedding of LAM cell clusters as a mechanism for dissemination in lymphangioleiomyomatosis. Am J Surg Pathol 2005;29(10):1356–66.
12. Ando H, Ogawa M, Watanabe Y, et al. Lymphangioleiomyoma of the Uterus and Pelvic Lymph Nodes: A Report of 3 Cases, Including the Potentially Earliest Manifestation of Extrapulmonary Lymphangioleiomyomatosis. Int J Gynecol Pathol 2020;39(3):227–32.
13. Guo M, Yu JJ, Perl AK, et al. Single-Cell Transcriptomic Analysis Identifies a Unique Pulmonary Lymphangioleiomyomatosis Cell. Am J Respir Crit Care Med 2020;202(10):1373–87.

14. Tobino K, Johkoh T, Fujimoto K, et al. Computed tomographic features of lymphangioleiomyomatosis: evaluation in 138 patients. Eur J Radiol 2015;84(3): 534–41.
15. Avila NA, Dwyer AJ, Rabel A, et al. Sporadic lymphangioleiomyomatosis and tuberous sclerosis complex with lymphangioleiomyomatosis: comparison of CT features. Radiology 2007;242(1):277–85.
16. Young LR, Inoue Y, McCormack FX. Diagnostic potential of serum VEGF-D for lymphangioleiomyomatosis. N Engl J Med 2008;358(2):199–200.
17. Young L, Lee HS, Inoue Y, et al. Serum VEGF-D a concentration as a biomarker of lymphangioleiomyomatosis severity and treatment response: a prospective analysis of the Multicenter International Lymphangioleiomyomatosis Efficacy of Sirolimus (MILES) trial. Lancet Respir Med 2013;1(6):445–52.
18. Yu JJ, Robb VA, Morrison TA, et al. Estrogen promotes the survival and pulmonary metastasis of tuberin-null cells. Proc Natl Acad Sci U S A 2009;106(8): 2635–40.
19. Prizant H, Sen A, Light A, et al. Uterine-specific loss of Tsc2 leads to myometrial tumors in both the uterus and lungs. Mol Endocrinol 2013;27(9):1403–14.
20. Prizant H, Taya M, Lerman I, et al. Estrogen maintains myometrial tumors in a lymphangioleiomyomatosis model. Endocr Relat Cancer 2016;23(4):265–80.
21. Liu HJ, Lizotte PH, Du H, et al. TSC2-deficient tumors have evidence of T cell exhaustion and respond to anti-PD-1/anti-CTLA-4 immunotherapy. JCI Insight 2018;3(8). https://doi.org/10.1172/jci.insight.98674.
22. Maisel K, Merrilees MJ, Atochina-Vasserman EN, et al. Immune Checkpoint Ligand PD-L1 Is Upregulated in Pulmonary Lymphangioleiomyomatosis. Am J Respir Cell Mol Biol 2018;59(6):723–32.
23. Gupta N, Lee HS, Ryu JH, et al. The NHLBI LAM Registry: Prognostic Physiologic and Radiologic Biomarkers Emerge From a 15-Year Prospective Longitudinal Analysis. Chest 2019;155(2):288–96.
24. Johnson SR, Tattersfield AE. Clinical experience of lymphangioleiomyomatosis in the UK. Thorax 2000;55(12):1052–7.
25. Almoosa KF, Ryu JH, Mendez J, et al. Management of pneumothorax in lymphangioleiomyomatosis: effects on recurrence and lung transplantation complications. Chest 2006;129(5):1274–81.
26. Gupta N, Finlay GA, Kotloff RM, et al. Lymphangioleiomyomatosis Diagnosis and Management: High-Resolution Chest Computed Tomography, Transbronchial Lung Biopsy, and Pleural Disease Management. An Official American Thoracic Society/Japanese Respiratory Society Clinical Practice Guideline. Am J Respir Crit Care Med 2017;196(10):1337–48.
27. Moua T, Olson EJ, Jean HC, et al. Resolution of chylous pulmonary congestion and respiratory failure in lymphangioleiomyomatosis with sirolimus therapy. Am J Respir Crit Care Med 2012;186(4):389–90.
28. Brook-Carter PT, Peral B, Ward CJ, et al. Deletion of the TSC2 and PKD1 genes associated with severe infantile polycystic kidney disease–a contiguous gene syndrome. Nat Genet 1994;8(4):328–32.
29. Avila NA, Kelly JA, Chu SC, et al. Lymphangioleiomyomatosis: abdominopelvic CT and US findings. Radiol 2000;216(1):147–53.
30. David M, Hansell DL, Page McAdams H, Alexander AB. Imaging of diseases of the chest. 5th edition. MOSBY, Elsevier; 2010.
31. Carrington CB, Cugell DW, Gaensler EA, et al. Lymphangioleiomyomatosis. Physiologic-pathologic-radiologic correlations. Am Rev Respir Dis 1977;116(6): 977–95.

32. Raoof S, Bondalapati P, Vydyula R, et al. Cystic Lung Diseases: Algorithmic Approach. Chest 2016;150(4):945–65.
33. AL K. Katzenstein and Askin's surgical pathology of non-neoplastic lung disease. 1997;(3rd Edition).
34. Bonetti F, Chiodera PL, Pea M, et al. Transbronchial biopsy in lymphangiomyomatosis of the lung. HMB45 for diagnosis. Am J Surg Pathol 1993;17(11):1092–102.
35. Miller WT, Cornog JL Jr, Lymphangiomyomatosis Sullivan MA. A clinical-roentgenologic-pathologic syndrome. Am J Roentgenol Radium Ther Nucl Med 1971;111(3):565–72.
36. Rappaport DC, Weisbrod GL, Herman SJ, et al. Pulmonary lymphangioleiomyomatosis: high-resolution CT findings in four cases. AJR Am J Roentgenol 1989;152(5):961–4.
37. Muller NL, Chiles C, Kullnig P. Pulmonary lymphangiomyomatosis: correlation of CT with radiographic and functional findings. Radiol 1990;175(2):335–9.
38. McCormack FX, Inoue Y, Moss J, et al. Efficacy and safety of sirolimus in lymphangioleiomyomatosis. N Engl J Med 2011;364(17):1595–606.
39. Taveira-DaSilva AM, Hathaway O, Stylianou M, et al. Changes in lung function and chylous effusions in patients with lymphangioleiomyomatosis treated with sirolimus. Ann Intern Med 2011;154(12):797–805. W-292-3.
40. Bissler JJ, Kingswood JC, Radzikowska E, et al. Everolimus for renal angiomyolipoma in patients with tuberous sclerosis complex or sporadic lymphangioleiomyomatosis: extension of a randomized controlled trial. Nephrol Dial Transpl 2016;31(1):111–9.
41. The LAM Foundation. Available at: https://wwwthelamfoundationorg/.
42. Hornstein OP, Knickenberg M. Perifollicular fibromatosis cutis with polyps of the colon–a cutaneo-intestinal syndrome sui generis. Arch Dermatol Res (1975) 1975;253(2):161–75.
43. Birt AR, Hogg GR, Dube WJ. Hereditary multiple fibrofolliculomas with trichodiscomas and acrochordons. Arch Dermatol 1977;113(12):1674–7.
44. Daccord C, Good JM, Morren MA, et al. Birt-Hogg-Dube syndrome. Eur Respir Rev 2020;29(157). https://doi.org/10.1183/16000617.0042-2020.
45. Khoo SK, Bradley M, Wong FK, et al. Birt-Hogg-Dube syndrome: mapping of a novel hereditary neoplasia gene to chromosome 17p12-q11.2. Oncogene 2001;20(37):5239–42.
46. Nickerson ML, Warren MB, Toro JR, et al. Mutations in a novel gene lead to kidney tumors, lung wall defects, and benign tumors of the hair follicle in patients with the Birt-Hogg-Dube syndrome. Cancer Cell 2002;2(2):157–64.
47. Schmidt LS, Nickerson ML, Warren MB, et al. Germline BHD-mutation spectrum and phenotype analysis of a large cohort of families with Birt-Hogg-Dube syndrome. Am J Hum Genet 2005;76(6):1023–33.
48. Pavlovich CP, Grubb RL 3rd, Hurley K, et al. Evaluation and management of renal tumors in the Birt-Hogg-Dube syndrome. J Urol 2005;173(5):1482–6.
49. Nahorski MS, Lim DH, Martin L, et al. Investigation of the Birt-Hogg-Dube tumour suppressor gene (FLCN) in familial and sporadic colorectal cancer. J Med Genet 2010;47(6):385–90.
50. Mota-Burgos A, Acosta EH, Marquez FV, et al. Birt-Hogg-Dube syndrome in a patient with melanoma and a novel mutation in the FCLN gene. Int J Dermatol 2013;52(3):323–6.
51. Lindor NM, Kasperbauer J, Lewis JE, et al. Birt-Hogg-Dube syndrome presenting as multiple oncocytic parotid tumors. Hered Cancer Clin Pract 2012;10(1):13.

52. Gupta N, BY Sunwoo, Kotloff RM. Birt-Hogg-Dube Syndrome. Clin Chest Med 2016;37(3):475–86.

53. Tong Y, Schneider JA, Coda AB, et al. Birt-Hogg-Dube Syndrome: A Review of Dermatological Manifestations and Other Symptoms. Am J Clin Dermatol 2018; 19(1):87–101.

54. Furuya M, Tanaka R, Koga S, et al. Pulmonary cysts of Birt-Hogg-Dube syndrome: a clinicopathologic and immunohistochemical study of 9 families. Am J Surg Pathol 2012;36(4):589–600.

55. Escalon JG, Richards JC, Koelsch T, et al. Isolated Cystic Lung Disease: An Algorithmic Approach to Distinguishing Birt-Hogg-Dube Syndrome, Lymphangioleiomyomatosis, and Lymphocytic Interstitial Pneumonia. AJR Am J Roentgenol 2019;19:1–5.

56. Toro JR, Pautler SE, Stewart L, et al. Lung cysts, spontaneous pneumothorax, and genetic associations in 89 families with Birt-Hogg-Dube syndrome. Am J Respir Crit Care Med 2007;175(10):1044–53.

57. Gupta N, Seyama K, McCormack FX. Pulmonary manifestations of Birt-Hogg-Dube syndrome. Fam Cancer 2013;12(3):387–96.

58. Hu X, Cowl CT, Baqir M, et al. Air travel and pneumothorax. Chest 2014;145(4): 688–94.

59. Gupta N, Vassallo R, Wikenheiser-Brokamp KA, et al. Diffuse Cystic Lung Disease. Part II. Am J Respir Crit Care Med 2015;192(1):17–29.

60. Stamatakis L, Metwalli AR, Middelton LA, et al. Diagnosis and management of BHD-associated kidney cancer. Fam Cancer 2013;12(3):397–402.

61. Benhammou JN, Vocke CD, Santani A, et al. Identification of intragenic deletions and duplication in the FLCN gene in Birt-Hogg-Dube syndrome. Genes Chromosomes Cancer 2011;50(6):466–77.

62. Cha SI, Fessler MB, Cool CD, et al. Lymphoid interstitial pneumonia: clinical features, associations and prognosis. Eur Respir J 2006;28(2):364–9.

63. Swigris JJ, Berry GJ, Raffin TA, et al. Lymphoid interstitial pneumonia: a narrative review. Chest 2002;122(6):2150–64.

64. Cosgrove GPFM, Schwarz MI. Lymphoplasmacytic infiltrations of the lung. Interstitial lung diseases. 4th edition. Hamilton, Canada: BC Decker; 2003.

65. Wick La. Practical pulmonary pathology. 2011.

66. Julsrud PR, Brown LR, Li CY, et al. Pulmonary processes of mature-appearing lymphocytes: pseudolymphoma, well-differentiated lymphocytic lymphoma, and lymphocytic interstitial pneumonitis. Radiology 1978;127(2):289–96.

67. Strimlan CV, Rosenow EC 3rd, Divertie MB, et al. Pulmonary manifestations of Sjögren's syndrome. Chest 1976;70(03):354–61.

68. Strimlan CV, Rosenow EC 3rd, Weiland LH, et al. Lymphocytic interstitial pneumonitis. Review of 13 cases. Ann Intern Med 1978;88(5):616–21. https://doi.org/10.7326/0003-4819-88-5-616.

69. Ichikawa Y, Kinoshita M, Koga T, et al. Lung cyst formation in lymphocytic interstitial pneumonia: CT features. J Comput Assist Tomogr 1994;18(5):745–8.

70. Silva CI, Flint JD, Levy RD, et al. Diffuse lung cysts in lymphoid interstitial pneumonia: high-resolution CT and pathologic findings. J Thorac Imaging 2006;21(3): 241–4.

71. Johkoh T, Muller NL, Pickford HA, et al. Lymphocytic interstitial pneumonia: thin-section CT findings in 22 patients. Radiology 1999;212(2):567–72.

72. Johkoh T, Ichikado K, Akira M, et al. Lymphocytic interstitial pneumonia: follow-up CT findings in 14 patients. J Thorac Imaging 2000;15(3):162–7.

73. Zhu C, Hu J, Wu J, et al. Transformation of lymphoid interstitial pneumonia (LIP) into malignant lymphoma in patients with Sjögren's syndrome: a case report and literature review. J Cardiothorac Surg 2022;17(1):79.
74. Carsons SE, Vivino FB, Parke A, et al. Treatment Guidelines for Rheumatologic Manifestations of Sjögren's Syndrome: Use of Biologic Agents, Management of Fatigue, and Inflammatory Musculoskeletal Pain. Arthritis Care Res (Hoboken) 2017;69(4):517–27.
75. Travis WD, Galvin JR. Non-neoplastic pulmonary lymphoid lesions. Thorax 2001; 56(12):964–71.
76. Ravichandran S, Lachmann HJ, Wechalekar AD. Epidemiologic and Survival Trends in Amyloidosis, 1987-2019. N Engl J Med 2020;382(16):1567–8.
77. Papa R, Lachmann HJ. Secondary, AA, Amyloidosis. Rheum Dis Clin North Am 2018;44(4):585–603.
78. Pozzi C, D'Amico M, Fogazzi GB, et al. Light chain deposition disease with renal involvement: clinical characteristics and prognostic factors. Am J Kidney Dis 2003;42(6):1154–63.
79. Zamora AC, White DB, Sykes AM, et al. Amyloid-associated Cystic Lung Disease. Chest 2016;149(5):1223–33.
80. Lantuejoul S, Moulai N, Quetant S, et al. Unusual cystic presentation of pulmonary nodular amyloidosis associated with MALT-type lymphoma. Eur Respir J 2007; 30(3):589–92.
81. Colombat M, Stern M, Groussard O, et al. Pulmonary cystic disorder related to light chain deposition disease. Am J Respir Crit Care Med 2006;173(7):777–80.
82. Travis WD, Borok Z, Roum JH, et al. Pulmonary Langerhans cell granulomatosis (histiocytosis X). A clinicopathologic study of 48 cases. Am J Surg Pathol 1993; 17(10):971–86.
83. Howarth DM, Gilchrist GS, Mullan BP, et al. Langerhans cell histiocytosis: diagnosis, natural history, management, and outcome. Cancer May 15 1999;85(10):2278–90.
84. Colby TV, Lombard C. Histiocytosis X in the lung. Hum Pathol Oct 1983;14(10): 847–56.
85. Vassallo R, Ryu JH, Colby TV, et al. Pulmonary Langerhans'-cell histiocytosis. N Engl J Med Jun 29 2000;342(26):1969–78.
86. Brauner MW, Grenier P, Tijani K, et al. Pulmonary Langerhans cell histiocytosis: evolution of lesions on CT scans. Radiology 1997;204(2):497–502.
87. Wick K. Practical pulmonary pathology: a diagnostic approach. 3rd edition. Philadelphia, PA: Elsevier; 2018.
88. Benattia A, Bugnet E, Walter-Petrich A, et al. Long-term outcomes of adult pulmonary Langerhans cell histiocytosis: a prospective cohort. Eur Respir J 2022;59(5). https://doi.org/10.1183/13993003.01017-2021.
89. Gupta N, Vassallo R, Wikenheiser-Brokamp KA, et al. Diffuse Cystic Lung Disease. Part I. Am J Respir Crit Care Med 2015;191(12):1354–66.
90. Heritier S, Emile JF, Barkaoui MA, et al. BRAF Mutation Correlates With High-Risk Langerhans Cell Histiocytosis and Increased Resistance to First-Line Therapy. J Clin Oncol 2016;34(25):3023–30.
91. Diamond EL, Subbiah V, Lockhart AC, et al. Vemurafenib for BRAF V600-Mutant Erdheim-Chester Disease and Langerhans Cell Histiocytosis: Analysis of Data From the Histology-Independent, Phase 2, Open-label VE-BASKET Study. JAMA Oncol 2018;4(3):384–8.
92. Gupta N, Meraj R, Tanase D, et al. Accuracy of chest high-resolution computed tomography in diagnosing diffuse cystic lung diseases. Eur Respir J Oct 2015; 46(4):1196–9.

Interstitial Lung Disease and Anti-Neutrophil Cytoplasmic Antibody–Associated Vasculitis

A Review

Matthew Steward, BMBS, MRCP[a,b,]*,
Hannah Thould, BA, BMBCh, MRCP[a], Aye Myat Noe Khin, MBBS[a],
Michael A. Gibbons, PhD, FRCP[a,b]

KEYWORDS

- MeSH headings • Vasculitis • Lung diseases • Interstitial
- Anti-neutrophil cytoplasmic antibody-associated vasculitis • Extracellular traps

KEY POINTS

- Interstitial lung disease (ILD) is a common complication of anti-neutrophil cytoplasmic antibody–associated vasculitis (AAV) and correlates with poorer outcomes and quality of life for patients.
- Myeloperoxidase anti-neutrophil cytoplasmic antibodies (MPO-ANCA) are implicated in the pathogenesis of fibrosis, and therefore, patients with a diagnosis of microscopic polyangiitis or MPO-ANCA positivity with granulomatous polyangiitis are most likely to develop ILD.
- AAV-ILD may be present at diagnosis of AAV, or develop thereafter, but precedes a diagnosis of renal vasculitis in a significant proportion of patients.
- Interstitial abnormalities are common findings in patients with AAV, and ground-glass changes may represent alveolar hemorrhage in some cases. AAV-ILD most commonly displays a usual interstitial pneumonia (UIP) pattern of fibrosis.
- Treatment of patients with systemic vasculitis and ILD includes immunosuppression, although evidence is limited. Immunosuppression is unlikely to improve outcomes and may be harmful in those with UIP pattern fibrosis who may instead benefit from antifibrotic therapy.

[a] Academic Department of Respiratory Medicine, Royal Devon University Healthcare NHS Foundation Trust, Exeter, UK; [b] Department of Clinical and Biomedical Sciences, University of Exeter Medical School, Exeter, UK
* Corresponding author. Department of Respiratory Medicine, Wonford Hospital, Barrack Road, Exeter, Devon EX2 5DW, UK.
E-mail address: matt.steward1@nhs.net

Immunol Allergy Clin N Am 43 (2023) 379–388
https://doi.org/10.1016/j.iac.2023.01.001
0889-8561/23/© 2023 Elsevier Inc. All rights reserved.
immunology.theclinics.com

INTRODUCTION

Vasculitis is a systemic autoimmune condition resulting in inflammation of blood vessels and consequently affects multiple organ systems. Interstitial lung disease (ILD), itself a condition resulting in inflammation and/or fibrosis of the lung, is a serious complication in patients with anti-neutrophil cytoplasmic antibody (ANCA) -associated vasculitis (AAV). AAV is an umbrella term and refers to 3 vasculitides: microscopic polyangiitis (MPA), granulomatosis with polyangiitis (GPA), and eosinophilic granulomatosis with polyangiitis (EGPA).

At a cellular level, the presence of ANCA causes destruction of proteins within the neutrophil. Proteins most commonly affected are myeloperoxidase (MPO), associated with perinuclear "p-ANCA," and proteinase 3 (PR3), associated with cytoplasmic "c-ANCA." AAV is classified on the basis of detection of these autoantibodies by enzyme-linked immunosorbent assay, often in combination with histologic assessment. MPO-ANCA is strongly associated with MPA and less strongly associated with EGPA, whereas PR3-ANCA is associated with GPA.[1]

ILD in association with vasculitis was first documented by Nada and colleagues[2] in 1990, with the link between ANCA and ILD first being made in 1995.[3] Since the role of ANCA was first implicated in the development of ILD, MPO-ANCA and hence MPA have been shown to be most strongly correlated with the development of ILD. In case series of AAV-ILD, ANCA positivity is largely and often exclusively for MPO-ANCA,[4] with PR3-ANCA positivity seen much less commonly.[5]

Development of ILD in the presence of MPO-ANCA, but in the absence of a clinical syndrome of vasculitis, is also well documented, implying a pathogenic mechanism relating to MPO-ANCA itself. A proportion of patients with MPA are also known to have interstitial abnormalities predating the development of vasculitis clinically,[6] which also raises the question of ILD itself resulting in MPO-ANCA formation.

Around 5% to 10% of patients labeled as having idiopathic pulmonary fibrosis (IPF) have ANCA-positivity documented at diagnosis,[7,8] with a further 10% developing ANCA-positivity during subsequent follow-up.[9] Notably, these patients are not included in the 2015 European Respiratory Society/American Thoracic Society definition of interstitial pneumonia with autoimmune features. Detection and early recognition of lung involvement are critical in AAV patients, as it has a significant impact on mortality and long-term outcome.[10]

In this review, the authors examine the pathobiology of development of ILD in patients with AAV, the clinical implications of AAV-ILD, and synthesize current evidence to provide practical pointers for clinical practice.

DISCUSSION
Prevalence

The prevalence of AAV-ILD appears to display geographic and ethnic variance. This appears to be linked to inherent variability in risk factors for development of AAV. Putative triggers for AAV include genetic predisposition,[11] smoking,[12] and exposure to drugs,[13] solvents, and environmental particles, such as silica.[14]

Japan has the highest global prevalence of AAV and demonstrates a predominance of MPO-ANCA vasculitis, which is also reflected in other Asian regions,[15] whereas European heritage is correlated with PR3-ANCA vasculitis. Given the correlation between MPO-ANCA and development of AAV-ILD, Asian regions therefore report higher rates of AAV-ILD, with 1 Japanese cohort reporting an ILD rate of 45% in their MPO-ANCA cohort.[16]

Diagnosis of AAV itself has increased, with improved definitions and recognition, but remains rare with an estimated prevalence of between 300 and 421 per million[17,18] and an estimated incidence of around 20 to 22 per million per year.[15]

Pathogenesis of Antibody-Associated Vasculitis–Interstitial Lung Disease

There are several proposed mechanisms for the pathogenesis of lung fibrosis in AAV-ILD (**Fig. 1**). Most relate directly to the effects of MPO-ANCA within the lung, but there are some similarities with other common ILDs, particularly those with a usual interstitial pneumonia (UIP) pattern of fibrosis, such as IPF or rheumatoid arthritis-ILD.

IPF is strongly correlated with a single-nucleotide polymorphism in the promoter region rs35705950 on MUC5B, which encodes mucin 5B. This results in mucous hypersecretion, impaired ciliary function, aberrant lung repair mechanisms, and chronic lung inflammation with subsequent fibrogenesis.[19–21] The association of MUC5B polymorphism has since been demonstrated to have a strong correlation with MPO-ANCA and ILD in a Japanese cohort. MUC5B polymorphisms were not seen in healthy controls, nor in PR3-ANCA patients, and were only seen in patients with MPO-ANCA who also had radiographic evidence of ILD.[22] This suggests a shared pathway in the development of UIP pattern fibrosis in MPO-ANCA ILD and IPF.

The pathogenicity of MPO-ANCA itself has been demonstrated in vitro[23] and in vivo. When activated, MPO has cytotoxic effects on neutrophils, resulting in release of reactive oxygen species (ROS) with consequent oxidative stress and fibroblast proliferation.[24] ROS alongside the presence of MPO itself[25] results in activated neutrophils

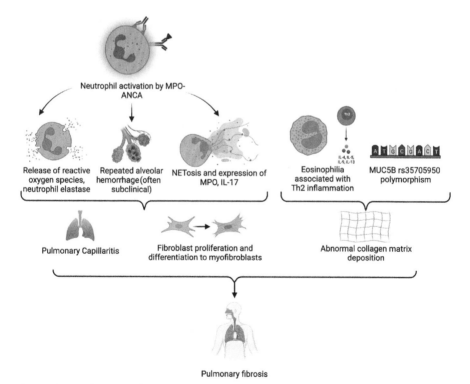

Fig. 1. The mechanisms of pathogenesis of fibrosis in AAV. IL-17, interleukin-17; Th2, T-helper cell 2. (Created with Biorender.com.)

releasing neutrophil extracellular traps (NETs). Release of these extracellular chromatin fiber networks is termed "NETosis" and was initially demonstrated as a mechanism of pathogen neutralisation,[26] but has since been shown to be pathogenic. NETs express proteins, such as interleukin-17[27] and neutrophil elastase (thereby activating transforming growth factor-β),[28] directly promote inflammation and differentiation of fibroblasts to myofibroblasts. The lung appears to be disproportionately affected by NET formation,[29] and the combination of these factors suggests why vasculitis patients with the presence of MPO-ANCA are predisposed to developing lung fibrosis.

The process of neutrophil activation, degranulation, and NETosis also results in destruction of the alveolar wall and pulmonary capillaritis.[30–32] Diffuse alveolar hemorrhage (DAH) is common in AAV and is seen across the spectrum of vasculitides,[33] and although half of patients with DAH have an underlying diagnosis of MPA, PR3-ANCA positivity is much more common when compared with rates seen with ILD.[34] DAH is a classic presentation of AAV and other pulmonary-renal syndromes and varies from being subclinical and identified on bronchoalveolar lavage or computed tomography (CT) scanning, to life-threatening hemoptysis and acute lung injury.

There is weak evidence to suggest that DAH may have a role in the development of ILD in a manner similar to pulmonary hemosiderosis owing to the inflammatory and oxidative effect of blood in the lung.[35] In addition, repeated episodes of subclinical DAH may also trigger aberrant lung repair mechanisms resulting in collagen and extracellular matrix deposition.[36]

Imaging

Pulmonary involvement (on imaging studies) is extremely common in AAV, with DAH and ILD being the most common findings seen on high-resolution computed tomography (HRCT). According to 1 retrospective study of 150 MPA patients in Japan, 97% had at least 1 lung abnormality on HRCT[37]; another retrospective study, which included 62 MPO-ANCA patients, had an 82% abnormal CT rate, with 94% of these abnormal scans suggesting interstitial involvement, such as ground-glass change.[38] In this context, ground-glass abnormalities are often thought to represent DAH. When compared with ANCA-negative vasculitis, pulmonary abnormalities were much more common with ANCA-positivity, again suggesting the pathogenicity of ANCA itself.[39]

Common parenchymal HRCT features of AAV include ground-glass opacities in most patients alongside reticular shadowing, interlobular septal thickening, consolidation, honeycombing, and bronchovascular bundle thickening.[6,37,40–42] Airway abnormalities are also reported in the form of bronchiolitis, bronchial wall thickening, and bronchiectasis.[6,37,41] Combined pulmonary fibrosis and emphysema has been recently reported in patients with MPA, suggesting the more complex picture of pulmonary involvement in MPA.[37,43,44]

Although a significant proportion of AAV-ILD patients will not have a definable pattern of ILD as per international consensus guidelines,[45] the predominant pattern of fibrosis in AAV-ILD is UIP.[6,46–51] This is the case for patients both with and without evidence of systemic vasculitis. Hallmarks of UIP include subpleural reticulation, honeycombing, and traction bronchodilatation, often heterogeneously interspersed with normal lung on histopathology and with a basal predominance.[45]

It should be mentioned that most studies looking at AAV-ILD include MPA or MPO-ANCA positivity in their inclusion criteria given the strong association with ILD development. As such, reporting of UIP as the predominant pattern of fibrosis is largely drawn from data for the MPA patient cohort. There are also studies reporting conflicting information, with 1 Chinese study reporting that only 9% of their AAV-ILD cohort had UIP compared with 64% with nonspecific interstitial pneumonia (NSIP).[10]

Imaging findings in AAV-ILD remains heterogeneous, with NSIP, desquamative interstitial pneumonia, and organizing pneumonia (OP) all being reported.[37,41,52,53]

Management

There have been no dedicated clinical trials to guide management of AAV-ILD. General principles for management should be guided by whether the patient has evidence of systemic vasculitis or an isolated ILD. Management of patients displaying systemic vasculitis is based on guidelines for the management of AAV itself, and evidence for use in AAV-ILD is limited to retrospective cohort studies and case reports. Where patients do not have systemic vasculitis, general principles of management for progressive fibrosing ILD (PF-ILD), idiopathic NSIP, or OP are recommended.

Immunosuppression

Management of AAV with lung involvement consists of induction of remission with a combination of glucocorticoids and rituximab/cyclophosphamide. Plasma exchange is often considered when DAH is present. Maintenance therapy thereafter is with weaning doses of glucocorticoids and the addition of steroid-sparing agents, such as azathioprine or mycophenolate mofetil.[54] Such therapy appears to have a positive impact on mortality.[42]

With respect to AAV-ILD, immunosuppression above that required for remission of vasculitis has no robust evidence. Some studies have suggested that additional cyclophosphamide or rituximab maintenance therapy confers a survival benefit at 5 years,[51] but other studies have failed to corroborate this.[37,55] Intense immunosuppression poses a serious risk of adverse events, including infection, and should be used with caution, particularly in the elderly, where there is some evidence of harm.[56] In patients with IPF, steroid use not only increases mortality but also is a risk factor as a trigger of an acute exacerbation of IPF,[57] and use should be avoided without a robust indication. Use of immunosuppression has additionally previously been associated with poorer outcomes for patients with IPF[58]; as such, in patients with AAV-ILD, a UIP pattern fibrosis on HRCT, and no evidence of a systemic vasculitis, immunosuppression is often avoided.

Antifibrotics

In the last few years, there has been discussion that the management of ILD may be better aligned to the pattern of disease, rather than the clinical syndrome.[59] Management of PF-ILD with nintedanib has been shown to be an effective treatment, regardless of clinical syndrome, in both the INBUILD and the RELIEF studies.[60,61] Extrapolation of this evidence to patients with AAV-ILD should be made with caution, but these investigators believe that treatment with nintedanib may be considered following discussion with the patient.

As previously discussed, MPO-ANCA ILD exhibits a predominance of UIP pattern fibrosis, and most patients also appear to have a PF-ILD phenotype.[62] Where fibrosis is seen, regardless of the pattern of disease, it is commonly suggested that these patients will have areas of UIP fibrosis histologically, and with time are likely to progress to a typical UIP pattern of fibrosis.[63]

In summary, evidence for treatment of AAV-ILD is limited, but immunosuppression for patients with systemic vasculitis is recommended, and continuation of immunosuppression may be considered for those with inflammatory-predominant AAV-ILD. For patients without vasculitis with a progressive fibrotic phenotype of ILD, and for those with UIP, antifibrotics may improve outcomes, whereas immunosuppression should be considered with caution.[64]

Clinical Outcomes

Poorer outcomes and increased mortality are seen in patients with AAV-ILD compared with those with AAV alone.[50] A meta-analysis of AAV-ILD has shown that respiratory failure and infective pneumonia were the most common causes of death, and that the risk of death for patients with AAV-ILD was 2.9 relative to controls. Importantly, this analysis did not demonstrate any survival benefit with the use of immunosuppression, but conclusions are difficult to draw given the heterogeneity of patterns of disease in AAV-ILD and the small numbers of patients in the included studies.[65]

Within AAV-ILD, the presence of UIP fibrosis is the single biggest factor negatively affecting mortality, and therefore, patients with MPA fare less well compared with GPA and EGPA cohorts.[6,37,49,66] Honeycombing on HRCT is a poor prognostic feature for all AAV-ILD,[63] as are elevated blood inflammatory markers, such as C-reactive protein and erythrocyte sedimentation rate.[10]

SUMMARY

AAV-ILD is a common complication of AAV and should be suspected in all patients with systemic vasculitis. It is most frequently seen in the presence of MPO-ANCA, and therefore in MPA, but the clinical course is heterogeneous, and ILD may predate (or antedate) vasculitis.

MPO-ANCA is implicated in the pathogenesis of pulmonary fibrosis. Treatment is based on expert consensus and limited data; prospective trials in this area would be beneficial given the potential for harm with immunosuppression in selected cases.

Antifibrotics are effective in the treatment of PF-ILD; their use in AAV-ILD is guided by limited data but may confer survival benefit for those patients with a progressive fibrotic phenotype, particularly those with a UIP pattern fibrosis.

CLINICS CARE POINTS

- Interstitial lung disease in antibody-associated vasculitis is common, affecting a quarter of patients. It is particularly common in patients with a diagnosis of microscopic polyangiitis.

- Myeloperoxidase–anti-neutrophil cytoplasmic antibody promotes lung inflammation, fibroblast proliferation, and differentiation. In combination with genetic susceptibility and extrinsic triggers, pulmonary fibrosis ensues.

- Imaging of antibody-associated vasculitis–interstitial lung disease commonly identifies ground-glass change, which may represent alveolar hemorrhage. Interstitial lung disease is heterogeneous, but usual interstitial pneumonia pattern fibrosis is the commonest pattern and is associated with poor outcomes.

- In patients with antibody-associated vasculitis–interstitial lung disease and systemic vasculitis, treatment is with standard immunosuppression for antibody-associated vasculitis ± antifibrotics.

- In patients with interstitial lung disease and anti-neutrophil cytoplasmic antibody positivity in the absence of vasculitis, treatment is guided by the predominant pattern of interstitial lung disease and should include consideration of antifibrotics for those with a progressive fibrotic phenotype.

DISCLOSURE

All authors confirm that they have no competing interests or financial disclosures to declare in relation to the writing of this article.

REFERENCES

1. Moiseev S, Bossuyt X, Arimura Y, et al. International Consensus on Antineutrophil Cytoplasmic Antibodies Testing in Eosinophilic Granulomatosis with Polyangiitis. Am J Respir Crit Care Med 2020;202(10):1360–72.
2. Nada AK, Torres VE, Ryu JH, et al. Pulmonary fibrosis as an unusual clinical manifestation of a pulmonary-renal vasculitis in elderly patients. Mayo Clin Proc 1990; 65:847–56.
3. Arimura Y, Minoshima S, Tanaka U, et al. Pulmonary involvement in patients with myeloperoxidase specific-antineutrophil cytoplasmic antibody. Ryumachi 1995; 35:46–55.
4. Alba MA, Flores-Suárez LF, Henderson AG, et al. Interstitial lung disease in ANCA vasculitis. Autoimmun Rev 2017;16(7):722–9.
5. Hozumi H, Enomoto N, Oyama Y, et al. Clinical Implication of Proteinase-3-antineutrophil Cytoplasmic Antibody in Patients with Idiopathic Interstitial Pneumonias. Lung 2016;194(2):235–42.
6. Tzelepis GE, Kokosi M, Tzioufas A, et al. Prevalence and outcome of pulmonary fibrosis in microscopic polyangiitis. Eur Respir J 2010;36(1):116–21.
7. Ando M, Miyazaki E, Ishii T, et al. Incidence of myeloperoxidase anti-neutrophil cytoplasmic antibody positivity and microscopic polyangiitis in the course of idiopathic pulmonary fibrosis. Respir Med 2013;107:608–15.
8. Liu GY, Ventura IB, Achtar-Zadeh N, et al. Prevalence and clinical significance of antineutrophil cytoplasmic antibodies in North American patients with idiopathic pulmonary fibrosis. Chest 2019;156:715–23.
9. Kagiyama N, Takayanagi N, Kanauchi T, et al. Anti-neutrophil cytoplasmic antibody-positive conversion and microscopic polyangiitis development in patients with idiopathic pulmonary fibrosis. BMJ Open Respir Res 2015;2:e000058.
10. Sun X, Peng M, Zhang T, et al. Clinical features and long-term outcomes of interstitial lung disease with anti-neutrophil cytoplasmic antibody. BMC Pulm Med 2021;21(1):88.
11. Lyons PA, Rayner TF, Trivedi S, et al. Genetically distinct subsets within ANCA-associated vasculitis. N Engl J Med 2012;367(3):214–23.
12. McDermott G, Fu X, Stone JH, et al. Association of Cigarette Smoking With Anti-neutrophil Cytoplasmic Antibody-Associated Vasculitis. JAMA Intern Med 2020; 180(6):870–6.
13. Kitching AR, Anders HJ, Basu N, et al. ANCA-associated vasculitis. Nat Rev Dis Primers 2020;6:71. https://doi.org/10.1038/s41572-020-0204-y.
14. Lane SE, Watts RA, Bentham G, et al. Are environmental factors important in primary systemic vasculitis? A case-control study. Arthritis Rheum 2003;48:814–23.
15. Fujimoto S, Watts RA, Kobayashi S, et al. Comparison of the epidemiology of antineutrophil cytoplasmic antibody-associated vasculitis between Japan and the U.K. Rheumatology 2011;50(10):1916–20.
16. Sada KE, Harigai M, Amano K, et al. Comparison of severity classification in Japanese patients with antineutrophil cytoplasmic antibody-associated vasculitis in a nationwide, prospective, inception cohort study. Mod Rheumatol 2016;26:730–7.
17. Berti A, Cornec D, Crowson CS. The Epidemiology of Antineutrophil Cytoplasmic Autoantibody-Associated Vasculitis in Olmsted County, Minnesota: A Twenty-Year US Population-Based Study. Arthritis Rheum 2017;69:2338–50.
18. Mohammad AJ, Jacobsson LT, Mahr AD, et al. Prevalence of Wegener's granulomatosis, microscopic polyangiitis, polyarteritis nodosa and Churg-Strauss

syndrome within a defined population in southern Sweden. Rheumatology 2007; 46:1329–37.

19. Seibold MA, Wise AL, Speer MC, et al. A common MUC5B promoter polymorphism and pulmonary fibrosis. N Engl J Med 2011;364(16):1503–12.

20. Stock CJ, Sato H, Fonseca C, et al. Mucin 5B promoter polymorphism is associated with idiopathic pulmonary fibrosis but not with development of lung fibrosis in systemic sclerosis or sarcoidosis. Thorax 2013;68(5):436–41.

21. Yang IV, Fingerlin TE, Evans CM, et al. MUC5B and Idiopathic Pulmonary Fibrosis. Ann Am Thorac Soc 2015;12(Suppl 2):S193–9.

22. Namba N, Kawasaki A, Sada K, et al. Ann Rheum Dis 2019;78:1144–6.

23. Foucher P, Heeringa P, Petersen AH, et al. Antimyeloperoxidase-associated lung disease. An experimental model. Am J Respir Crit Care Med 1999;160(3): 987–94.

24. Guilpain P, Chereau C, Goulvestre C, et al. The oxidation induced by antimyeloperoxidase antibodies triggers fibrosis in microscopic polyangiitis. Eur Respir J 2011;37(6):1503–13.

25. Metzler KD, Fuchs TA, Nauseef WM, et al. Myeloperoxidase is required for neutrophil extracellular trap formation: implications for innate immunity. Blood 2011; 117(3):953–9.

26. Thiam HR, Wong SL, Wagner DD, et al. Cellular Mechanisms of NETosis. Annu Rev Cell Dev Biol 2020 Oct 6;36:191–218.

27. Chrysanthopoulou A, Mitroulis I, Apostolidou E, et al. Neutrophil extracellular traps promote differentiation and function of fibroblasts. J Pathol 2014;233(3): 294–307.

28. Lee KY, Ho SC, Lin HC, et al. Neutrophil-derived elastase induces TGF-beta1 secretion in human airway smooth muscle via NF-kappaB pathway. Am J Respir Cell Mol Biol 2006;35(4):407–14.

29. Cheng OZ, Palaniyar N. NET balancing: a problem in inflammatory lung diseases. Front Immunol 2013 Jan 24;4:1.

30. Schwarz MI. Rare diseases bullet 10: Small vessel vasculitis of the lung. Thorax 2000;55(6):502–10.

31. Lee AS, Specks U. Pulmonary capillaritis. Semin Respir Crit Care Med 2004; 25(5):547–55.

32. Schwarz MI, Zamora MR, Hodges TN, et al. Isolated pulmonary capillaritis and diffuse alveolar hemorrhage in rheumatoid arthritis and mixed connective tissue disease. Chest 1998;113(6):1609–15.

33. Nasser M, Cottin V. Alveolar Hemorrhage in Vasculitis (Primary and Secondary). Semin Respir Crit Care Med 2018;39(4):482–93.

34. Gallagher H, Kwan JT, Jayne DR. Pulmonary renal syndrome: a 4-year, single-center experience. Am J Kidney Dis 2002;39(1):42–7.

35. Saha BK. Idiopathic pulmonary hemosiderosis: A state of the art review. Respir Med 2021;176:106234.

36. Magro CM, Allen J, Pope-Harman A, et al. The role of microvascular injury in the evolution of idiopathic pulmonary fibrosis. Am J Clin Pathol 2003;119:556–67.

37. Arulkumaran N, Periselneris N, Gaskin G, et al. Interstitial lung disease and ANCA-associated vasculitis: a retrospective observational cohort study. Rheumatology 2011;50(11):2035–43.

38. Ando Y, Okada F, Matsumoto S, et al. Thoracic manifestation of myeloperoxidase/ antineutrophil cytoplasmic antibody (MPO-ANCA)-related disease. CT findings in 51 patients. J Comput Assist Tomogr 2004;28:710–6.

39. Suarez-Cuartin G, Molina-Molina M. Clinical implications of ANCA positivity in idiopathic pulmonary fibrosis patients. Breathe 2020;16(1):190321.

40. Baqir M, Yi EE, Colby TV, et al. Radiologic and pathologic characteristics of myeloperoxidase-antineutrophil cytoplasmic antibody-associated interstitial lung disease: a retrospective analysis. Sarcoidosis Vasc Diffuse Lung Dis 2019;36:195–201.

41. Kwon M, Lee AS, Mira-Avendano I, et al. Interstitial Lung Disease in Antineutrophil Cytoplasmic Antibody-Associated Vasculitis Patients: Comparison With Idiopathic Pulmonary Fibrosis. J Clin Rheumatol 2021;27(8):324–30.

42. Huang H, Wang YX, Jiang CG, et al. A retrospective study of microscopic polyangiitis patients presenting with pulmonary fibrosis in China. BMC Pulm Med 2014;14(1):8.

43. Tzouvelekis A, Zacharis G, Oikonomou A, et al. Combined pulmonary fibrosis and emphysema associated with microscopic polyangiitis. Eur Respir J 2012;40:505–7.

44. Gocho K, Sugino K, Sato K, et al. Microscopic polyangiitis preceded by combined pulmonary fibrosis and emphysema. Respir Med Case Rep 2015;15:128–32.

45. Raghu G, Remy-Jardin M, Richeldi L, et al. Idiopathic Pulmonary Fibrosis (an Update) and Progressive Pulmonary Fibrosis in Adults: An Official ATS/ERS/JRS/ALAT Clinical Practice Guideline. Am J Respir Crit Care Med 2022;205(9):e18–47.

46. Watanabe T, Minezawa T, Hasegawa M, et al. Prognosis of pulmonary fibrosis presenting with a usual interstitial pneumonia pattern on computed tomography in patients with myeloperoxidase anti-neutrophil cytoplasmic antibody-related nephritis: a retrospective single-center study. BMC Pulm Med 2019;19(1):194.

47. Wurmann P, Sabugo F, Elgueta F, et al. Interstitial lung disease and microscopic polyangiitis in Chilean patients. Sarcoidosis Vasc Diffuse Lung Dis 2020;37(1):37–42.

48. Suzuki A, Sakamoto S, Kurosaki A, et al. Chest High-Resolution CT Findings of Microscopic Polyangiitis: A Japanese First Nationwide Prospective Cohort Study. AJR Am J Roentgenol 2019;213(1):104–14.

49. Yamagata M, Ikeda K, Tsushima K, et al. Prevalence and Responsiveness to Treatment of Lung Abnormalities on Chest Computed Tomography in Patients With Microscopic Polyangiitis: A Multicenter, Longitudinal, Retrospective Study of One Hundred Fifty Consecutive Hospital-Based Japanese Patients. Arthritis Rheumatol 2016;68(3):713–23.

50. Doliner B, Rodriguez K, Montesi SB, et al. Interstitial lung disease in ANCA-associated vasculitis: associated factors, radiographic features, and mortality. Rheumatology 2022;keac339 [published online ahead of print, 2022 Jun 14].

51. Comarmond C, Crestani B, Tazi A, et al. Pulmonary fibrosis in antineutrophil cytoplasmic antibodies (ANCA)-associated vasculitis: a series of 49 patients and review of the literature. Medicine (Baltim) 2014;93(24):340–9. Published correction appears in Medicine (Baltimore).

52. Imokawa S, Uehara M, Uto T, et al. Organizing pneumonia associated with myeloperoxidase anti-neutrophil cytoplasmic antibody. Respirol Case Rep 2015;3(4):122–4.

53. Takada K, Miyamoto A, Nakahama H, et al. Myeloperoxidase anti-neutrophil cytoplasmic antibody-associated vasculitis with a unique imaging presentation of organizing pneumonia: A case report. Respir Med Case Rep 2020;31:101294.

54. Yates M, Watts RA, Bajema IM, et al. EULAR/ERA-EDTA recommendations for the management of ANCA-associated vasculitis. Annals of the. Rheumatic Diseases 2016;75:1583–94.
55. Hervier B, Pagnoux C, Agard C, et al. Pulmonary fibrosis associated with ANCA-positive vasculitides. Retrospective study of 12 cases and review of the literature. Ann Rheum Dis 2009;68(3):404–7.
56. Yamaguchi K, Yamaguchi A, Itai M, et al. Interstitial lung disease with myeloperoxidase-antineutrophil cytoplasmic antibody-associated vasculitis in elderly patients. Rheumatol Int 2021;41(9):1641–50.
57. Kawamura K, Ichikado K, Ichiyasu H, et al. Acute exacerbation of chronic fibrosing interstitial pneumonia in patients receiving antifibrotic agents: incidence and risk factors from real-world experience. BMC Pulm Med 2019;19(1):113.
58. Idiopathic Pulmonary Fibrosis Clinical Research Network, Raghu G, Anstrom KJ, et al. Prednisone, azathioprine, and N-acetylcysteine for pulmonary fibrosis. N Engl J Med 2012;366(21):1968–77.
59. Morisset J, Lee JS. New trajectories in the treatment of interstitial lung disease: treat the disease or treat the underlying pattern? Curr Opin Pulm Med 2019; 25(5):442–9.
60. Wells AU, Flaherty KR, Brown KK, et al. Nintedanib in patients with progressive fibrosing interstitial lung diseases-subgroup analyses by interstitial lung disease diagnosis in the INBUILD trial: a randomised, double-blind, placebo-controlled, parallel-group trial. Lancet Respir Med 2020;8(5):453–60.
61. Behr J, Prasse A, Kreuter M, et al. Pirfenidone in patients with progressive fibrotic interstitial lung diseases other than idiopathic pulmonary fibrosis (RELIEF): a double-blind, randomised, placebo-controlled, phase 2b trial. Lancet Respir Med 2021;9(5):476–86.
62. Kishaba T. Current perspective of progressive-fibrosing interstitial lung disease. Respir Investig 2022;60(4):503–9.
63. Adegunsoye A, Oldham JM, Bellam SK, et al. Computed tomography honeycombing identifies a progressive fibrotic phenotype with increased mortality across diverse interstitial lung diseases. Ann Am Thorac Soc 2019;16:580–8.
64. Yamakawa H, Toyoda Y, Baba T, et al. Anti-Inflammatory and/or Anti-Fibrotic Treatment of MPO-ANCA-Positive Interstitial Lung Disease: A Short Review. J Clin Med 2022;11(13):3835.
65. Zhou P, Ma J, Wang G. Impact of interstitial lung disease on mortality in ANCA-associated vasculitis: A systematic literature review and meta-analysis. Chron Respir Dis 2021;18. 1479973121994562.
66. Hozumi H, Kono M, Hasegawa H, et al. Clinical Significance of Interstitial Lung Disease and Its Acute Exacerbation in Microscopic Polyangiitis. Chest 2021; 159(6):2334–45.

Post-COVID Interstitial Lung Disease—The Tip of the Iceberg

Namrata Kewalramani, MD[a,b,*], Kerri-Marie Heenan, MB Bch, BAO[c],
Denise McKeegan, MB Bch, BAO, MSc[c], Nazia Chaudhuri, MD, PhD[d]

KEYWORDS

- COVID-19 • Post-COVID-19 condition (long COVID) • Interstitial lung disease
- Post-COVID fibrosis • Long-term impact

KEY POINTS

- Some patients have persistent symptoms, lung function impairment, and radiological abnormalities post-severe acute respiratory syndrome coronavirus 2 infection.
- Post-COVID-fibrotic changes have shown resolution at 12 months, however, in a cohort of patients, the changes persist.
- The long-term impact of post-COVID fibrosis remains unknown and ongoing studies are aimed at assessing the frequency and consequences of this new disease entity.
- Post-COVID interstitial lung disease may represent a significant burden on the health care systems.

INTRODUCTION

On the March 11, 2020, the World Health Organization (WHO) declared the outbreak of severe acute respiratory syndrome coronavirus 2 (SARS-CoV-2) as a global pandemic, commonly referred to as coronavirus 2019 (COVID-19).[1] The first documented case was recognized in Wuhan, China, in December 2019.[2] As of November 2022, there have been over 550 million cases worldwide and over 6 million deaths associated with COVID-19.[3] The spectrum of presentations and symptoms of COVID-19 can vary widely from asymptomatic carriers to life-threatening respiratory and multi-organ failure. The risk factors for the severity of COVID-19 are thought to

[a] Department for BioMedical Research DBMR, Inselspital, Bern University Hospital, University of Bern, Switzerland; [b] Department of Pulmonary Medicine, Inselspital, Bern University Hospital, University of Bern, Switzerland; [c] Department of Respiratory Medicine, Antrim Area Hospital, Northern Health and Social Care Trust, Antrim, Northern Ireland, UK; [d] University of Ulster Magee Campus, Northland Road, Londonderry, Northern Ireland, UK
* Corresponding author. Department of Biomedical Research, Lung Precision Medicine, Room 340, Murtenstrasse 24, Bern 3008. Switzerland
E-mail address: Namrata.kewalramani@gmail.com

Immunol Allergy Clin N Am 43 (2023) 389–410
https://doi.org/10.1016/j.iac.2023.01.004
0889-8561/23/© 2023 Elsevier Inc. All rights reserved.

correlate with increasing age, body mass index (BMI), and comorbidities such as diabetes, obesity, cardiovascular disease, hypertension, and chronic kidney disease.[4-7]

The widespread collaborative efforts of governments, public health, pharmaceutical industry, and researchers have led to a wealth of expertise in tackling the pandemic over a relatively short time. We have effective therapies that can reduce the symptom burden and risk of hospitalization and in-hospital mortality with COVID-19. Antivirals, monoclonal antibodies, and immunomodulatory drugs have emerged through robust trials as treatments for SARS-CoV-2 infection.[8,9] Several therapies have been shown to reduce the risk of hospitalization in patients with mild to moderate disease. Treatment of symptomatic COVID-19 with Paxlovid, a SARS-CoV-2 protease inhibitor consisting of nirmatrelvir and ritonavir, has led to a reduction of severe COVID-19 by 89%, without evident safety concerns.[10] In non-hospitalized patients with mild to moderate COVID-19 disease, Molnupiravir reduces the risk of hospitalization or death by approximately 50%.[11-13] Coupled with the rollout of mass vaccination programs worldwide, we have seen the mortality from COVID-19 declining despite continued high rates of infection.[14,15]

Although we are grappling with the changing nature of the virus and attempting to rebuild our lives and economies, we are now faced with an emerging yet unquantifiable health epidemic –post-COVID-19 condition (long COVID). This review will discuss the emerging evidence for the development of post-COVID interstitial lung disease (PC-ILD) focusing on the pathophysiological mechanisms, incidence, diagnosis, and impact of this potentially new and emerging respiratory disease.

PATHOPHYSIOLOGY OF POST-COVID INTERSTITIAL LUNG DISEASE

Data from previous coronavirus outbreaks of Middle East respiratory syndrome (MERS) and SARS suggest that between 25% and 35% of survivors will experience long-term respiratory complications with lung function and radiographic abnormalities consistent with the development of pulmonary fibrosis, therefore, raising the suspicion that persistent respiratory symptoms post-SARS-CoV-2 infection may have similar pathophysiological mechanisms to MERS and SARS infections.[7,16-20]

Several histopathological findings have been identified among COVID-19 cases. Gross examination of postmortem specimens revealed that tissue damage was more severe in the lung peripheries, where fibrous tissue proliferation in the alveolar septa and alveolar destruction was remarkably abundant. In the central areas, the alveolar structure was roughly preserved with only focal fibrosis.[21] The most commonly reported histological pattern of lung injury is diffuse alveolar damage (DAD) with two identifiable stages; an acute stage, defined by scattered or diffuse hyaline membranes, associated with alveolar edema, an alveolar eosinophil exudate, and few vacuolated macrophages, and a more organized stage of parenchymal collapse, enlargement of alveolar septa, alveolar fibrin deposits, hyperplasia of type-2 pneumocytes, sparse multinucleated giant cells, and minor fibroblast proliferation[22,23] A lung cryobiopsy study performed in patients with a mean disease duration of 31.3 days observed marked fibrotic lung parenchymal remodeling, characterized by fibroblast proliferation, airspace obliteration, and micro-honeycombing.[24]

According to a meta-analysis of COVID-19 inpatients, 14.8% developed acute respiratory distress syndrome (ARDS).[25] DAD has long been considered the hallmark histologic finding in acute ARDS.[26] Pulmonary fibrosis (PF) subsequent to ARDS is well-recognized and given the relatively high incidence of ARDS among COVID-19 patients,[25,27] PC-ILD as a potential long-term outcome of COVID-19 is concerning. Distinct from the idiopathic form of PF or other progressive ILD, fibrosis resulting from ARDS is largely stable. However, whereas some patients with fibrosis post-ARDS may fully recover, some may have lasting symptoms of decreased lung function.[28] In postmortem studies of those with COVID-19 features suggestive of a fibrotic phase, such as mural fibrosis and microcystic honeycombing, these findings were observed to be focal, rather than widespread. This may be due to the short duration of the disease at the time of death.[22]

The underlying pathology of ARDS is complex, and the inflammatory response and immune system play a critical role.[29] In general, there is conflicting evidence regarding the possibility that viral infection may predispose one to the development of fibrosis. It is postulated that chronic viral infection may contribute to the fibrotic response through the promotion of a state of mild but chronic inflammation, which disrupts homeostasis and healing, thereby leading to increased susceptibility to a secondary insult. The coronavirus infection tends to have an acute duration; however, there is evidence from ARDS that even a duration of less than 1 week can lead to fibrosis.[30] Inflammation promotes viral clearance, but excessive cytokine response can be damaging.[31]

Viruses can upregulate the expression of critical host cell surface receptors, signaling pathways, and production of growth factors. The angiotensin-converting enzyme 2 (ACE2) receptor, which is engaged by the S1 subunit of the SARS-CoV-2 spike protein, acts as a regulator of the renin-angiotensin system (RAS), which activates a broad range of signaling pathways including proinflammatory and profibrotic effects. Inflammation promotes viral clearance, but excessive cytokine response can be damaging.[31] Cytokines such as transforming growth factor (TGF)-β, interleukin (IL)-6, tumor necrosis factor (TNF)-α, and chemokines promote activation of immune populations that clear infection and promote immunity through T-cell and B-cell recruitment. They also activate macrophage populations that clear apoptotic cellular debris. In acute lung injury, activated macrophages also contribute to the induction of neutrophil recruitment and activation.[32] Neutrophilic infiltrate, in turn, contributes to the generation of reactive oxygen species (ROS) and both neutrophilic infiltrate and ROS may contribute to tissue injury.[33,34] In response to injury, the alveolar epithelial cells recruit fibroblast and inflammatory cells to initiate wound healing by reshaping the extracellular environment to restore tissue integrity and promote the replacement of parenchymal cells.[35] Usually, this pro-fibrotic process is turned off once the tissue heals. However, repeated damage and repair, such as that seen in SARS-CoV-2 infection, can lead to the imbalance of this process, resulting in excessive pathological deposition of extracellular matrix protein, accompanied by upregulation of myofibroblast activity, resulting in a chronic inflammatory environment of macrophage and immune cell infiltration. This is supported by a study on lung samples from individuals who succumbed to COVID-19 and control individuals using single-nucleus RNA sequencing. They noted a reduction in the epithelial cell compartment, of both alveolar type 1 and 2 cells, and an increase in monocytes/macrophages and fibroblasts in COVID-19 patients as compared with control lungs.[36] Furthermore, in a multi-omics study of postmortem COVID-19 patients, there was hyperinflammation, alveolar epithelial cell exhaustion, vascular changes and fibrosis, and parenchymal lung senescence as a molecular state of COVID-19 pathology. A forkhead transcription factor, FOXO3A suppression was implicated as a potential mechanism underlying the fibroblast-to-myofibroblast transition associated with PC-ILD.[37] In this cellular environment, massive proinflammatory and profibrotic cytokines are released, thus, activating fibrosis-related pathways including the TGF-β signal pathway, wingless/integrated (WNT), signal pathway and yes-associated protein/transcriptional cofactor with PDZ binding motif signal pathways.[38,39]

Fig. 1 illustrates how viruses can upregulate the expression of critical host cell surface receptors, signaling pathways, and production of growth factors. The ACE2 receptor acts as a regulator of the RAS which activates a broad range of signaling pathways including proinflammatory and profibrotic effects.

A significant proportion of patients with severe COVID-19 required invasive mechanical ventilation (IMV). IMV can induce stretch force injury and alveolar injury and may contribute to ARDS. Increased lung stretch can induce oxidative injury, increase cytokine production, increase epithelial-mesenchymal transition (EMT),[40,41] and increase collagen deposition in the lungs which contributes to the development of PF. Careful ventilation of injured lungs, or lungs that may have increased stiffness, could potentially help to minimize ventilator-induced profibrotic signaling.[40]

PERSISTENT SYMPTOMS POST-COVID

Although the majority of patients' symptoms recover within 4 to 8 weeks of a SARS-CoV-2 infection, some find their symptoms will persist beyond 12 weeks, leading to the term "long COVID".[42,43] The WHO has defined "post-COVID-19 (long COVID)" as a condition occurring in individuals with a history of probable or confirmed SARS-CoV-2 infection, usually 3 months from the onset of COVID-19 with symptoms that last for at least 2 months and cannot be explained by an alternative diagnosis. Studies have shown up to 48.8% of individuals reporting not feeling fully recovered from COVID-19 with a median of nine persistent symptoms 1 year following the SARS-CoV-2 infection (**Box 1**) with the most reported symptoms being breathlessness and fatigue.[44–47] Female gender, being middle age (40–59 years), having two or more self-reported comorbidities and experiencing a more severe form of COVID-19 at the time of diagnosis and resultant hospitalization had a lower rate of self-reported recovery[6,44,45]

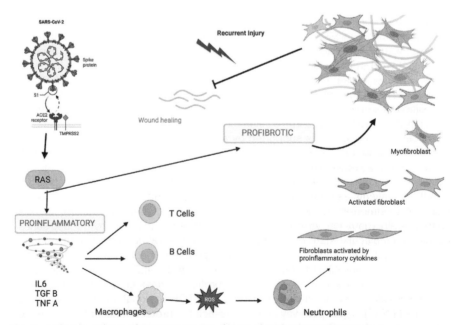

Fig. 1. Pathophysiology of Post-COVID ILD. (Created with BioRender.com.)

Box 1
Commonly reported persistent symptoms post-COVID-19

- Breathlessness
- Fatigue
- Impaired sleep quality
- Aching of muscles (pain)
- Physical slowing down
- Joint pain or swelling
- Limb weakness
- Pain
- Short-term memory loss
- Slowing down in thinking

Data from Refs.[44–47]

Persistent symptoms of COVID-19 have been reported in the early phases and late phases of follow-up (**Table 1**). As time has elapsed since the emergence of the novel SARS-CoV-2 infection, we are beginning to appreciate the long-term symptom burden. Two large prospective observational studies looking at long-term outcomes after SARS-CoV-2 infection, the Lung Injury COVID-19 study and the Post-Hospitalization COVID-19 study (PHOSP-COVID) have followed up 305 Spanish and 1077 UK patients, respectively.[46,48] The Lung Injury COVID-19 study stratified patients according to the severity of SARS-CoV-2 infection as a moderate disease (features of pneumonia with oxygen saturations above 90% requiring supplemental oxygen, n = 162) or severe disease (patients who required either non-invasive ventilation, high flow oxygen, or intubation and IMV, n = 143). At medium term follow-up classed as less than 180 days from the initial symptoms, 55.5% of patients with severe disease and 44.1% of patients with moderate disease had persistent dyspnea with a modified Medical Research Council (mMRC) dyspnea scale of above 2. Dyspnea was significantly more prevalent in the severe group than in the moderate group ($P = 0.042$). At this time point, only 13.5% of patients had symptom resolution and other persistent symptoms included chest pain, fatigue, and cough with no differences in frequency between the moderate and severe groups.[48] Beyond 10 months, one-third of patients' symptoms had resolved; however, breathlessness (mMRC>2) remained in 18.4 and 20% of the moderate and severe groups, respectively. Intriguingly, patients with moderate disease severity had a higher symptom burden at this later time point than those with severe disease, including cough (11.9% vs 3%; $P = 0.03$), chest pain (14% vs 4.4%; $P = 0.025$), and fatigue (20% vs 7.7%; $P = 0.017$). This suggests that the ongoing symptoms do not correlate with the severity of the acute COVID-19 illness.[49] In the PHOSP-COVID study only 239 of 830 (28.8%) individuals described themselves as fully recovered at a median of 5.9 months (interquartile range 4.9–6.5) post-hospital discharge; 632 of 855 (92.8%) individuals had at least one persistent symptom with a median of nine symptoms (see **Table 1**).[45]

A persistence of respiratory symptoms at 1-year follow-up in a subset of patients after acute COVID-19 highlights the potential for ongoing respiratory sequelae and the need for continued monitoring of this group of patients. With over 550 million people affected worldwide,[3] up to 20% may have continued respiratory symptoms in a

Table 1
Published reports on symptoms post-severe acute respiratory syndrome coronavirus 2 infection

	Mandel et al,[44] 2021	Carfi et al,[47] 2020	Willi et al,[50] 2021	Froidure et al,[51] 2021	Boari et al,[52] 2021	Robery et al,[53] 2021	Faverio et al,[54] 2021	Han et al,[55] 2021	Hama Amin et al,[56] 2022	Zangrillo et al,[57] 2022	Huang et al,[58] 2021	Faverio et al,[59] 2022	Evans et al,[45,46]
Type of study	Cross-sectional study	Prospective cohort	Systematic literature search of 31 studies	Single-center cohort study	Prospective Cohort	Retrospective analysis	Multicenter prospective observational cohort	Prospective longitudinal study	Meta-analysis of 618 articles	Prospective observational study	Ambidirectional cohort study	Multicenter prospective observational cohort	Prospective, longitudinal cohort study
Country	UK	Italy	Switzerland	Belgium	Italy	UK	Northern Italy	China	Worldwide	Italy	Wuhan, China	Northern Italy	Multicenter, UK
Duration of follow-up	Median 54 days (IQR 47–59)	Mean 60.3 days (SD 13.6)	9–90 days	Median 95 days	Average 4 months	8–18 weeks	6 months	6 months	Up to 7 months	12 months	6 and 12 months	11–13 months	2–14 months post-discharge
Number of patients	384	142	48,258	134	94	221	312	114	2018	116	1276	287	2320 at 5 months 807 at 1 year
Persistent symptoms	71.9%	87.4%	66%–87.4%	-	-	100%[d] 21%[e]	-	-	-	-	68%[h] 49%[i]	-	54.9%[h] 48.8%[i]
Specific symptoms													
Fatigue	67.3%[a] 73.3%[b] 76.9%[c]	53.1%	16.36%–72%	25%	52%	-	-	-	38.7%[f] 80%[g]	-	52%[h] 20%[i]	-	-
Dyspnea	54.8%[a] 63.3%[b] 57.7%[c]	43.4%	14.55%–74.3%	35%	36%	-	38%	6.1%	26.6%[f] 50%[g]	7% (at rest) 46% (on exertion)	26%[h] 30%[i]	40%	-
Cough	32.2%[a] 36.7%[b] 46.2%[c]	-	61%	10%	-	-	-	10%	15.5%[f] 31.6%[g]	-	-	-	-
Joint/muscle pain	-	27.3%	27.3%	-	-	-	-	-	15.4%[f] 58.3%[g]	-	11%[h] 12%[i]	-	-
Chest pain	-	21.7%	21.7%	-	-	-	-	-	8%[f] 30.5%[g]	39%	5%[h] 7%[i]	-	-
Poor sleep quality	61.1%[a] 93.3%[b] 76.9%[c]	-	24%	-	31%	-	-	-	-	-	27%[h] 17%[i]	-	-

Headache	-	18.18%–61%	-	-	-	-	2%[h] 5%[i]
GI symptoms	-	31%	-	-	-	-	1%[h] 1%[i]
Physiological distress	-	23.5%–46.9%	-	21%	-	36%	23%[h] 26%[i]
Comments	-	11 prospective cohort 11 retrospective cohort 4 cross-sectional 5 case reports	-	-	-	13 studies used	-

Abbreviations: CPAP, continuous positive airway pressure; ICU, intensive care unit; IMV, invasive mechanical ventilation; IQR, inter quartile range; SD, standard deviation.

[a] Oxygen alone.
[b] CPAP.
[c] IMV.
[d] Required ICU.
[e] Did not require ICU.
[f] Non-fibrotic group.
[g] Fibrotic group.
[h] 6 months.
[i] 12 months.
[j] 5 months.

year equating to a staggering 110 million people. This proportion of symptomatic patients with post-COVID-19 condition (long COVID) represents a significant burden on the individual as well as on the health care systems. A greater understanding of the natural evolution of symptoms over a longer period and the impacts of interventions will improve our understanding of the long-term impacts of the COVID-19 disease. Persistent respiratory symptoms have a complex etiology and are not always attributable to the underlying parenchymal disease. Although the natural assumption is that these symptomatic patients may have underlying structural changes such as PF, one needs to be mindful that deconditioning. overall well-being such as the presence of anxiety and depression and muscle weakness/fatigue may also be contributing to ongoing breathlessness. Objective evidence of pulmonary abnormalities with pulmonary physiology and advanced radiology is therefore paramount.

Pulmonary Function Impairment Post-COVID-19

Pulmonary function abnormalities are seen as early as 2 weeks post-discharge of an acute SARS-CoV-2 infection. In a retrospective observational study of 137 patients from China, 81% of patients demonstrated an inspiratory vital capacity of less than 80% predicted and 24.1% of patients had a forced vital capacity (FVC) of less than 80% predicted. The degree of restrictive ventilatory impairment correlates with the severity of acute SARS-CoV-2 infection[60,61] and impairment was greatest in those patients who required intensive care unit (ICU) admission, of which 50% required intubation and IMV.[49] Lung function impairment had poor correlation with the presence of respiratory symptoms, however, a correlation between biomarkers involved in host defense reflecting neutrophil activation (lipocalin-2), fibrosis signaling (matrix metalloproteinase-7) and alveolar repair (hepatocyte growth factor), and reduction in FVC and diffusing capacity for carbon monoxide (DLCO) was found.[49]

Several studies have shown persistent lung function abnormalities at 3 and 4 months follow-up[20,51,53,62–65](**Tables 2**). The principal study out of Wuhan, China, showed that in 83 patients who did not require IMV, 55% of patients had a DLCO less than 80% predicted and 23% had an FVC of less than 80% predicted at 3 months post-discharge.[20] Similar findings in DLCO and FVC decline were seen in Canadian, Belgian, French, and UK cohorts.[51,53,62,63] Impairments in lung function do not correlate with persistent symptoms,[51] however, were related to the severity of COVID-19 as defined as the need for IMV,[63,65] ICU admission,[51,53,63] percentage inspired oxygen,[53,65] and days on inspired oxygen.[62] Correlations were also seen with age and severity of initial lung involvement.[63]

Longitudinal follow-up has shown that lung function impairments improve over time.[20,54,59,66,67] However, even after a year post-COVID-19, a proportion of patients will continue to have lung function impairment, raising the suspicion of long-term pulmonary complications such as the development of PF. In a Chinese study of 83 patients, 33% of patients had a DLCO less than 80% predicted at 12 months compared with 55% at 3 months and 11% of patients had an FVC less than 80% predicted at 12 months compared with 23% at 3 months.[20] Similar improvements albeit persistent impairments in lung function parameters were observed in a Dutch study of 92 patients where the frequency of impaired FVC improved from 25% at 6 weeks to 11% at 6 months, and for DLCO, this percentage improved from 63% to 46%.[66] Larger multicenter prospective studies have corroborated these findings and have identified risk factors for persistent lung function impairment as having asthma as a comorbidity,[54,59] female gender,[67] and age.[48,67] Persistent lung function abnormalities highlight underlying structural lung involvement as a mechanism of ongoing respiratory symptoms post-COVID and necessitate further radiological assessment.

Table 2
Published reports on pulmonary function testing post-severe acute respiratory syndrome coronavirus 2 infection

Study	Type of Study	Country	Population/ Data	Duration of the Study	DLCO % Predicted	Alterations in DLCO (<80% Predicated)	FVC % Predicted	Alterations in FVC (<80% Predicated)	Comments
LV et al,[61] 2020	Retrospective analysis	Taizhou, China	137 patients	2 weeks following discharge	-	-	-	55.6%	The degree of restrictive ventilatory impairment correlated with the severity of acute SARS-CoV-2 infection. Evidence of small airway dysfunction at a much lower frequency
Froidure et al,[51] 2021	Single-center cohort study	Belgium	134 patients	Median 95-day interval	Median 74%	46%	Median 88%	-	Impairments in lung function do not correlate with persistent symptoms. Impairments in lung function correlated with ICU admission
Robey et al,[53] 2021	Retrospective analysis	United Kingdom	221 patients	8–18 weeks	Mean 76.6%	53%	Mean 86.5%	-	Alterations more common in patients requiring ICU. DLCO alterations more frequent with abnormal CT findings

(continued on next page)

Table 2
(continued)

Study	Type of Study	Country	Population/ Data	Duration of the Study	DLCO % Predicted	Alterations in DLCO (<80% Predicated)	FVC % Predicted	Alterations in FVC (<80% Predicated)	Comments
Frija-Masson et al,[63] 2021	Retrospective study	Paris, France	137 patients	3 months after symptom onset	Median 49%	-	Median 98%	-	Alterations in PFT correlated to age, degree of initial lung involvement, and endotracheal intubation
Guler et al,[64] 2021	Multicenter prospective cohort	Switzerland	113 patients	4 months	Mean 73.2	-	Mean 86.6%	-	Alterations more pronounced in patients who had severe/critical COVID-19 vs mild/moderate COVID-19
Safont et al,[67] 2022	Multicenter prospective cohort	Spain	313 patients	2 months (mean 63 ± 12 days) and 6 (mean 181 ± 10 days) months after discharge	Mean 77.25% (2 months) 81.50 (6 months)	54.63% at 2 months 46.96% at 6 months	Mean 99.02 (2 months) Mean 100.59 (6 months)	14.38% (2 months) 9.27% (6 months)	FVC % predicted improved over time. Increased risk of DLCO impairment at 6 months was age D-dimer peak value, female sex, and peak RALE score
Faverio et al,[54] 2021	multicenter, prospective, observational cohort study	Northern Italy	312 patients	6 months from discharge	Median 76.0% vs 84.0% vs 77.4% (oxygen vs CPAP vs IMV.)	58% vs 36% vs 54% (oxygen vs CPAP vs IMV.)	Median 107.2% vs 106.4% vs 102% (oxygen vs CPAP vs IMV.	-	Patients with COVID-19 who required oxygen have less impairment on PFT compared with patients requiring CPAP and patients requiring IMV

| Faverio et al,[59] 2022 | multicenter, prospective, observational cohort study | Northern Italy | 287 patients 11–13 months from discharge | Median 79.0 vs 80% (oxygen vs CPAP vs IMV. | 53% vs 29% vs 49% (oxygen vs CPAP vs IMV. | Median 108.0%, 110.0% vs 106.5% (oxygen vs CPAP vs IMV. | – | Improvement from 6 to 12 months. Patients who required less respiratory support had fewer alterations in PFT |
| Tarraso et al,[68] 2022 | Multicenter prospective observational cohort study | Spain | 284 patients 12 months | – | 53.8% vs 46.8% 39.8% 60 days vs 180 days vs 365 days | – | 14.32% vs 9.29% 6.69% 60 days vs 180 days vs 365 days | Age, female sex, and BMI risk of DLCO impairment at 365 days |

Abbreviations: CPAP, continuous positive airway pressure; CT, computed tomography; DLCO, diffusing capacity for carbon monoxide; FVC, forced vital capacity; ICU, intensive care unit; IMV, invasive mechanical ventilation; RALE, radiological assessment of lung edema.

Radiological features post-COVID-19

Radiology has been a very helpful tool in helping us understand the disease process[44, 70, 73, 63, 53, 50, 71, 54, 67, 59, 74] **(Table 3)**.[68] In a retrospective study out of the Lombardy region in Italy, the worst hit region in Europe, 90 consecutive hospitalized patients had computerized tomography (CT) performed on admission and 60 days post-discharge. On admission, 90% of patients had bilateral lung disease with an 80% peripheral and 63% mid-zone and lower-zone predominance; 54.4% demonstrated diffuse ground glass opacities (GGO) and 46.6% had both GGO and consolidation. CT images were reported as fibrotic based on the presence of reticulation, architectural distortion, traction bronchiectasis, and honeycombing. Twenty-three (25.5%) patients were defined as having a non-specific interstitial pneumonia (NSIP) pattern by two thoracic radiologists with over 30 years of experience. Patients with features of fibrosis on their imaging were older and had evidence of systemic inflammation with statistically higher lactate dehydrogenase (LDH), c-reactive protein, erythrocyte sedimentation rate (ESR), D-dimer, evidence of bone marrow suppression with reduced hemoglobin, white cell counts and platelets, and corresponding reductions in lung function parameters (FVC and DLCO) compared with individuals without features of fibrosis on their imaging[69] These findings were similar to studies out of Wuhan, China, where 46% of patients at a median of 56 days follow-up had CT evidence of fibrotic changes manifesting as parenchymal bands (76%), irregular interface (32%), traction bronchiectasis (38%), lung distortion (25%), and honeycombing (9%). The fibrosis was predominantly peripheral in distribution (89%), corresponding with the areas of acute COVID-19 changes, and the overall burden of fibrosis was minimal or mild in the majority (84%) of patients[70] In 50% of this cohort, initial features of lung distortion attributed to improved fibrosis, suggesting a reversible element to these changes. On multivariate analysis, fibrosis was associated with higher ESR, eosinophil counts, and advancing age. More patients in the fibrosis cohort required non-invasive ventilation and 77% of the overall cohort was defined as having severe SARS-CoV-2 infection.[70] A further study of 216 discharged patients found that 85.1% had CT abnormalities at 3 months and these were more frequent in patients defined as severe/critical or required IMV or high-flow oxygen. There was also a significant negative correlation between total lung capacity (TLC) and residual volume and a weaker correlation to DLCO on lung function testing ($P < 0.05$).[71] These early studies raised several questions as to whether features defined as fibrotic during early imaging are reversible over time and thus highlighted the need for longer follow-up studies, or whether the severity of COVID-19 or the need for IMV is driving the development of fibrosis. One such study found that at 4 months follow-up, 44.4% of patients had a multi-disciplinary diagnosis of ILD on CT imaging; 56% had evidence of architectural distortion and this correlated with reductions in DLCO. The majority of patients with ILD at 4 months were admitted to ICU (6.3% vs 93.8%; $P = 0.001$) and required IMV, high flow oxygen, or underwent prone ventilation, and also had more complications of venous thromboembolism (VTE) and ARDS during their acute illness.[65] Highlighting a potential role of severity of infection and IMV as risk factors and contributors to the development of fibrosis. Furthermore, in a study of 220 patients with 20% incomplete CT resolution at 6 months, predicators of persistent CT abnormalities were older age, prolonged hospital stay, a lower PaO2/FiO2 at hospital admission, a higher degree of support, and higher oxygen requirements.[72] The presence of reticulations and consolidation on CT at hospital admission predicted the persistence of radiological abnormalities during follow-up.[72]

Table 3
Published reports on radiology findings post-severe acute respiratory syndrome coronavirus infection

	Mandel et al,[44] 2021	Yang et al,[70] 2020	Zhang et al,[73] 2021	Frija-Masson et al,[63] 2021	Robey et al,[53] 2021	Willi et al,[50] 2021	Zhou et al,[71] 2021	Faverio et al,[54] 2021	Safont et al,[67] 2022	Faverio et al,[59] 2022	Besutti et al,[74] 2022	Tarraso et al,[68] 2022
Type of study	Cross-sectional study	Retrospective study	Retrospective longitudinal study	Retrospective study	Retrospective analysis	Systematic literature search of 31 studies	Prospective cohort study	Multicenter prospective observational cohort	Multicenter prospective cohort	Multicenter prospective observational cohort	Retrospective study	Multicenter prospective observational cohort study
Country	UK	Greece	China	Paris, France	UK	Switzerland	Wuhan, China	Northern Italy	Spain	Northern Italy	Italy	Spain
Duration of follow-up	Median 54 days (IQR 47–59)	Median 56 days after symptom onset	Various time points up to 12 weeks	3 months	8–18 weeks	9–90 days	4 months	6 months	2 months and 6 months after discharge	11–13 months	12 months	2 months and 12 months
Number of patients	384	116	310	137	221	48,258	216	312	313	287	65	325[a] 156[b]
Abnormal radiology	38% CXR remained abnormal 9% CXR deteriorating	46% with CT evidence of fibrotic changes	60.7% of CT had abnormalities after 12 weeks	Overall % of abnormalities on CT not declared	65% of CT scans had abnormalities	54.3–83% had CT abnormalities	Abnormalities on CT scans 85.1%[a] 68.0%[b] 22.2%[c] (P-value <0.001)	Abnormalities on CT scans 25%[a] 24%[b] 44%[c] (P < 0.001)	Abnormalities on CT scans 52.38%[a] 91.14%[b] (P-value 0.001>)	Abnormalities on CT scans 46%[a] 65%[b] 80%[c] (P < 0.001)	86.2% had ongoing CT abnormalities Residual non-fibrotic abnormalities (37.5%)[a] Residual fibrotic abnormalities (4.4%)[b] Post-ventilatory abnormalities (2.5%)[c]	At 2 months 61.6% (200/325) had CT abnormalities and at 12 months 78.8% (123/156)
Specific findings on CT scans												
GGO			51.6%	75%	44%		79.3%[a] 60.0%[b] 22.2%[c] (P-value <0.001)	16%[a] 7%[b] 12%[c] (P = 00186)	36.73%[a] 68.35%[b] (P = 0.001)	30%[a] 48%[b] 71%[c] (P < 0.001)	32.1% at 5–7 months[a] 3.5% at 5–7 months[b] 2.2% at 5–7 months[c]	73.5%[a] (32% of cohort) 45.5%[b] (15.8% of cohort)
Parenchymal bands	76%		32%		-			13.60%[a] 38.46%[b] (P = 0.001)			2.7% at 5–7 months[a]	33.4%[b] (11.6% of cohort)

(continued on next page)

Table 3
(continued)

	Mandel et al,[44] 2021	Yang et al,[70] 2020	Zhang et al,[73] 2021	Frija-Masson et al,[63] 2021	Robey et al,[53] 2021	Willi et al,[50] 2021	Zhou et al,[71] 2021	Faverio et al,[54] 2021	Safont et al,[67] 2022	Faverio et al,[59] 2022	Besutti et al,[74] 2022	Tarraso et al,[68] 2022
Bronchiectasis		32%	11.5%		-		4.6%[a] 0.0%[b] 0.0%[c]		8.16%[a] 44.30%[b] (P = 0.001)	4%[a] 2%[b] 11%[c] (P = 0.03)	12.8% at 5–7 months[a] 4.0% at 5–7 months[b] 2.2% at 5–7 months[c]	30.8%[b] (10.7% of entire cohort)
Lung distortion		25%		-	-							
Honeycombing		9%			-					0%[a] 2%[b] 1%[c]	0.5% at 5–7 months[b] 0.2% at 5–7 months[c]	
Reticulation			5.7%	30%			11.5%[a] 16.0%[b] 0.0%[c] (P-value = 0.019)	19%[a] 19%[b] 34%[c] (P < 0.042)	10.88%[a] 34.17%[b] (P = 0.001)	27%[a] 42%[b] 29%[c] (P < 0.001)	3.7% at 5–7 months[b] 1.7% at 5–7 months[c]	33.9%[b] (11.8% of entire cohort)
Fibrotic changes		89%	36.1%	18%	21%	1.8%–47%					4.4%	65.4%[b] (22.7% of entire cohort)
Comments	Patients more likely to have fibrotic changes were older and had a more severe form of COVID-19		Severe COVID-19 more likely to cause CT changes which persist longer	Patients with fibrosis on Ct also had impairments in PFT	Features of fibrosis on CT felt to be significant to patients who required ICU (P = 0.0259)		Severe/critical[a] Mild/moderate[b] Asymptomatic[c]	a = Oxygen alone b = CPAP c = IMV Abnormalities on CT were more frequent in patients requiring higher respiratory support	Moderate[a] Severe[b]	a = Oxygen alone b = CPAP c = IMV	70.8%[a] at 5–7 months[a] of which 20 (30.8%) had residual changes. The remaining 10 (15.4%) with fibrotic[c] abnormalities remained unchanged at 12 months	2 months[a] 12 months[b]

A systematic review of 31 studies found abnormal CT findings in 39 to 83% of patients with five studies describing PF at 3 months.[50] Longitudinal serial CT studies over 3 and 6 months showed that fibrosis-like findings were more prominent with severe SARS-CoV-2 infection (24.3% (17/70) vs 52.0% (53/102)), and that even with severe disease, these findings could improve over time with 24% and 52% improvement seen in severe and moderate disease, respectively. Radiological abnormalities persisted and were slower to resolve in the severe group.[73] A further large retrospective Italian study of 405 patients with follow-up between 5 and 7 months showed CT resolution in 55.6% of patients. Residual non-fibrotic and fibrotic abnormalities were noted in 37.5% and 6.9% of patients, respectively. Non-fibrotic changes were described as overt GGO (4.9% of whole population) or barely visible GGO (27.2% of whole population), peripheral predominant bronchiectasis (12.8%), peri lobular opacities (7.9%), and peripheral parenchymal bands (2.7%), resembling an NSIP pattern with or without organizing pneumonia features. Residual fibrotic abnormalities were found in 6.9% of patients of which a third were attributed to post-ventilatory abnormalities. Fibrotic abnormalities included subpleural reticulation (3.7%), bronchiectasis (4%), and volume loss (2.2%).[74] A subset of 65 patients had further CT imaging at 12 months follow-up. Nine (13.8%) had complete resolution at 12 months, 46 had non-fibrotic residual abnormalities at 5 to 7 months, of which 26 (40%) completely resolved and 20 (30.8%) had improvement but with residual changes. The remaining 10 (15.4%) with fibrotic abnormalities remained unchanged at 12 months.[75] In multivariate analysis, length of hospital admission, smoking history, and obesity have been identified as risk factors for persistent radiological abnormalities.[75]

The Emergence of Post-COVID Interstitial Lung Disease

Persistent symptoms, lung function, and radiological abnormalities have been reported post-COVID-19 (see **Box 1**, **Table 1, 2 and 3**). Several studies have demonstrated the gradual resolution of these findings over time including improvements in lung function impairment and radiological abnormalities.[20,48,54,56,58,59,68,76] The COVID-FIBROTIC study of 448 patients demonstrated ongoing radiological abnormalities in 27.4% of the patients at 12 months, with GGO being the most common abnormality (15.8%) followed by reticular pattern (11.8%), traction bronchiectasis (10.7%), and parenchymal bands (11.6%). Overall residual fibrotic changes were noted at 12 months in 22.7% of the cohort. Residual fibrotic features have been noted at varying time points in studies extending out to a year.[68] Risk factors for developing PC-ILD include increasing age (mean age 59 in fibrotic group vs 48.5 non-fibrotic group), chronic obstructive pulmonary disease (HR 2.88; 95% CI 1.27, 6.52), and severity of COVID-19 stratified according to baseline CT, a requirement for non-invasive or IMV and prolonged length of stay.[51,53,54,56,58,59,63,65,71,72,74,76,77]

A systematic review and meta-analysis of 46 studies assessing radiological features in 2811 CT images within 12 months found great heterogeneity in fibrotic findings between studies with a mean estimate of 29% (95% CI 22–37%).[77] Other meta-analyses have described the presence of fibrosis as high as 45%.[56]

There remain several unanswered questions regarding PC-ILD. There is little doubt that a cohort of individuals have residual fibrotic changes at 12 months ranging from 1 to 29% in studies,[48,59,78] however, pathologically whether that is related to fibrosis promoted by coronavirus itself or sequelae of severe infection and IMV remains to be determined. Certainly, studies have shown the presence of fibrosis being highest among those mechanically ventilated.[54,58,59,65] Similarly, it is unclear if COVID-19 unmasks and accelerates an undiagnosed pre-existing ILD or if it acts as a provoking viral agent triggering ILD.[79] Long-term studies are also needed to ascertain whether the fibrotic changes observed at a year, and consequently pulmonary function impairment and symptoms, continue to improve or remain static (similar to that seen in ARDS) over time. One such study, The UK Interstitial Lung Disease Long COVID study (UKILD-Long COVID) aims to investigate the prevalence and risk factors for PC-ILD looking at clinical, functional, and imaging parameters over time.[7]

Treatment of Post COVID Interstitial Lung Disease

A greater understanding of the pathophysiological mechanisms by which COVID-19 contributes to the development of lung fibrosis is key to our understanding of the natural history and development of PC-ILD. This, in turn, may lead us to the development of therapies that could ameliorate or hasten resolution.

The beneficial role of Dexamethasone in acutely unwell COVID-19 patients has been demonstrated in a randomized controlled trial.[80] There is limited trial evidence of therapy for PC-ILD. The majority of data are from observational cohorts. In a study of 837 patients followed up 4 weeks after discharge, 325 had ongoing symptoms and were offered further investigations and assessment; 35 (4.8%) patients were given the diagnosis of PC-ILD–predominantly an organizing pneumonia pattern; 30 patients were treated with corticosteroid therapy at day 61 ($\pm$ 19) post-COVID which was weaned over a period of 3 weeks. Patients reported symptomatic (median MRC improved from 3 (±2) to 2 (±1); P = 0.002), physiological (mean relative increase in FVC of 9.6% (±13.6); P = 0.004 and mean increase in Tl_{CO} of 31.49% (±27.7); P < 0.001), and radiological improvements. There was no observation of the progression of CT findings or change to fibrosis after treatment with corticosteroids. This study was limited due to the lack of randomization and control arm.[81]

Furthermore, the potential role of antifibrotics has been studied in a small retrospective, matched case-control study of 21 patients who received nintedanib therapy. There were improvements in SpO2/FiO2 ratio (P = 0.006) with no differences in chest imaging or oxygenation between the nintedanib and the control group.[82] To date, only a few observational studies have investigated the role of immunomodulatory and antifibrotic therapies highlighting the great need for randomized control trials.[83]

Novel therapies targeting histone deacetylase 88 and hepatocyte growth factor secreted by mesenchymal stem cells have been proposed due to their antifibrotic effects.[84,85] A phase 1 clinical trial in 27 patients with COVID-19 PF using human embryonic stem cell-derived immunity and matrix-regulatory cells during the SARS-CoV-2 outbreak in Wuhan City showed improvements in exercise capacity and resolution of fibrotic changes on CT.[86] There are ongoing trials of Sirolimus, Pirfenidone, and Colchicine assessing the impact on the development of PC-ILD[83,87,88] and we eagerly await robust trials investigating therapies in PC-ILD.

SUMMARY

The long-term impact of the COVID-19 pandemic remains to be elucidated. The SARS-CoV-2 virus triggers a significant inflammatory and immune response, which causes lung damage. Though the majority of patients will improve and recover fully, some have persistent symptoms, reduced lung function, and radiological abnormalities at 12 months. With over 550 million people affected worldwide, the significance of persistent pulmonary abnormalities in the form of PF cannot be underestimated in terms of ongoing morbidity. The incidence of PC-ILD is very heterogenous and varies from study to study, according to varied factors including the duration of follow-up, severity of SARS-CoV-2 infection, and need for IMV. as well as other potential risk factors. Further studies are eagerly awaited that will glean more light on the risk factors for developing PC-ILD, the role of therapies in preventing or treating PC-ILD, and give a greater understanding of the clinical significance of this new disease.

CLINICS CARE POINTS

- Persistent pulmonary symptoms are commonly reported post-SARS-CoV-2 infection and risk factors include increased length of stay in hospital with COVID-19, severe COVID-19 pneumonitis on initial CT, the need for higher respiratory support, female gender, and increasing age.
- Lung function impairment improves over time, however, can persist in a proportion of patients post-SARS-CoV-2 infection.
- CT abnormalities at 1 year include mostly non-fibrotic changes (like GGO, bronchiectasis, peri lobular opacities, and parenchymal bands), and less commonly, peripheral fibrotic changes.
- The long-term consequences of persistent fibrotic changes post-COVID-19 remain to be elucidated and studies need to assess the significance of these findings.

DISCLOSURE

N. Kewalramani reports grant and nonfinancial support from CSL Behring, Bern (Switzerland) outside the submitted work. K.-M. Heenan has nothing to disclose. D. McKeegan has nothing to disclose. N. Chaudhuri has nothing to disclose.

REFERENCES

1. Ghebreyesus TA. WHO Director-General's opening remarks at the media briefing on COVID-19. In: World Health Organization. 2020. Available at WHO Director-General's opening remarks at the media briefing on COVID-19-11 March 2020. Accessed September 9, 2022.
2. Zhu N, Zhang D, Wang W, et al. A Novel Coronavirus from Patients with Pneumonia in China, 2019. N Engl J Med 2020;382(8):727–33.
3. World Health Organization. WHO Coronavirus (COVID-19) Dashboard | WHO Coronavirus (COVID-19) Dashboard With Vaccination Data. In: World Health Organization 2022. Available at WHO Coronavirus (COVID-19) Dashboard | WHO Coronavirus (COVID-19) Dashboard With Vaccination Data. Accessed September 9, 2022.
4. Gao Y, Ding M, Dong X, et al. Risk factors for severe and critically ill COVID-19 patients: A review. Allergy 2021;76(2):428–55.
5. Zhou F, Yu T, Du R, et al. Clinical course and risk factors for mortality of adult inpatients with COVID-19 in Wuhan, China: a retrospective cohort study. Lancet 2020;395(10229):1054–62.
6. Wu Z, McGoogan JM. Characteristics of and important lessons from the coronavirus disease 2019 (COVID-19) outbreak in China. JAMA 2020;323(13):1239.
7. Wild JM, Porter JC, Molyneaux PL, et al. Understanding the burden of interstitial lung disease post-COVID-19: the UK Interstitial Lung Disease-Long COVID Study (UKILD-Long COVID). BMJ Open Respiratory Research 2021;8(1):e001049.
8. Drożdżal S, Rosik J, Lechowicz K, et al. An update on drugs with therapeutic potential for SARS-CoV-2 (COVID-19) treatment. Drug Resist Updates 2021;59:100794.

9. Parums D. v. Editorial: current status of oral antiviral drug treatments for SARS-CoV-2 Infection in non-hospitalized patients. Med Sci Mon Int Med J Exp Clin Res 2022;28:e935952.

10. Hammond J, Leister-Tebbe H, Gardner A, et al. Oral Nirmatrelvir for high-risk, nonhospitalized adults with Covid-19. N Engl J Med 2022;386(15):1397–408.

11. Fischer WA 2nd, Eron JJ Jr, et al. A phase 2a clinical trial of molnupiravir in patients with COVID-19 shows accelerated SARS-CoV-2 RNA clearance and elimination of infectious virus. Sci Transl Med 2022;14(628):eabl7430.

12. Mohd I, Kumar Arora M, Asdaq SMB, et al. Discovery, development, and patent trends on molnupiravir: a prospective oral treatment for COVID-19. Molecules 2021;26(19):5795.

13. Mahase E. Covid-19: Molnupiravir reduces risk of hospital admission or death by 50% in patients at risk, MSD reports. BMJ 2021;375:n2422.

14. Office for National Statistics. Coronavirus (COVID-19) latest insights. In:Office for National Statistics 2022. Available at Coronavirus (COVID-19) latest insights - Office for National Statistics (ons.gov.uk). Accessed September 10, 2022.

15. Centers for Disease Control and Prevention. CDC COVID Data Tracker: Daily and Total Trends. In: Centers for Disease Control and Prevention 2022. Available at CDC COVID Data Tracker: Daily and Total Trends. Accessed August 25, 2022.

16. George PM, Wells AU, Jenkins RG. Pulmonary fibrosis and COVID-19: the potential role for antifibrotic therapy. Lancet Respir Med 2020;8(8):807–15.

17. George PM, Barratt SL, Condliffe R, et al. Respiratory follow-up of patients with COVID-19 pneumonia. Thorax 2020;75(11):1009–16.

18. Das KM, Lee EY, Singh R, et al. Follow-up chest radiographic findings in patients with MERS-CoV after recovery. Indian J Radiol Imag 2017;27(03):342–9.

19. Xie L, Liu Y, Fan B, et al. Dynamic changes of serum SARS-Coronavirus IgG, pulmonary function and radiography in patients recovering from SARS after hospital discharge. Respir Res 2005;6(1):5.

20. Wu X, Liu X, Zhou Y, et al. 3-month, 6-month, 9-month, and 12-month respiratory outcomes in patients following COVID-19-related hospitalisation: a prospective study. Lancet Respir Med 2021;9(7):747–54.

21. Zhao L, Wang X, Xiong Y, et al. Correlation of autopsy pathological findings and imaging features from 9 fatal cases of COVID-19 pneumonia. Medicine 2021;100(12):e25232.

22. Carsana L, Sonzogni A, Nasr A, et al. Pulmonary post-mortem findings in a series of COVID-19 cases from northern Italy: a two-centre descriptive study. Lancet Infect Dis 2020;20(10):1135–40.

23. Ducloyer M, Gaborit B, Toquet C, et al. Complete post-mortem data in a fatal case of COVID-19: clinical, radiological and pathological correlations. Int J Legal Med 2020;134(6):2209–14.

24. Grillo F, Barisione E, Ball L, et al. Lung fibrosis: an undervalued finding in COVID-19 pathological series. Lancet Infect Dis 2021;21(4):e72.

25. Sun P, Qie S, Liu Z, et al. Clinical characteristics of hospitalized patients with SARS-CoV-2 infection: A single arm meta-analysis. J Med Virol 2020;92(6):612–7.

26. Sinha P, Bos LD. Pathophysiology of the acute respiratory distress syndrome. Crit Care Clin 2021;37(4):795–815.

27. Lai CC, Shih TP, Ko WC, et al. Severe acute respiratory syndrome coronavirus 2 (SARS-CoV-2) and coronavirus disease-2019 (COVID-19): The epidemic and the challenges. Int J Antimicrob Agents 2020;55(3):105924.

28. Mcdonald LT. Healing after COVID-19: are survivors at risk for pulmonary fibrosis? Am J Physiol Lung Cell Mol Physiol 2021;320(2):L257–65.

29. Ware LB, Matthay MA. The Acute Respiratory Distress Syndrome. N Engl J Med 2000;342(18):1334–49.
30. Thille AW, Esteban A, Fernández-Segoviano P, et al. Chronology of histological lesions in acute respiratory distress syndrome with diffuse alveolar damage: a prospective cohort study of clinical autopsies. Lancet Respir Med 2013;1(5): 395–401.
31. Moore JB, June CH. Cytokine release syndrome in severe COVID-19. Science 2020;368(6490):473–4.
32. Ye C, Li H, Bao M, et al. Alveolar macrophage - derived exosomes modulate severity and outcome of acute lung injury. Aging 2020;12(7):6120–8.
33. Deng Y, Herbert JA, Robinson E, et al. Neutrophil-airway epithelial interactions result in increased epithelial damage and viral clearance during respiratory syncytial virus infection. J Virol 2020;94(13). 021611–e2219.
34. Herbert JA, Deng Y, Hardelid P, et al. β_2-integrin LFA1 mediates airway damage following neutrophil transepithelial migration during respiratory syncytial virus infection. Eur Respir J 2020;56(2):1902216.
35. John AE, Joseph C, Jenkins G, et al. COVID-19 and pulmonary fibrosis: a potential role for lung epithelial cells and fibroblasts. Immunol Rev 2021;302(1):228–40.
36. Melms JC, Biermann J, Huang H, et al. A molecular single-cell lung atlas of lethal COVID-19. Nature 2021;595(7865):114–9.
37. Wang S, Yao X, Ma S, et al. A single-cell transcriptomic landscape of the lungs of patients with COVID-19. Nat Cell Biol 2021;23(12):1314–28.
38. Zhang C, Zhao W, Li JW, et al. Discharge may not be the end of treatment: pay attention to pulmonary fibrosis caused by severe COVID-19. J Med Virol 2021;93: 1378–86.
39. Piersma B, Bank RA, Boersema M. Signaling in Fibrosis: TGF-β, WNT, and YAP/TAZ Converge. Front Med (Lausanne) 2015;2:59.
40. Cabrera-Benítez NE, Parotto M, Post M, et al. Mechanical stress induces lung fibrosis by epithelial–mesenchymal transition*. Crit Care Med 2012;40(2):510–7.
41. Zhang R, Pan Y, Fanelli V, et al. Mechanical stress and the induction of lung fibrosis via the midkine signaling pathway. Am J Respir Crit Care Med 2015; 192(3):315–23.
42. Wei J, Yang H, Lei P, et al. Analysis of thin-section CT in patients with coronavirus disease (COVID-19) after hospital discharge. J X Ray Sci Technol 2020;28(3): 383–9.
43. National Institute for Health and Care Excellence. COVID-19 rapid guideline: managing the long-term effects of COVID-19 (NG188). In:London: National Institute for Health and Care Excellence (NICE). 2021. Available at Overview | COVID-19 rapid guideline: managing the long-term effects of COVID-19 | Guidance | NICE. Accessed September 10, 2022.
44. Mandal S, Barnett J, Brill SE, et al. 'Long-COVID': a cross-sectional study of persisting symptoms, biomarker and imaging abnormalities following hospitalization for COVID-19. Thorax 2021;76(4):396–8.
45. Evans RA, McAuley H, Harrison EM, et al. Physical, cognitive, and mental health impacts of COVID-19 after hospitalisation (PHOSP-COVID): a UK multicentre, prospective cohort study. Lancet Respir Med 2021;9(11):1275–87.
46. Evans RA, Leavy OC, Richardson M, et al. Clinical characteristics with inflammation profiling of long COVID and association with 1-year recovery following hospitalisation in the UK: a prospective observational study. Lancet Respir Med 2022;10(8):761–75.

47. Carfì A, Bernabei R, Landi F. Persistent symptoms in patients after acute COVID-19. JAMA 2020;324(6):603.
48. Vargas Centanaro G, Calle Rubio M, Álvarez-Sala Walther JL, Martinez-Sagasti F, Albuja Hidalgo A, Herranz Hernández R, Rodríguez Hermosa JL. Long-term Outcomes and Recovery of Patients who Survived COVID-19: LUNG INJURY COVID-19 Study. Open Forum Infect Dis 2022;9(4):ofac098.
49. Chun HJ, Coutavas E, Pine AB, et al. Immunofibrotic drivers of impaired lung function in postacute sequelae of SARS-CoV-2 infection. JCI Insight 2021;6(14):e148476.
50. Willi S, Lüthold R, Hunt A, et al. COVID-19 sequelae in adults aged less than 50 years: a systematic review. Trav Med Infect Dis 2021;40:101995.
51. Froidure A, Mahsouli A, Liistro G, et al. Integrative respiratory follow-up of severe COVID-19 reveals common functional and lung imaging sequelae. Respir Med 2021;181:106383.
52. Boari GEM, Bonetti S, Braglia-Orlandini F, et al. Short-Term Consequences of SARS-CoV-2-Related Pneumonia: A Follow Up Study. High Blood Pres Cardiovasc Prev 2021;28(4):373–81.
53. Robey RC, Kemp K, Hayton P, et al. Pulmonary sequelae at 4 months After COVID-19 infection: a single-centre experience of a COVID Follow-Up Service. Adv Ther 2021;38(8):4505–19.
54. Faverio P, Luppi F, Rebora P, et al. Six-month pulmonary impairment after severe COVID-19: a prospective, multicentre follow-up study. Respiration 2021;100(11):1078–87.
55. Han X, Fan Y, Alwalid O, et al. Six-month follow-up chest CT Findings after severe COVID-19 pneumonia. Radiology 2021;299(1):E177–86.
56. Hama Amin BJ, Kakamad FH, Ahmed GS, et al. Post COVID-19 pulmonary fibrosis; a meta-analysis study. Annals of Medicine and Surgery 2022;77:103590.
57. Zangrillo A, Belletti A, Palumbo D, et al. One-Year Multidisciplinary Follow-Up of Patients With COVID-19 Requiring Invasive Mechanical Ventilation. J Cardiothorac Vasc Anesth 2022;36(5):1354–63.
58. Huang L, Yao Q, Gu X, et al. 1-year outcomes in hospital survivors with COVID-19: a longitudinal cohort study. Lancet 2021;398(10302):747–58.
59. Faverio P, Luppi F, Rebora P, et al. One-year pulmonary impairment after severe COVID-19: a prospective, multicenter follow-up study. Respir Res 2022;23(1):65.
60. Eksombatchai D, Wongsinin T, Phongnarudech T, et al. Pulmonary function and six-minute-walk test in patients after recovery from COVID-19: A prospective cohort study. PLoS One 2021;16(9):e0257040.
61. Lv D, Chen X, Wang X, et al, Pulmonary function of patients with 2019 novel coronavirus induced-pneumonia: a retrospective cohort study. Ann Palliat Med 2020;9(5):3447–52.
62. Shah AS, Wong AW, Hague CJ, et al. A prospective study of 12-week respiratory outcomes in COVID-19-related hospitalisations. Thorax 2021;76(4):402–4.
63. Frija-Masson J, Debray MP, Boussouar S, et al. Residual ground glass opacities three months after Covid-19 pneumonia correlate to alteration of respiratory function: The post Covid M3 study. Respir Med 2021;184:106435.
64. Guler SA, Ebner L, Aubry-Beigelman C, et al. Pulmonary function and radiological features 4 months after COVID-19: first results from the national prospective observational Swiss COVID-19 lung study. Eur Respir J 2021;57(4):2003690.
65. Noel-Savina E, Viatgé T, Faviez G, et al. Severe SARS-CoV-2 pneumonia: clinical, functional and imaging outcomes at 4 months. Respiratory Medicine and Research 2021;80:100822.

66. Hellemons ME, Huijts S, Bek LM, et al. Persistent health problems beyond pulmonary recovery up to 6 months after hospitalization for COVID-19: a longitudinal study of respiratory, physical, and psychological outcomes. Annals of the American Thoracic Society 2022;19(4):551–61.

67. Safont B, Tarraso J, Rodriguez-Borja E, et al. Lung function, radiological findings and biomarkers of fibrogenesis in a cohort of COVID-19 patients six months after hospital discharge. Arch Bronconeumol 2022;58(2):142–9.

68. Tarraso J, Safont B, Carbonell-Asins JA, et al. Lung function and radiological findings 1 year after COVID-19: a prospective follow-up. Respir Res 2022;23(1):242.

69. Marvisi M, Ferrozzi F, Balzarini L, et al. First report on clinical and radiological features of COVID-19 pneumonitis in a Caucasian population: Factors predicting fibrotic evolution. Int J Infect Dis 2020;99:485–8.

70. Yang ZL, Chen C, Huang L, et al. Fibrotic changes depicted by thin-section CT in patients With COVID-19 at the early recovery stage: preliminary experience. Front Med 2020;7:605088.

71. Zhou M, Xu J, Liao T, et al. Comparison of residual pulmonary abnormalities 3 months after discharge in patients who recovered from COVID-19 of Different severity. Front Med 2021;8:682087.

72. Cocconcelli E, Bernardinello N, Giraudo C, et al. Characteristics and prognostic factors of pulmonary fibrosis After COVID-19 pneumonia. Front Med 2022;8:823600.

73. Zhang D, Zhang C, Li X, et al. Thin-section computed tomography findings and longitudinal variations of the residual pulmonary sequelae after discharge in patients with COVID-19: a short-term follow-up study. Eur Radiol 2021;31(9):7172–83.

74. Besutti G, Monelli F, Schirò S, et al. Follow-Up CT patterns of residual lung abnormalities in severe COVID-19 pneumonia survivors: a multicenter retrospective study. Tomography 2022;8(3):1184–95.

75. Wallis TJM, Heiden E, Horno J, et al. Risk factors for persistent abnormality on chest radiographs at 12-weeks post hospitalisation with PCR confirmed COVID-19. Respir Res 2021;22(1):157.

76. Caruso D, Guido G, Zerunian M, et al. Post-acute sequelae of COVID-19 pneumonia: six-month chest CT follow-up. Radiology 2021;301(2):E396–405.

77. Fabbri L, Moss S, Khan FA, et al. Parenchymal lung abnormalities following hospitalisation for COVID-19 and viral pneumonitis: a systematic review and meta-analysis. Thorax 2022;78(2):191–201.

78. Bocchino M, Lieto R, Romano F, et al. Chest CT-based assessment of 1-year outcomes after moderate COVID-19 pneumonia. Radiology 2022;305(2):479–85.

79.. Mehta P, Rosas IO, Singer M. Understanding post-COVID-19 interstitial lung disease (ILD): a new fibroinflammatory disease entity. Intensive Care Med 2022;48(12):1803–6.

80. RECOVERY Collaborative Group, Horby P, Lim WS, et al. Dexamethasone in hospitalized patients with Covid-19. N Engl J Med 2021;384(8):693–704.

81. Myall KJ, Mukherjee B, Castanheira AM, et al. Persistent post–COVID-19 interstitial lung disease. An observational study of corticosteroid treatment. Annals of the American Thoracic Society 2021;18(5):799–806.

82. Saiphoklang N, Patanayindee P, Ruchiwit P. The effect of NINTEDANIB in Post-COVID-19 lung fibrosis: an observational study. Critical Care Research and Practice 2022;2022:1–7.

83. Molina M. Pirfenidone Compared to Placebo in Post-COVID19 Pulmonary Fibrosis COVID-19. In: ClinicalTrials.gov. 2021. Available at Pirfenidone

Compared to Placebo in Post-COVID19 Pulmonary Fibrosis COVID-19-Full Text View - ClinicalTrials.gov. Accessed October 10, 2022.

84. Krishna Murthy P, Sivashanmugam K, Kandasamy M, et al. Repurposing of histone deacetylase inhibitors: a promising strategy to combat pulmonary fibrosis promoted by TGF-β signalling in COVID-19 survivors. Life Sci 2021;266:118883.

85. Vishnupriya M, Naveenkumar M, Manjima K, et al. Post-COVID pulmonary fibrosis: therapeutic efficacy using with mesenchymal stem cells - How the lung heals. Eur Rev Med Pharmacol Sci 2021;25(6):2748–51.

86. Wu J, Zhou X, Tan Y, et al. Phase 1 trial for treatment of COVID-19 patients with pulmonary fibrosis using hESC-IMRCs. Cell Prolif 2020;53(12):e12944.

87. University of Chicago. Assessing the Efficacy of Sirolimus in Patients with COVID-19 Pneumonia for Prevention of Post-COVID Fibrosis. In:ClinicalTrials.gov. 2021, Available at Assessing the Efficacy of Sirolimus in Patients With COVID-19 Pneumonia for Prevention of Post-COVID Fibrosis - Full Text View - ClinicalTrials.gov. Accessed October 10, 2022.

88. Issak ER. Colchicine and Post-COVID-19 Pulmonary Fibrosis. In: ClinicalTrials.gov, 2021. Available at Colchicine and Post-COVID-19 Pulmonary Fibrosis - Full Text View - ClinicalTrials.gov. Accessed October 10, 2022.

Clinically Relevant Biomarkers in Connective Tissue Disease-Associated Interstitial Lung Disease

Janelle Vu Pugashetti, MD, MS[a],*, Dinesh Khanna, MD, MS[b],
Ella A. Kazerooni, MD, MS[a,c], Justin Oldham, MD, MS[a,d]

KEYWORDS

- Connective tissue disease • Interstitial lung disease • Computed tomography
- Biomarkers

KEY POINTS

- Blood-based biomarkers that reflect lung epithelial cell dysfunction, aberrant immunity, and abnormal lung remodeling may discriminate the presence of interstitial lung disease in patients with connective tissue diseases.
- High-resolution computed tomography (HRCT) is the current best diagnostic tool for ILD and may have prognostic value in CTD-ILD.
- Texture-based and volumetric HRCT analysis show promise as prognostic biomarkers in CTD-ILD.
- Composite biomarkers improve risk prediction compared with stand-alone biomarkers, showing high promise in the diagnosis and prognosis of patients with connective tissue-associated interstitial lung disease.
- The combination of large blood-based platforms, radiomic algorithms, and use of machine learning is expected to advance the study of CTD-ILD in coming years.

INTRODUCTION

Interstitial lung disease (ILD) is a common manifestation of connective tissue disease (CTD), most often affecting patients with rheumatoid arthritis (RA), systemic sclerosis (SSc), idiopathic inflammatory myopathy (IIM), and mixed CTD.[1–5] ILD can also develop

[a] Division of Pulmonary and Critical Care Medicine, Department of Internal Medicine, University of Michigan; [b] Scleroderma Program, Division of Rheumatology, Department of Internal Medicine, University of Michigan; [c] Division of Cardiothoracic Radiology, Department of Radiology, University of Michigan; [d] Department of Epidemiology, University of Michigan
* Corresponding author. 1150 West Medical Center Drive, 6220 MSRB III / SPC 5642, Ann Arbor, MI 48109.
E-mail address: vupugash@med.umich.edu

Immunol Allergy Clin N Am 43 (2023) 411–433
https://doi.org/10.1016/j.iac.2023.01.012
0889-8561/23/Published by Elsevier Inc.

immunology.theclinics.com

in patients with Sjögren syndrome (SS) and systemic lupus erythematosus, but is less common with these disorders.[6,7] Among patients who do develop CTD-ILD, a subset will develop a progressive phenotype, leading to parenchymal destruction, lung function decline, and early mortality.[8–21] Early and accurate diagnosis is essential for effectively managing patients with CTD-ILD, particularly because effective treatments exist to stabilize disease and sometimes improve lung function.[13–15,22–24] Diagnosing ILD is often nuanced and difficult, as many patients with CTD-ILD have no respiratory symptoms, and symptoms are nonspecific when they do develop.[25,26] Pulmonary function testing (PFT) can help raise suspicion for ILD in patients with CTD, but test performance characteristics are modest.[25,27] Once ILD is diagnosed, the inability to discriminate patients likely to progress remains elusive. Clinical prediction models have been developed to predict ILD progression in patients with CTD, but many are CTD specific, reducing generalizability to the larger CTD-ILD population. The ability to predict CTD-ILD progression would empower patients and clinicians to make better informed decisions about treatment, lung transplantation, and goals of care.

Biomarkers, defined as indicators of normal biological processes and pathogenic processes, hold promise for improving our ability to accurately diagnose ILD and predict disease trajectory.[28] The ideal biomarker should be noninvasive or minimally invasive, with high accuracy for predicting the end point of interest. Biomarkers most likely to inform clinical decision making in patients with CTD are those that predict early disease before the development of respiratory symptoms and a progressive phenotype. In the past decade, numerous studies have identified candidate blood-based and high-resolution computed tomography (HRCT) biomarkers, and recent -omics investigations have added composite biomarkers to the list of potentially clinically relevant biomarkers in the CTD-ILD population. However, barriers to clinical implementation remain. This review provides an overview of recent advances in CTD-ILD biomarker investigation, focusing on blood-based and HRCT biomarkers, and highlights strategies to advance these biomarkers toward clinical implementation in patients with CTD-ILD.

BLOOD-BASED DIAGNOSTIC BIOMARKERS

Blood-based biomarkers carry high promise for diagnosing ILD in patients with CTD and providing prognostic information for these patients, because many reflect molecular pathways involved in fibrogenesis and can signal early disease before the development of overt fibrosis and respiratory symptoms. Furthermore, the minimally invasive nature of peripheral blood acquisition better positions this class of biomarkers for clinical implementation when compared with more invasive procedures such as bronchoalveolar lavage and surgical lung biopsy. Blood-based biomarkers include clinically approved autoantibodies and inflammatory markers, and research biomarkers identified through targeted and unbiased analysis. The major challenge remaining with blood-based biomarkers, however, is achieving adequate test performance to justify clinical implementation; this is particularly difficult in patients with CTD, because many blood-based biomarkers may reflect systemic and extrapulmonary processes.

The detection of autoantibodies serves a critical role in the diagnosis of CTD-ILD, and autoantibodies are the only blood biomarkers available for clinical use. There are a number of autoantibodies found in patients with CTD that are associated with higher risk of ILD. In patients with SSc, antitopoisomerase I antibody (anti-Scl70) has repeatedly been associated with ILD across cohorts.[29–33] Anti-Th/To ribonucleoprotein antibodies and anti-PM/Scl have also been shown to be associated with ILD, although they are more rarely detected in patients with SSc.[34,35] In addition, in 2 large SSc cohorts, the presence of anti-SSA/Ro was found to be associated with at least a 2-fold increased odds of SSc-ILD.[36,37] Conversely, the absence of anticentromere antibodies is associated with decreased likelihood of ILD.[30,38] In patients with RA, anti-citrullinated cyclic peptide (CCP) antibodies and high-titer rheumatoid factor predict ILD, with some studies demonstrating a correlation between anti-CCP titers and HRCT severity.[39–42] In patients with IIM, anti-tRNA synthetase antibodies are commonly detected, most frequently anti-Jo-1, anti-PL-7, and PL-12 antibodies. These antisynthetase antibodies are the hallmark of antisynthetase syndrome, which carries high risk of developing ILD, with reports of ILD in more than 90% of antisynthetase antibody-positive patients.[43,44] Another antibody found in patients with IIM is the (anti-MDA5/CADM-140), which characterizes a subset with clinically amyopathic myositis and high risk of ILD.[45–50] Unfortunately, many of these antibodies tend to signal overall disease extent and risk of ILD, rather than the presence of ILD.

Beyond clinically approved autoantibodies, multiple investigations have focused on molecular markers of lung epithelial cell dysfunction, aberrant immunity (cytokines and chemokines), and abnormal lung remodeling (collagen peptides/extracellular matrix biomarkers) in patients with CTD-ILD. Among those with the best described test performance characteristics is Krebs von den Lungen 6 (KL-6), which is strongly expressed on regenerating type II pneumocytes and thought to be a marker of epithelial injury.[51] At various cutoff points, the sensitivity of KL-6 ranges from 73% to 87% and specificity ranges from 70% to 100% for discriminating CTD-ILD among patients with CTD.[52–60] The area under the curve (AUC), which describes global discrimination without a cutoff threshold, ranges from 0.86 to 0.90, depending on the cohort in which the test is applied. Another well-studied marker of lung epithelial damage and turnover is surfactant protein D (SP-D). As a biomarker of ILD in patients with CTD, sensitivity ranges from 68% to 89.4% and specificity ranges from 70% to 83% depending on the dichotomization threshold used, with an AUC of 0.72 to 0.983.[41,52,53,61] In studies comparing KL-6 and SP-D in the same cohort, the specificity of SP-D is generally lower than that of KL-6.[52,53,62]

Other well-studied blood-based biomarkers are described in **Table 1** and include SP-A[62,63]; club cell secreted protein 16[54]; pulmonary and activation-regulated chemokine (PARC)[41]; interleukin (IL)-6, 8, and 10[64]; tumor necrosis factor-α[64]; metalloproteinase (MMP)-7[41]; and Wnt Family member 5a (Wnt5a).[65] Although test performance characteristics are not reported for all biomarkers listed, studies have shown that circulating concentration of these biomarkers are higher in patients with CTD-ILD compared with those with CTD without ILD. Despite the advances made studying these blood-based biomarkers, none have been implemented clinically. Given the complexity of ILD pathogenesis, it is likely that biomarkers from multiple pathways are needed to achieve sufficient test performance to justify clinical implementation. Doyle and colleagues[41] demonstrated the promise of this approach in detecting RA-ILD. A model composed of clinical factors including demographics and autoantibodies, combined with a biomarker signature composed of MMP-7, PARC, and SP-D, outperformed the clinical signature alone or any of the standalone biomarkers.

The emergence of machine learning has further improved risk prediction and is likely to become an important tool in the diagnosis of CTD-ILD. Machine learning comprises mathematical algorithms that build, train, and self-evaluate iterative models to self-improve predictive power.[66] Kass and colleagues[67] demonstrated the promise of machine-learning in patients with RA, showing that biomarker signatures derived

Table 1
Novel blood-based diagnostic CTD-ILD biomarkers

Biomarker	Reference(s)	Diagnostic Test Performance (CTD-ILD from CTD Without ILD)
Lung epithelial cell dysfunction		
CA 125	RA[128]	RA[128]: cutoff 35 U/mL, sens 60.71%, spec 79.52%, AUC 0.78
CC16	SSc[54]	SSc[54]: cutoff 46.0 ng/mL, sens 51.8%, spec 88.8%, AUC 0.76
CCL18	SSc[129]	
E-Selectin	SSc[130,131] RA[132] IIM & SSc[133]	
ET-1	SSc[130]	
ICAM-1	SSc[134]	
KL-6	SSc[52–54,135,136] RA[55,56,137,57] IIM[62,58,138,139,60,140] SS[141] CTD[59]	SSc[52]: cutoff 602 U/mL, sens 73%, spec 70% SSc[53]: cutoff 500 U/mL, sens 78.8%, spec 90.0%, AUC 0.90 SSc[54]: cutoff 302 U/mL, sens 85.5%, spec 85.3%, AUC 0.89 RA[55]: cutoff 277.5 U/mL, sens 86.7%, spec 88%, AUC 0.88 RA[56]: cutoff 399 U/mL, sens 85.71%, spec 90.91%, AUC 0.92 RA[57]: AUC 0.81 IIM[58]: cutoff 437 U/mL, sens 87%, spec 96%, AUC 0.97 CTD[59]: cutoff 275.1 U/mL, sens 79.4%, spec 79.9%, AUC 0.86 IIM[60]: cutoff 549 U/mL, sens 83%, spec 100%
SP-A	SSc[63] IIM[62]	SSc[63]: Cutoff 43.8 ng/mL, sens 33%, spec 100% IIM[62]: Cutoff 39.5 ng/mL, PPV = 70%
SP-D	SSc[52–54] RA[41,137] IIM[62]	SSc[52]: cutoff 62.2 ng/mL, sens 68%, spec 70% SSc[53]: cutoff 90 ng/mL, sens 89.4%, spec 80.0%, AUC 0.983 Ssc[54]: cutoff 91.0 ng/mL, sens 71.4%, spec 77.2%, AUC 0.72 SSc: cutoff 110 ng/mL, sens 77%, spec 83% RA[41]: AUC 0.75 RA[41]: AUC 0.91
VEGF	SSc[130]	
Aberrant immunity		
CCL2	IIM[62,142] SSc[61]	
CX3CL1	SSc[143]	
CXCL10/IP-10	SSc[144,145] RA[146] IIM[147,142] CTD[148]	
CXCL11	CTD[148] IIM[142]	

(continued on next page)

Table 1
(continued)

Biomarker	Reference(s)	Diagnostic Test Performance (CTD-ILD from CTD Without ILD)
CXCL12		
CXCL13	SS[149]	
CXCL16	SSc[150]	
CXCL4	SSc[151]	
CXCL9/MIG	SSc[67] CTD[148]	
IL-04	SSc[152]	
IL-06	SS[64] IIM[147]	SS[64]: cutoff 7.109 pg/mL, sens 90.88%, spec 62.75%, AUC 0.67
IL-08	SS[64,153] IIM[147]	SS[64]: cutoff 20.094 pg/mL, sens 90.9%, spec 62.8%, AUC 0.71
IL-10	SS[64]	SS[64]: cutoff 5.162 pg/mL, sens 87.54%, spec 78.63%, AUC 0.89
IL-15		
IL-23	SSc[154]	
IL-33	SSc[155]	
IL-35	SSc[156]	
PARC	SSc[135] RA[41]	RA[41]: AUC 0.80 RA[41]: AUC 0.70
TNF-α	SS[64] IIM[147]	SS[64]: cutoff 9.116 pg/mL, sens 80.6%, spec 73.2%, AUC 0.73
Wnt5a	RA[65]	RA[65]: cutoff 4.49, sens 55.6%, spec 4.9%, AUC 0.75
Abnormal lung remodeling		
MMP-7	SSc[157,158] RA[41,146,137] IIM[159]	RA[41]: AUC 0.86, RA[41]: AUC 0.83
MMP-12	SSc[160]	
TIMP-1	SSc[161]	
CCN2/CTGF	RA[162] SSc[163]	
GDF-15	SSc[164–166]	
YKL-40	SSc[167]	

Abbreviations: CC16, club cell secreted protein 16; CCL18, C-C motif chemokine ligand 18; IL, interleukin; MMP, metalloproteinase; PARC, pulmonary and activation-regulated chemokine; sens, sensitivity; spec, specificity; TNF, tumor necrosis factor; YKL-40, chitinase-3-like-1.

using this method could effectively discriminate ILD in these patients with higher sensitivity and specificity than stand-alone proteins. Although this approach can result in a highly in-sample predictive classifier, overfitting remains an issue and out-of-sample validation is required. Kass and colleagues[67] demonstrated this challenge, showing that the highly predictive diagnostic signatures developed in independent RA cohorts differed greatly, with little overlap in covariates. Qin and colleagues[57] pursued a similar approach in patients with RA, showing that 3 machine learning algorithms discriminated ILD with AUC of at least 0.95. These results have yet to be externally validated, however.

BLOOD-BASED PROGNOSTIC BIOMARKERS

As with diagnosis, the use of peripheral blood-based biomarkers holds promise as a prognostic tool in CTD-ILD. The outcomes of progression in CTD-ILD studies have generally been survival, lung function decline including forced vital capacity (FVC) and diffusing capacity of carbon monoxide (DLCO), or a composite end point of these measures (**Table 2**). With the recent publication of consensus definitions to define progressive pulmonary fibrosis,[68] substantial research is expected in the coming years to optimally define progression in this population.

Clinically approved autoantibodies have been studied in the prognosis of patients with CTD. In a large SSc outcome study, the presence of anti-Scl-70 antibody in patients predicted a faster rate of FVC decline.[31] Conversely, presence of anti-PM/Scl antibodies has been associated with less FVC decline and better survival compared with patients with anti-Scl-70.[69] In patients with anti-Jo or anti-MDA-5 antibody, the concurrent positivity with anti-SSA/Ro portends worse ILD and mortality compared with patients without dual antibodies.[70,71] Patients with IIM with anti-MDA-5 positivity have been well described to have rapidly progressive and fatal ILD among Japanese cohorts, with 33% to 66% experiencing 6-month and antibody positivity portending a 6-fold risk of death.[45–48] However, in predominantly Caucasian cohorts in the United States, patients with ILD with anti-MDA5 did not have the rapidly progressive ILD described in Japanese cohorts.[50]

Several studies of novel biomarkers have also evaluated prognosis in CTD-ILD. KL-6 again is among the best studied across common CTD-ILD subtypes.[59,72–74] Among 82 patients with SSc-ILD in the Genetics versus Environment Scleroderma Outcome Study (GENISOS), higher baseline KL-6 levels were predictive of faster progression, with patients averaging 7% more decline in annualized percent change of FVC when baseline KL-6 was greater than the cutoff value.[75] Chitinase-3-like-1 (YKL-40), C-C motif chemokine ligand 18 (CCL18), and IL-6, along with several other biomarkers previously linked to progression in idiopathic pulmonary fibrosis (IPF), have also been shown to predict worse outcome among patients with CTD-ILD (see **Table 2**). Like diagnostic biomarker studies, investigators have just begun to harness the power of composite biomarkers in risk prediction. In a multicenter retrospective cohort of Japanese patients with IIM-ILD, Gono and colleagues[76] showed that a prediction model based on anti-MDA-5 status, C-reactive protein level, and KL-6 level differentiated survival more effectively than anti-MDA-5 antibody testing alone. In the tocilizumab phase 3 trial, elevated acute phase reactants, as an entry criterion, were associated with marked decline in FVC during 1 year in the placebo group in those with ILD (257 mL in placebo group vs 6.5 mL in active group).[22]

Our group recently completed the first proteomic analysis of patients with non-IPF ILD, which included 245 patients with CTD-ILD across 3 centers.[77] Relative plasma concentration of 368 biomarkers was determined using a medium-throughput proteomic platform, 31 of which were found to be associated with near-term ILD progression, defined as death, lung transplant, or 10% or greater relative FVC decline within 1 year of blood draw. Of these 31 proteins identified in the derivation cohort, 17 maintained association in an independent validation cohort, with consistent outcome association in each of the ILD subgroups assessed. Using machine learning, we then derived a 12-analyte proteomic signature, which discriminated 1-year ILD progression with good sensitivity and negative predictive value across cohorts, suggesting this tool could effectively identify patients at low risk of ILD progression, justifying a conservative strategy in this population. Notably, those with a low-risk proteomic signature experienced an increase in FVC over 1 year, whereas those with a high-risk signature

Table 2
Novel blood-based prognostic CTD-ILD biomarkers

Biomarker	Prognostic
	CTD-ILD subtype (reference): outcome of progression
Lung epithelial cell dysfunction	
CA 125	CTD[168]: composite FVC and survival
CC16	SSc[169]: composite FVC and survival
CCL18	SSc[170]: FVC, D$_{LCO}$, and survival
	SSc[136]: FVC and radiologic progression
ICAM-1	SSc[134]: FVC
IGFBP-2	SSc[171]: D$_{LCO}$
KL-6	SSc[75]: FVC
	SSc[172]: composite FVC, oxygen supplementation, survival
	IIM[72]: survival
	SS[73]: survival
	CTD[74]: survival
	CTD[59]: HRCT progression
SP-D	CTD[168]: composite (lung function and survival)
	SSc[173]: FVC
Aberrant immunity	
CCL2	Ssc[174]: FVC, survival
	IIM[142]: survival
CX3CL1	SSc[143]: composite survival, FVC, and HRCT
CXCL10/IP-10	IIM[142]: survival
CXCL11	IIM[142]: survival
CXCL12	CTD[168]: composite FVC and survival
CXCL13	CTD[168]: composite FVC and survival
CXCL4	SSc[175]: FVC
	SSc[151]: D$_{LCO}$
IL-06	SSc[176]: FVC, D$_{LCO}$, survival
	IIM[177]: survival
	CTD[178]: survival
IL-08	IIM[147]: survival
IL-10	Ssc[174]: FVC
	IIM[179]: survival
IL-15	IIM[179]: survival
	IIM[180]: exacerbation, survival
Neopterin	IIM[181]: survival
Abnormal lung remodeling	
MMP-7	SSc[158]: survival
	IIM[159]: survival
YKL-40	CTD[168]: composite FVC and survival
	IIM[182]: survival
	IIM[183]: survival

experienced an FVC loss of 227 mL, which mirrored that of placebo-treated patients from IPF clinical trials[78,79] (**Fig. 1**). Prospective validation of these findings could result in a clinically actionable biomarker to inform clinical decision making in patients with CTD-ILD and other fibrosing ILDs.

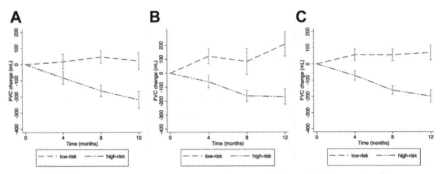

Fig. 1. Longitudinal plots comparing 1-year change in forced vital capacity between patients with high-risk and low-risk proteomic signature in the derivation (*A*), validation (*B*), and combined cohorts (*C*). (*Reprinted with permission from* Elsevier. The Lancet Respiratory Medicine, June 2022, 10 (6), 593-602.)

HIGH-RESOLUTION COMPUTED TOMOGRAPHY: CONNECTIVE TISSUE DISEASE-INTERSTITIAL LUNG DISEASE DIAGNOSIS AND PROGNOSIS

HRCT is a crucial component of the diagnostic evaluation of CTD-ILD, with thin slices and reconstruction algorithms tailored to the detection of patterns and distributions of interstitial, parenchymal, and airway abnormalities.[80,81] With the poor sensitivity of chest radiography [82,83] and PFT,[25,27] reliance on these measures to diagnose or rule out ILD in a patient with CTD is inadequate. An interdisciplinary expert consensus panel recently recommended that all patients with SSc be screened with HRCT at baseline, and the authors recommend a similar approach for all CTDs in which ILD commonly manifests. Major educational efforts have been undertaken to promote HRCT screening,[84,85] which will be critical to reduce the well-described diagnostic delays that occur in patients with ILD.[86,87]

With HRCT as our best tool for diagnosing ILD in patients with CTD, several groups have also investigated the role of HRCT as a predictor of CTD-ILD outcome. Extent of fibrotic disease on baseline HRCT, including the extent of reticulation, traction bronchiectasis, and honeycombing, is consistently associated with worse survival across CTD-ILD subtypes.[40,88–93] Walsh and colleagues[94] evaluated HRCTs and pulmonary function variables in 168 patients with CTD-ILD, and identified severity of traction bronchiectasis and extent of honeycombing as indices independently predictive of mortality. In patients with SSc-ILD, a higher extent of fibrosis on baseline HRCT was associated with subsequent lung function decline in the placebo group of the Scleroderma Lung Study.[95] A cutoff of 20% fibrotic extent has been proposed as an optimal predictor of mortality in patients with SSc-ILD, forming the basis of the Goh simple staging system for mortality risk.[96,97] It should be noted that by combining HRCT and PFTs in this staging system by using an FVC threshold when HRCT fibrotic extent was indeterminate, the risk prediction considerably improved beyond either HRCT or PFTs alone.

An additional question has been the role of the HRCT pattern of abnormality. There are many patterns described in CTD-ILD, with the 2 important patterns being that of nonspecific interstitial pneumonia (NSIP) and usual interstitial pneumonia (UIP).[98] The radiologic pattern of NSIP, characterized by bibasilar ground-glass opacities, is well recognized in patients with CTD-ILD, and is the most common pattern in patients with SSc-ILD and IIM-ILD.[99,100] In contrast, the radiologic pattern of UIP, with bibasilar reticulation and fibrotic architectural distortion, is most commonly observed among patients with RA-ILD.[40,101,102] The radiologic pattern of UIP is classically associated with IPF, the prototypic ILD characterized by poor prognosis, so naturally the question of whether UIP portends worse prognosis in the setting of non-IPF ILD arises. Several groups have found that a UIP pattern is associated with worse survival in patients with CTD-ILD.[40,88,94,103–106] In a cohort of patients with RA-ILD evaluated at National Jewish Health, Solomon and colleagues[107] also found that patients with UIP pattern had a shorter survival time than those with radiologic NSIP. However, in all multivariate Cox models that included key clinical variables or pulmonary physiology, baseline HRCT pattern was no longer a predictor of survival.[107] Rather, baseline FVC and evidence of FVC decline were independent predictors of worse survival. It remains unclear what additional information UIP pattern on HRCT provides, other than being a by-product of pulmonary fibrosis.

Although HRCT in cross-section may predict outcome, serial acquisition of HRCT may provide more clues about disease trajectory. Patients with SSc who had an increase in fibrotic extent on serial HRCT were more likely to experience further fibrotic progression and lung function decline[92]; this is congruent with our findings that worsening fibrosis extent on HRCT is a poor prognostic sign, with patients experiencing near-term FVC decline and a 2-fold increased risk of mortality after showing radiologic progression.[108,109] However, the radiation exposure of serial HRCT remains a consideration, especially among younger individuals with CTD-ILD, and in particular women due to radiation exposure to the breast tissue.

RADIOMICS AND QUANTITATIVE HIGH-RESOLUTION COMPUTED TOMOGRAPHY

The widespread use of visual HRCT assessment as biomarker in patients with CTD-ILD is currently limited due to low interobserver agreement.[110,111] Although semiquantitative scoring classifications have been proposed to judge the extent of fibrosis, discrepancy has been observed between radiologists' scoring, even after training.[97] Furthermore, the best studied candidate predictors of progression on HRCT—fibrotic extent and the UIP pattern—are both by-products of progressive pulmonary fibrosis. Tools that more effectively predict CTD-ILD progression before progression has occurred are more likely to be of clinical value.

One possible strategy to obviate interobserver variation is computer-based radiomic analysis. Radiomics is an emerging field that converts medical images into high-dimensional quantitative data and has high potential to serve as a novel avenue for ILD subphenotyping and outcome prediction. Quantification of HRCT features, density, and texture, along with algorithms developed by machine learning, has the potential to not only standardize the role of HRCT interpretation but also detect diagnostic and prognostic data not visually detectable by humans. Deep learning, which is a unique machine learning algorithm that incorporates multiple layers of learning architecture to create increasingly complex schema to improve autonomously, has emerged as a useful approach to modeling radiomic data.

In 2016, Anthimopoulos and colleagues[112] trained and tested a deep learning algorithm using HRCT examinations in 120 patients to detect ground-glass opacity, reticulation, consolidation, micronodules, and honeycombing, which had been manually labeled by 2 thoracic radiologists. This deep learning algorithm had an accuracy of 85% in classifying these imaging features. Using a similar approach, Kim and colleagues[113] employed a deep learning algorithm that achieved 95% accuracy for classifying these features of interest on HRCT images of patients with ILD. Advancing beyond individual HRCT features and toward HRCT pattern recognition, Walsh and colleagues[114] used a deep learning algorithm to detect classification of UIP based on the 2011 consensus guidelines. Their algorithm showed an accuracy of 76.4% for the classification of UIP in the derivation cohort, and an accuracy of 73.3% in an external validation cohort. Although promising, these investigations continue to rely on visual assessment as the gold standard, limiting their use to what can be detected by the human eye.

Evaluation of HRCT using density histogram analysis evaluates the lung according to simple density characteristics, deriving metrics of histogram skewness and kurtosis. Although Ash and colleagues[115] demonstrated a 3-fold increased risk of death or transplant in patients with IPF with higher mean lung density, the addition of quantitative HRCT density did not significantly augment prognostication beyond visual assessment of baseline lung fibrosis.[116] A more complex approach is texture-based analysis, which incorporates morphologic features. A quantitative lung fibrosis score can be generated using automated computer-aided diagnosis systems developed for assessing ILD using texture features. In patients with IPF, this texture-based score correlated with longitudinal FVC change, whereas HRCT density alone did not.[117] Kim and colleagues[118] applied this score to the HRCT examinations of 129 patients with SSc-ILD and showed good accuracy for detecting fibrosis when compared with visual assessment. Oh and colleagues[119] applied the quantitative lung fibrosis score to HRCT images of 144 patients with RA-ILD, and found that it predicted 5-year mortality. At a cutoff of 12% of total lung volume, higher quantitative lung fibrosis scores predicted survival similar to patients with IPF.[119] In addition, use of texture-based radiomic features in cluster analysis can predict different disease stages with moderate sensitivity and excellent specificity in patients with SSc-ILD.[120] In a recent study of 90 patients with SSc, texture-based radiomic features were extracted and cluster analysis performed to reveal 2 distinct patient clusters. Despite similar scores on the Goh simple staging system between clusters (based on visual assessment of HRCT and FVC), one texture-based radiomic cluster had significantly more impaired lung function. A radiomic risk score predicted faster disease progression and worse survival.[121]

For well over a decade, advances in CT scanner acquisition speed have led to the increase of volumetric HRCT scans, which can be acquired in a single breath-hold of 5 to 10 seconds, which bypasses the traditional issue of interspaced HRCT images with gaps of 1 cm or more between images, and allows for more precise evaluation of patterns such as honeycombing. Computer Aided Lung Informatics for Pathology Evaluation and Rating (CALIPER) is a tool that employs volumetric structural and textural analysis of the lung, trained to label and measure volumetric HRCT data as normal, ground glass, reticulation, low-attenuation, honeycombing, and vessel-related structures.[122] Jacob and colleagues[119] applied this tool in a study of 203 patients with CTD-ILD, with the CALIPER variable of vessel-related structure volume being the one most strongly associated with mortality (**Fig. 2**).[123] This same CALIPER variable has been shown to best predict mortality in patients with IPF.[122,124,125] Given that IPF mortality is worse than CTD-ILD mortality, Chung and colleagues[126] postulated that CALIPER may be able to differentiate CTD-ILD from IPF in the setting of a UIP pattern, finding that the vessel-related structure volume was greater in patients with IPF than patients with CTD-ILD, potentially showing its promise as a marker to differentiate CTD-ILD from IPF.[126]

CALIPER variables can be integrated into current classification schemes for prognosis in CTD-ILD. The CALIPER algorithm allows unbiased identification of CTD-ILD patient phenotypes using automated stratification. The substitution of this automated CALIPER model in place of pulmonary function variables in the ILD-GAP score, a validated staging score in ILD, resulted in a more sensitive predictor of 1- and 2-year

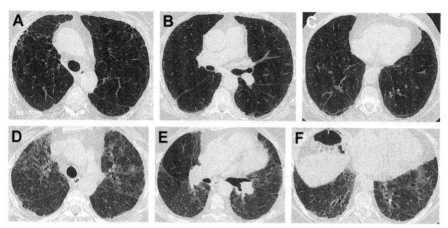

Fig. 2. Axial HRCT image color maps demonstrating CALIPER-derived vessel-related structures (VRS; red). VRS represent pulmonary arteries and veins (excluding hilar vessels) and connected tubular structures, the latter primarily reflecting adjoining regions of fibrosis. (*A–C*) Axial sections in a 71-year-old female 30-pack-year exsmoker with upper lobe emphysema and fibrosis visible in the lower lobes (VRS 2.1%); (*D–F*) axial sections in a 62-year-old female never smoker with upper lobe-predominant fibrosis (VRS 7.0%). Nonvascular region captures in the VRS signal are visible in the upper lobes (*D*) and adjacent to the right hemidiaphragm (*F*). (Reproduced with permission of the © ERS 2022: European Respiratory Journal 53 (1) 1800869; https://doi.org/10.1183/13993003.00869-2018 Published 3 January 2019.)

mortality.[123] In addition, Jacob and colleagues[127] conducted a study of 157 patients with RA-ILD to compare 3 prediction models based on HRCT: the Goh scleroderma simple staging system, the Fleischner Society IPF diagnostic guidelines, and CALIPER scores of vessel-related structures. Although all 3 models strongly predicted outcome, combining the CALIPER vessel-related structures threshold with the visual scoring from the Goh and Fleischner systems improved outcome modeling, predicting 4-year survival indistinguishable from a comparator group of patients with IPF.[127]

Although early, these studies are promising and suggest that radiomics has high potential to inform clinical decision making once widespread automation of one or more of these algorithms becomes possible. With machine learning, data extracted from quantitative HRCT carries the potential to develop new imaging biomarkers not discernible by humans and bypass the inherent problems of visual assessment. Radiomics is likely to provide complementary diagnostic and prognostic information with exciting potential for outcome prediction.

UNMET RESEARCH NEEDS AND STRATEGIES FOR BIOMARKER OPTIMIZATION

Although there has been impressive progress in biomarker discovery, unmet needs remain. At present, there are few biomarkers reliably predicting the presence of ILD in patients with CTD, and even fewer have been validated to predict CTD-ILD progression before it occurs. Although we reviewed emerging blood-based and HRCT biomarkers, none have been incorporated into clinical practice, reflecting modest test performance characteristics for most; this stems in large part from a paucity of validation testing for most biomarkers, because most candidate studies have been performed in retrospective single-center studies. Validation of these promising biomarkers in external cohorts will be key in biomarker investigation going forward. Equally important will be the assessment of test performance characteristics, which will allow clinicians to weigh the clinical utility of any biomarker advanced for clinical implementation. Furthermore, before clinical application, it will be essential that well-designed, prospective, multicenter studies be conducted.

As multicohort investigations become standard in biomarker investigation, it will be essential to ensure that the outcomes chosen in future studies are uniform and well-defined, particularly in studies of prognostic biomarkers. Understandably, survival should remain to be an important outcome. However, near-term progression should also be prioritized in future biomarker investigation. Near-term lung function decline has clinical implications, because patients may necessitate earlier intervention, as well as implications for drug development in clinical trials. At present, large sample sizes are required to ensure adequate power to detect differences in lung function decline, so the ability to predict near-term progression would allow clinical trial enrichment and more efficient recruitment.

Last, there is increased potential when modeling biomarkers in aggregate. The combination of multiple biomarkers across multiple modalities, perhaps combining clinical, blood-based, and radiomic biomarkers, holds high potential in CTD-ILD risk prediction. Machine learning can seamlessly tackle increasingly large datasets and the rapidly growing number of candidate biomarkers. After deriving and validating candidate signatures retrospectively, it will be necessary to quantify identified biomarkers and to prospectively validate specific thresholds that define individual risk most precisely.

SUMMARY

A number of biomarkers have been proved to be informative in patients with CTD-ILD, derived from blood-based and HRCT data. The development of large blood-based platforms, the refinement of radiomic algorithms, and the use of machine learning have shown early promise in the diagnosis and prognosis of CTD-ILD. A rapid expansion of investigation with aggregate biomarkers is expected in the coming years, making precision medicine closer to reality and improving outcomes in patients with CTD-ILD.

CLINICS CARE POINTS

- HRCT is the screening and diagnostic tool of choice for patients with CTDs. When screening for ILD, PFT and chest radiography are insufficient and an HRCT should be ordered.
- There are no single blood-based biomarkers validated for the diagnosis or prognosis of CTD-associated ILD. When caring for patients with CTD-ILD, making clinical decisions based on single laboratory tests should be avoided.
- The best prognostic radiographic markers are extent of fibrosis and evidence of progression on serial HRCT. When a patient has a large extent of fibrosis or shows worsening fibrosis on HRCT, the likelihood of future ILD progression is high.

FUNDING

NHLBI T32 HL007749 (Pugashetti).

REFERENCES

1. Juge PA, Lee JS, Ebstein E, et al. MUC5B Promoter Variant and Rheumatoid Arthritis with Interstitial Lung Disease. N Engl J Med 2018;379(23):2209–19.

2. Gabbay E, Tarala R, Will R, et al. Interstitial lung disease in recent onset rheumatoid arthritis. Am J Respir Crit Care Med 1997;156(2 Pt 1):528–35.
3. Walker UA, Tyndall A, Czirjak L, et al. Clinical risk assessment of organ manifestations in systemic sclerosis: a report from the EULAR Scleroderma Trials And Research group database. Ann Rheum Dis 2007;66(6):754–63.
4. Fathi M, Dastmalchi M, Rasmussen E, et al. Interstitial lung disease, a common manifestation of newly diagnosed polymyositis and dermatomyositis. Ann Rheum Dis 2004;63(3):297–301.
5. Reiseter S, Gunnarsson R, Mogens Aalokken T, et al. Progression and mortality of interstitial lung disease in mixed connective tissue disease: a long-term observational nationwide cohort study. Rheumatology (Oxford) 2018;57(2): 255–62.
6. Flament T, Bigot A, Chaigne B, et al. Pulmonary manifestations of Sjogren's syndrome. Eur Respir Rev 2016;25(140):110–23.
7. Castelino FV, Varga J. Interstitial lung disease in connective tissue diseases: evolving concepts of pathogenesis and management. Arthritis Res Ther 2010; 12(4):213.
8. Flaherty KR, Wells AU, Cottin V, et al. Nintedanib in Progressive Fibrosing Interstitial Lung Diseases. The New Engl J Med 2019. https://doi.org/10.1056/NEJMoa1908681.
9. Cottin V, Wollin L, Fischer A, et al. Fibrosing interstitial lung diseases: knowns and unknowns. Eur Respir Rev 2019;28(151). https://doi.org/10.1183/16000617.0100-2018.
10. Adegunsoye A, Oldham JM, Bellam SK, et al. Computed Tomography Honeycombing Identifies a Progressive Fibrotic Phenotype with Increased Mortality across Diverse Interstitial Lung Diseases. Ann Am Thorac Soc 2019;16(5): 580–8.
11. Tashkin DP, Elashoff R, Clements PJ, et al. Cyclophosphamide versus placebo in scleroderma lung disease. N Engl J Med 2006;354(25):2655–66.
12. Tashkin DP, Roth MD, Clements PJ, et al. Mycophenolate mofetil versus oral cyclophosphamide in scleroderma-related interstitial lung disease (SLS II): a randomised controlled, double-blind, parallel group trial. Lancet Respir Med 2016;4(9):708–19.
13. Fischer A, Brown KK, Du Bois RM, et al. Mycophenolate mofetil improves lung function in connective tissue disease-associated interstitial lung disease. J Rheumatol 2013;40(5):640–6.
14. Oldham JM, Lee C, Valenzi E, et al. Azathioprine response in patients with fibrotic connective tissue disease-associated interstitial lung disease. Respir Med 2016;121:117–22.
15. Huapaya JA, Silhan L, Pinal-Fernandez I, et al. Long-Term Treatment With Azathioprine and Mycophenolate Mofetil for Myositis-Related Interstitial Lung Disease. Chest 2019;156(5):896–906.
16. Sharma N, Putman MS, Vij R, et al. Myositis-associated Interstitial Lung Disease: Predictors of Failure of Conventional Treatment and Response to Tacrolimus in a US Cohort. J Rheumatol 2017;44(11):1612–8.
17. Witt LJ, Demchuk C, Curran JJ, et al. Benefit of adjunctive tacrolimus in connective tissue disease-interstitial lung disease. Pulm Pharmacol Ther 2016;36: 46–52.
18. Duarte AC, Cordeiro A, Fernandes BM, et al. Rituximab in connective tissue disease-associated interstitial lung disease. Clin Rheumatol 2019;38(7):2001–9.

19. Keir GJ, Maher TM, Hansell DM, et al. Severe interstitial lung disease in connective tissue disease: rituximab as rescue therapy. Eur Respir J 2012;40(3):641–8.

20. Koduri G, Norton S, Young A, et al. Interstitial lung disease has a poor prognosis in rheumatoid arthritis: results from an inception cohort. Rheumatology (Oxford) 2010;49(8):1483–9.

21. Steen VD, Medsger TA. Changes in causes of death in systemic sclerosis, 1972-2002. Ann Rheum Dis 2007;66(7):940–4.

22. Khanna D, Lin CJF, Furst DE, et al. Tocilizumab in systemic sclerosis: a randomised, double-blind, placebo-controlled, phase 3 trial. The Lancet Respir Med 2020;8(10):963–74.

23. Tashkin DP, Elashoff R, Clements PJ, et al. Cyclophosphamide versus placebo in scleroderma lung disease. The New Engl J Med 2006;354(25):2655–66.

24. Tashkin DP, Roth MD, Clements PJ, et al. Mycophenolate mofetil versus oral cyclophosphamide in scleroderma-related interstitial lung disease (SLS II): a randomised controlled, double-blind, parallel group trial. Lancet Respir Med 2016;4(9):708–19.

25. Pugashetti JV, Kitich A, Alqalyoobi S, et al. Derivation and Validation of a Diagnostic Prediction Tool for Interstitial Lung Disease. Chest 2020. https://doi.org/10.1016/j.chest.2020.02.044.

26. Bilgici A, Ulusoy H, Kuru O, et al. Pulmonary involvement in rheumatoid arthritis. Rheumatol Int 2005;25(6):429–35.

27. Suliman YA, Dobrota R, Huscher D, et al. Brief Report: Pulmonary Function Tests: High Rate of False-Negative Results in the Early Detection and Screening of Scleroderma-Related Interstitial Lung Disease. Arthritis Rheumatol 2015; 67(12):3256–61.

28. Wu AC, Kiley JP, Noel PJ, et al. Current Status and Future Opportunities in Lung Precision Medicine Research with a Focus on Biomarkers. An American Thoracic Society/National Heart, Lung, and Blood Institute Research Statement. Am J Respir Crit Care Med 2018;198(12):e116–36.

29. Reveille JD, Solomon DH. American College of Rheumatology Ad Hoc Committee of Immunologic Testing G. Evidence-based guidelines for the use of immunologic tests: anticentromere, Scl-70, and nucleolar antibodies. Arthritis Rheum 2003;49(3):399–412.

30. Nihtyanova SI, Schreiber BE, Ong VH, et al. Prediction of Pulmonary Complications and Long-Term Survival in Systemic Sclerosis. Arthritis Rheumatol 2014; 66(6):1625–35.

31. Jandali B, Salazar GA, Hudson M, et al. The Effect of Anti-Scl -70 Antibody Determination Method on Its Predictive Significance for Interstitial Lung Disease Progression in Systemic Sclerosis. ACR Open Rheumatol 2022;4(4):345–51.

32. Walker UA, Tyndall A, Czirjak L, et al. Clinical risk assessment of organ manifestations in systemic sclerosis: a report from the EULAR Scleroderma Trials And Research group database. Ann Rheum Dis 2007;66(6):754–63.

33. Liaskos C, Marou E, Simopoulou T, et al. Disease-related autoantibody profile in patients with systemic sclerosis. Autoimmunity 2017;50(7):414–21.

34. Mitri GM, Lucas M, Fertig N, et al. A comparison between anti-Th/To- and anti-centromere antibody-positive systemic sclerosis patients with limited cutaneous involvement. Arthritis Rheum 2003;48(1):203–9.

35. Lazzaroni M-G, Marasco E, Campochiaro C, et al. The clinical phenotype of systemic sclerosis patients with anti-PM/Scl antibodies: results from the EUSTAR cohort. Rheumatology 2021;60(11):5028–41.

36. Hudson M, Pope J, Mahler M, et al. Clinical significance of antibodies to Ro52/TRIM21 in systemic sclerosis. Arthritis Res Ther 2012;14(2):R50.
37. Mierau R, Moinzadeh P, Riemekasten G, et al. Frequency of disease-associated and other nuclear autoantibodies in patients of the German network for systemic scleroderma: correlation with characteristic clinical features. Arthritis Res Ther 2011;13(5):R172.
38. Wangkaew S, Euathrongchit J, Wattanawittawas P, et al. Incidence and predictors of interstitial lung disease (ILD) in Thai patients with early systemic sclerosis: Inception cohort study. Mod Rheumatol 2016;26(4):588–93.
39. Kamiya H, Panlaqui OM. Systematic review and meta-analysis of the risk of rheumatoid arthritis-associated interstitial lung disease related to anti-cyclic citrullinated peptide (CCP) antibody. BMJ Open 2021;11(3):e040465.
40. Kelly CA, Saravanan V, Nisar M, et al. Rheumatoid arthritis-related interstitial lung disease: associations, prognostic factors and physiological and radiological characteristics–a large multicentre UK study. Rheumatology (Oxford) 2014;53(9):1676–82.
41. Doyle TJ, Patel AS, Hatabu H, et al. Detection of Rheumatoid Arthritis–Interstitial Lung Disease Is Enhanced by Serum Biomarkers. Am J Respir Crit Care Med 2015;191(12):1403–12.
42. Giles JT, Danoff SK, Sokolove J, et al. Association of fine specificity and repertoire expansion of anticitrullinated peptide antibodies with rheumatoid arthritis associated interstitial lung disease. Ann Rheum Dis 2014;73(8):1487–94.
43. Richards TJ, Eggebeen A, Gibson K, et al. Characterization and peripheral blood biomarker assessment of anti-Jo-1 antibody-positive interstitial lung disease. Arthritis Rheum 2009;60(7):2183–92.
44. Marie I, Josse S, Decaux O, et al. Comparison of long-term outcome between anti-Jo1- and anti-PL7/PL12 positive patients with antisynthetase syndrome. Autoimmun Rev 2012;11(10):739–45.
45. Sato S, Hirakata M, Kuwana M, et al. Autoantibodies to a 140-kd polypeptide, CADM-140, in Japanese patients with clinically amyopathic dermatomyositis. Arthritis Rheum 2005;52(5):1571–6.
46. Tsuji H, Nakashima R, Hosono Y, et al. Multicenter Prospective Study of the Efficacy and Safety of Combined Immunosuppressive Therapy With High-Dose Glucocorticoid, Tacrolimus, and Cyclophosphamide in Interstitial Lung Diseases Accompanied by Anti–Melanoma Differentiation–Associated Gene 5–Pos. Arthritis Rheumatol 2020;72(3):488–98.
47. Hamaguchi Y, Kuwana M, Hoshino K, et al. Clinical Correlations With Dermatomyositis-Specific Autoantibodies in Adult Japanese Patients With Dermatomyositis. Arch Dermatol 2011;147(4):391.
48. Koga T, Fujikawa K, Horai Y, et al. The diagnostic utility of anti-melanoma differentiation-associated gene 5 antibody testing for predicting the prognosis of Japanese patients with DM. Rheumatology (Oxford) 2012;51(7):1278–84.
49. Fiorentino D, Chung L, Zwerner J, et al. The mucocutaneous and systemic phenotype of dermatomyositis patients with antibodies to MDA5 (CADM-140): A retrospective study. J Am Acad Dermatol 2011;65(1):25–34.
50. Hall JC, Casciola-Rosen L, Samedy L-A, et al. Anti-Melanoma Differentiation-Associated Protein 5-Associated Dermatomyositis: Expanding the Clinical Spectrum. Arthritis Care Res 2013;65(8):1307–15.
51. Ishikawa N, Hattori N, Yokoyama A, et al. Utility of KL-6/MUC1 in the clinical management of interstitial lung diseases. Respir Investig 2012;50(1):3–13.

52. Asano Y, Ihn H, Yamane K, et al. Clinical significance of surfactant protein D as a serum marker for evaluating pulmonary fibrosis in patients with systemic sclerosis. Arthritis Rheum 2001;44(6):1363–9.

53. Hant FN, Ludwicka-Bradley A, Wang H-J, et al. Surfactant Protein D and KL-6 as Serum Biomarkers of Interstitial Lung Disease in Patients with Scleroderma. The J Rheumatol 2009;36(4):773–80.

54. Hasegawa M, Fujimoto M, Hamaguchi Y, et al. Use of Serum Clara Cell 16-kDa (CC16) Levels as a Potential Indicator of Active Pulmonary Fibrosis in Systemic Sclerosis. The J Rheumatol 2011;38(5):877–84.

55. Fotoh DS, Helal A, Rizk MS, et al. Serum Krebs von den Lungen-6 and lung ultrasound B lines as potential diagnostic and prognostic factors for rheumatoid arthritis–associated interstitial lung disease. Clin Rheumatol 2021;40(7): 2689–97.

56. Zheng M, Lou A, Zhang H, et al. Serum KL-6, CA19-9, CA125 and CEA are Diagnostic Biomarkers for Rheumatoid Arthritis-Associated Interstitial Lung Disease in the Chinese Population. Rheumatol Ther 2021;8(1):517–27.

57. Qin Y, Wang Y, Meng F, et al. Identification of biomarkers by machine learning classifiers to assist diagnose rheumatoid arthritis-associated interstitial lung disease. Arthritis Res Ther 2022;24(1). https://doi.org/10.1186/s13075-022-02800-2.

58. Takanashi S, Nishina N, Nakazawa M, et al. Usefulness of serum Krebs von den Lungen-6 for the management of myositis-associated interstitial lung disease. Rheumatology 2019;58(6):1034–9.

59. Lee JS, Lee EY, Ha Y-J, et al. Serum KL-6 levels reflect the severity of interstitial lung disease associated with connective tissue disease. Arthritis Res Ther 2019; 21(1). https://doi.org/10.1186/s13075-019-1835-9.

60. Fathi M, Barbasso Helmers S, Lundberg IE. KL-6: a serological biomarker for interstitial lung disease in patients with polymyositis and dermatomyositis. J Intern Med 2012;271(6):589–97.

61. Hasegawa M, Fujimoto M, Matsushita T, et al. Serum chemokine and cytokine levels as indicators of disease activity in patients with systemic sclerosis. Clin Rheumatol 2011;30(2):231–7.

62. Chen F, Lu X, Shu X, et al. Predictive value of serum markers for the development of interstitial lung disease in patients with polymyositis and dermatomyositis: a comparative and prospective study. Intern Med J 2015;45(6):641–7.

63. Takahashi H, Kuroki Y, Tanaka H, et al. Serum levels of surfactant proteins A and D are useful biomarkers for interstitial lung disease in patients with progressive systemic sclerosis. Am J Respir Crit Care Med 2000;162(1):258–63.

64. Yang H. Cytokine expression in patients with interstitial lung disease in primary Sjogren's syndrome and its clinical significance. Am J Transl Res 2021;13(7): 8391–6.

65. Yu M, Guo Y, Zhang P, et al. Increased circulating Wnt5a protein in patients with rheumatoid arthritis-associated interstitial pneumonia (RA-ILD). Immunobiology 2019;224(4):551–9.

66. Maher TM, Nambiar AM, Wells AU. The role of precision medicine in interstitial lung disease. Eur Respir J 2022;60(3):2102146.

67. Kass DJ, Nouraie M, Glassberg MK, et al. Comparative Profiling of Serum Protein Biomarkers in Rheumatoid Arthritis-Associated Interstitial Lung Disease and Idiopathic Pulmonary Fibrosis. Arthritis Rheumatol 2020;72(3):409–19.

68. Raghu G, Remy-Jardin M, Richeldi L, et al. Idiopathic Pulmonary Fibrosis (an Update) and Progressive Pulmonary Fibrosis in Adults: An Official ATS/ERS/

JRS/ALAT Clinical Practice Guideline. Am J Respir Crit Care Med 2022;205(9): e18–47.

69. Guillen-Del Castillo A, Pilar Simeon-Aznar C, Fonollosa-Pla V, et al. Good outcome of interstitial lung disease in patients with scleroderma associated to anti-PM/Scl antibody. Semin Arthritis Rheum 2014;44(3):331–7.

70. Xu A, Ye Y, Fu Q, et al. Prognostic values of anti-Ro52 antibodies in anti-MDA5-positive clinically amyopathic dermatomyositis associated with interstitial lung disease. Rheumatology (Oxford) 2021;60(7):3343–51.

71. Bauhammer J, Blank N, Max R, et al. Rituximab in the Treatment of Jo1 Antibody-associated Antisynthetase Syndrome: Anti-Ro52 Positivity as a Marker for Severity and Treatment Response. J Rheumatol 2016;43(8):1566–74.

72. Arai S, Kurasawa K, Maezawa R, et al. Marked increase in serum KL-6 and surfactant protein D levels during the first 4 weeks after treatment predicts poor prognosis in patients with active interstitial pneumonia associated with polymyositis/dermatomyositis. Mod Rheumatol 2013;23(5):872–83.

73. Kamiya Y, Fujisawa T, Kono M, et al. Prognostic factors for primary Sjögren's syndrome-associated interstitial lung diseases. Respir Med 2019;159:105811.

74. Satoh H, Kurishima K, Ishikawa H, et al. Increased levels of KL-6 and subsequent mortality in patients with interstitial lung diseases. J Intern Med 2006; 260(5):429–34.

75. Salazar GA, Kuwana M, Wu M, et al. KL-6 But Not CCL-18 Is a Predictor of Early Progression in Systemic Sclerosis-related Interstitial Lung Disease. The J Rheumatol 2018;45(8):1153–8.

76. Gono T, Masui K, Nishina N, et al. Risk Prediction Modeling Based on a Combination of Initial Serum Biomarker Levels in Polymyositis/Dermatomyositis–Associated Interstitial Lung Disease. Arthritis Rheumatol 2021;73(4):677–86.

77. Bowman WS, Newton CA, Linderholm AL, et al. Proteomic biomarkers of progressive fibrosing interstitial lung disease: a multicentre cohort analysis. Lancet Respir Med 2022. https://doi.org/10.1016/S2213-2600(21)00503-8.

78. Noble PW, Albera C, Bradford WZ, et al. Pirfenidone in patients with idiopathic pulmonary fibrosis (CAPACITY): two randomised trials. Comparative Study Multicenter Study Randomized Controlled Trial Research Support. Non-U.S Gov't Lancet 2011;377(9779):1760–9.

79. Richeldi L, Du Bois RM, Raghu G, et al. Efficacy and Safety of Nintedanib in Idiopathic Pulmonary Fibrosis. New Engl J Med 2014;370(22):2071–82.

80. Mayo JR. CT evaluation of diffuse infiltrative lung disease: dose considerations and optimal technique. J Thorac Imaging 2009;24(4):252–9.

81. Kazerooni EA. High-resolution CT of the lungs. AJR Am J Roentgenol 2001; 177(3):501–19.

82. Ghodrati S, Pugashetti JV, Kadoch MA, et al. Diagnostic Accuracy of Chest Radiography for Detecting Fibrotic Interstitial Lung Disease. Ann Am Thorac Soc 2022. https://doi.org/10.1513/AnnalsATS.202112-1377RL.

83. Schurawitzki H, Stiglbauer R, Graninger W, et al. Interstitial lung disease in progressive systemic sclerosis: high-resolution CT versus radiography. Radiology 1990;176(3):755–9. https://doi.org/10.1148/radiology.176.3.2389033.

84. Hoffmann-Vold A-M, Maher TM, Philpot EE, et al. The identification and management of interstitial lung disease in systemic sclerosis: evidence-based European consensus statements. Lancet Rheumatol 2020;2(2):e71–83. https://doi.org/10.1016/s2665-9913(19)30144-4.

85. Bruni C, Chung L, Hoffmann-Vold AM, et al. High-resolution computed tomography of the chest for the screening, re-screening and follow-up of systemic

sclerosis-associated interstitial lung disease: a EUSTAR-SCTC survey. Clin Exp Rheumatol 2022. https://doi.org/10.55563/clinexprheumatol/7ry6zz.

86. Pritchard D, Adegunsoye A, Lafond E, et al. Diagnostic test interpretation and referral delay in patients with interstitial lung disease. Respir Res 2019;20(1): 253. https://doi.org/10.1186/s12931-019-1228-2.

87. Cano-Jiménez E, Vázquez Rodríguez T, Martín-Robles I, et al. Diagnostic delay of associated interstitial lung disease increases mortality in rheumatoid arthritis. Scientific Rep 2021;11(1). https://doi.org/10.1038/s41598-021-88734-2.

88. Kim EJ, Elicker BM, Maldonado F, et al. Usual interstitial pneumonia in rheumatoid arthritis-associated interstitial lung disease. Eur Respir J 2010;35(6): 1322–8.

89. Nurmi HM, Kettunen H-P, Suoranta S-K, et al. Several high-resolution computed tomography findings associate with survival and clinical features in rheumatoid arthritis-associated interstitial lung disease. Respir Med 2018;134:24–30.

90. Yamakawa H, Sato S, Tsumiyama E, et al. Predictive factors of mortality in rheumatoid arthritis-associated interstitial lung disease analysed by modified HRCT classification of idiopathic pulmonary fibrosis according to the 2018 ATS/ERS/JRS/ALAT criteria. J Thorac Dis 2019;11(12):5247–57.

91. Winstone TA, Assayag D, Wilcox PG, et al. Predictors of mortality and progression in scleroderma-associated interstitial lung disease: a systematic review. Chest 2014;146(2):422–36.

92. Hoffmann-Vold A-M, Aaløkken TM, Lund MB, et al. Predictive Value of Serial High-Resolution Computed Tomography Analyses and Concurrent Lung Function Tests in Systemic Sclerosis. Arthritis Rheumatol 2015;67(8):2205–12.

93. Kocheril SV, Appleton BE, Somers EC, et al. Comparison of disease progression and mortality of connective tissue disease-related interstitial lung disease and idiopathic interstitial pneumonia. Arthritis Rheum 2005;53(4):549–57.

94. Walsh SLF, Sverzellati N, Devaraj A, et al. Connective tissue disease related fibrotic lung disease: high resolution computed tomographic and pulmonary function indices as prognostic determinants. Thorax 2014;69(3):216–22.

95. Khanna D, Tseng C-H, Farmani N, et al. Clinical course of lung physiology in patients with scleroderma and interstitial lung disease: Analysis of the Scleroderma Lung Study Placebo Group. Arthritis Rheum 2011;63(10):3078–85.

96. Moore OA, Goh N, Corte T, et al. Extent of disease on high-resolution computed tomography lung is a predictor of decline and mortality in systemic sclerosis-related interstitial lung disease. Rheumatology 2013;52(1):155–60.

97. Goh NS, Desai SR, Veeraraghavan S, et al. Interstitial lung disease in systemic sclerosis: a simple staging system. Am J Respir Crit Care Med 2008;177(11): 1248–54.

98. Raghu G, Remy-Jardin M, Myers JL, et al. Diagnosis of Idiopathic Pulmonary Fibrosis. An Official ATS/ERS/JRS/ALAT Clinical Practice Guideline. Am J Respir Crit Care Med 2018;198(5):e44–68.

99. Desai SR, Veeraraghavan S, Hansell DM, et al. CT features of lung disease in patients with systemic sclerosis: comparison with idiopathic pulmonary fibrosis and nonspecific interstitial pneumonia. Radiology 2004;232(2):560–7.

100. Travis WD, Costabel U, Hansell DM, et al. An official American Thoracic Society/European Respiratory Society statement: Update of the international multidisciplinary classification of the idiopathic interstitial pneumonias. Am J Respir Crit Care Med 2013;188(6):733–48.

101. Bendstrup E, Moller J, Kronborg-White S, et al. Interstitial Lung Disease in Rheumatoid Arthritis Remains a Challenge for Clinicians. J Clin Med 2019;8(12). https://doi.org/10.3390/jcm8122038.

102. Tanaka N, Kim JS, Newell JD, et al. Rheumatoid arthritis-related lung diseases: CT findings. Radiology 2004;232(1):81–91.

103. Assayag D, Lubin M, Lee JS, et al. Predictors of mortality in rheumatoid arthritis-related interstitial lung disease. Respirology 2014;19(4):493–500.

104. Liu H, Xie S, Liang T, et al. Prognostic factors of interstitial lung disease progression at sequential HRCT in anti-synthetase syndrome. Eur Radiol 2019;29(10):5349–57.

105. Maillet T, Goletto T, Beltramo G, et al. Usual interstitial pneumonia in ANCA-associated vasculitis: A poor prognostic factor. J Autoimmun 2020;106:102338. https://doi.org/10.1016/j.jaut.2019.102338.

106. Kim HC, Lee JS, Lee EY, et al. Risk prediction model in rheumatoid arthritis-associated interstitial lung disease. Respirology 2020;25(12):1257–64.

107. Solomon JJ, Chung JH, Cosgrove GP, et al. Predictors of mortality in rheumatoid arthritis-associated interstitial lung disease. Eur Respir J 2016;47(2):588–96.

108. Pugashetti JV, Adegunsoye A, Wu Z, et al. Validation of Proposed Criteria for Progressive Pulmonary Fibrosis. Am J Respir Crit Care Med 2023;207(1):69–76.

109. Oldham JM, Lee CT, Wu Z, et al. Lung function trajectory in progressive fibrosing interstitial lung disease. Eur Respir J 2021. https://doi.org/10.1183/13993003.01396-2021.

110. Watadani T, Sakai F, Johkoh T, et al. Interobserver variability in the CT assessment of honeycombing in the lungs. Radiology 2013;266(3):936–44.

111. Nathan SD, Pastre J, Ksovreli I, et al. HRCT evaluation of patients with interstitial lung disease: comparison of the 2018 and 2011 diagnostic guidelines. Ther Adv Respir Dis 2020;14. 175346662096849.

112. Anthimopoulos M, Christodoulidis S, Ebner L, et al. Lung Pattern Classification for Interstitial Lung Diseases Using a Deep Convolutional Neural Network. IEEE Trans Med Imaging 2016;35(5):1207–16.

113. Kim GB, Jung K-H, Lee Y, et al. Comparison of Shallow and Deep Learning Methods on Classifying the Regional Pattern of Diffuse Lung Disease. J Digital Imaging 2018;31(4):415–24.

114. Walsh SLF, Calandriello L, Silva M, et al. Deep learning for classifying fibrotic lung disease on high-resolution computed tomography: a case-cohort study. Lancet Respir Med 2018;6(11):837–45.

115. Ash SY, Harmouche R, Vallejo DLL, et al. Densitometric and local histogram based analysis of computed tomography images in patients with idiopathic pulmonary fibrosis. Respir Res 2017;18(1). https://doi.org/10.1186/s12931-017-0527-8.

116. Best AC, Meng J, Lynch AM, et al. Idiopathic pulmonary fibrosis: physiologic tests, quantitative CT indexes, and CT visual scores as predictors of mortality. Radiology 2008;246(3):935–40.

117. Kim HJ, Brown MS, Chong D, et al. Comparison of the quantitative CT imaging biomarkers of idiopathic pulmonary fibrosis at baseline and early change with an interval of 7 months. Acad Radiol 2015;22(1):70–80.

118. Kim HG, Tashkin DP, Clements PJ, et al. A computer-aided diagnosis system for quantitative scoring of extent of lung fibrosis in scleroderma patients. Clin Exp Rheumatol 2010;28(5 Suppl 62):S26–35.

119. Oh JH, Kim GHJ, Cross G, et al. Automated quantification system predicts survival in rheumatoid arthritis-associated interstitial lung disease. Rheumatology (Oxford) 2022. https://doi.org/10.1093/rheumatology/keac184.

120. Martini K, Baessler B, Bogowicz M, et al. Applicability of radiomics in interstitial lung disease associated with systemic sclerosis: proof of concept. Eur Radiol 2021;31(4):1987–98.

121. Schniering J, Maciukiewicz M, Gabrys HS, et al. Computed tomography-based radiomics decodes prognostic and molecular differences in interstitial lung disease related to systemic sclerosis. Eur Respir J 2022;59(5):2004503.

122. Jacob J, Bartholmai BJ, Rajagopalan S, et al. Automated Quantitative Computed Tomography Versus Visual Computed Tomography Scoring in Idiopathic Pulmonary Fibrosis: Validation Against Pulmonary Function. J Thorac Imaging 2016;31(5):304–11.

123. Jacob J, Bartholmai BJ, Rajagopalan S, et al. Evaluation of computer-based computer tomography stratification against outcome models in connective tissue disease-related interstitial lung disease: a patient outcome study. BMC Med 2016-12-01 2016;14(1). https://doi.org/10.1186/s12916-016-0739-7.

124. Jacob J, Bartholmai BJ, Rajagopalan S, et al. Mortality prediction in idiopathic pulmonary fibrosis: evaluation of computer-based CT analysis with conventional severity measures. Eur Respir J 2017;49(1):1601011.

125. Jacob J, Bartholmai BJ, Rajagopalan S, et al. Predicting Outcomes in Idiopathic Pulmonary Fibrosis Using Automated Computed Tomographic Analysis. Am J Respir Crit Care Med 2018;198(6):767–76.

126. Chung JH, Adegunsoye A, Cannon B, et al. Differentiation of Idiopathic Pulmonary Fibrosis from Connective Tissue Disease-Related Interstitial Lung Disease Using Quantitative Imaging. J Clin Med 2021;10(12):2663.

127. Jacob J, Hirani N, Van Moorsel CHM, et al. Predicting outcomes in rheumatoid arthritis related interstitial lung disease. Eur Respir J 2019;53(1):1800869.

128. Wang T, Zheng XJ, Ji YL, et al. Tumour markers in rheumatoid arthritis-associated interstitial lung disease. Clin Exp Rheumatol 2016;34(4):587–91.

129. Prasse A, Pechkovsky DV, Toews GB, et al. CCL18 as an indicator of pulmonary fibrotic activity in idiopathic interstitial pneumonias and systemic sclerosis. Arthritis Rheum 2007;56(5):1685–93.

130. Kuryliszyn-Moskal A, Klimiuk PA, Sierakowski S. Soluble adhesion molecules (sVCAM-1, sE-selectin), vascular endothelial growth factor (VEGF) and endothelin-1 in patients with systemic sclerosis: relationship to organ systemic involvement. Clin Rheumatol 2005;24(2):111–6.

131. Ihn H, Sato S, Fujimoto M, et al. Increased serum levels of soluble vascular cell adhesion molecule-1 and E-selectin in patients with systemic sclerosis. Br J Rheumatol 1998;37(11):1188–92.

132. Ates A, Kinikli G, Turgay M, et al. Serum-Soluble Selectin Levels in Patients with Rheumatoid Arthritis and Systemic Sclerosis. Scand J Immunol 2004;59(3):315–20.

133. Kumanovics G, Minier T, Radics J, et al. Comprehensive investigation of novel serum markers of pulmonary fibrosis associated with systemic sclerosis and dermato/polymyositis. Clin Exp Rheumatol 2008;26(3):414–20.

134. Hasegawa M, Asano Y, Endo H, et al. Serum Adhesion Molecule Levels as Prognostic Markers in Patients with Early Systemic Sclerosis: A Multicentre, Prospective, Observational Study. PLoS ONE 2014;9(2):e88150.

135. Kodera M, Hasegawa M, Komura K, et al. Serum pulmonary and activation-regulated chemokine/CCL18 levels in patients with systemic sclerosis: A sensitive indicator of active pulmonary fibrosis. Arthritis Rheum 2005;52(9):2889–96.

136. Elhai M, Hoffmann-Vold AM, Avouac J, et al. Performance of Candidate Serum Biomarkers for Systemic Sclerosis–Associated Interstitial Lung Disease. Arthritis Rheumatol 2019;71(6):972–82.

137. Moon J, Lee JS, Yoon YI, et al. Association of Serum Biomarkers With Pulmonary Involvement of Rheumatoid Arthritis Interstitial Lung Disease: From KORAIL Cohort Baseline Data. J Rheum Dis 2021;28(4):234–41.

138. Bandoh S. Sequential changes of KL-6 in sera of patients with interstitial pneumonia associated with polymyositis/dermatomyositis. Ann Rheum Dis 2000; 59(4):257–62.

139. Kubo M, Ihn H, Yamane K, et al. Serum KL-6 in adult patients with polymyositis and dermatomyositis. Rheumatology 2000;39(6):632–6.

140. Wang Y, Chen S, Lin J, et al. Lung ultrasound B-lines and serum KL-6 correlate with the severity of idiopathic inflammatory myositis-associated interstitial lung disease. Rheumatology 2020;59(8):2024–9.

141. Chiu Y-H, Chu C-C, Lu C-C, et al. KL-6 as a Biomarker of Interstitial Lung Disease Development in Patients with Sjögren Syndrome: A Retrospective Case–Control Study. J Inflamm Res 2022;15:2255–62.

142. Oda K, Kotani T, Takeuchi T, et al. Chemokine profiles of interstitial pneumonia in patients with dermatomyositis: a case control study. Scientific Rep 2017;7(1). https://doi.org/10.1038/s41598-017-01685-5.

143. Hoffmann-Vold A-M, Weigt SS, Palchevskiy V, et al. Augmented concentrations of CX3CL1 are associated with interstitial lung disease in systemic sclerosis. PLOS ONE 2018;13(11):e0206545.

144. Tiev KP, Chatenoud L, Kettaneh A, et al. [Increase of CXCL10 serum level in systemic sclerosis interstitial pneumonia]. Rev Med Interne 2009;30(11):942–6. Augmentation de CXCL10 dans le serum au cours de la pneumopathie interstitielle de la sclerodermie systemique.

145. Antonelli A, Ferri C, Fallahi P, et al. CXCL10 (alpha) and CCL2 (beta) chemokines in systemic sclerosis–a longitudinal study. Rheumatology (Oxford) 2008; 47(1):45–9.

146. Chen J, Doyle TJ, Liu Y, et al. Biomarkers of Rheumatoid Arthritis-Associated Interstitial Lung Disease. Arthritis Rheumatol 2015;67(1):28–38.

147. Gono T, Kaneko H, Kawaguchi Y, et al. Cytokine profiles in polymyositis and dermatomyositis complicated by rapidly progressive or chronic interstitial lung disease. Rheumatology (Oxford) 2014;53(12):2196–203.

148. Kameda M, Otsuka M, Chiba H, et al. CXCL9, CXCL10, and CXCL11; biomarkers of pulmonary inflammation associated with autoimmunity in patients with collagen vascular diseases–associated interstitial lung disease and interstitial pneumonia with autoimmune features. PLOS ONE 2020;15(11):e0241719.

149. Nishikawa A, Suzuki K, Kassai Y, et al. Identification of definitive serum biomarkers associated with disease activity in primary Sjögren's syndrome. Arthritis Res Ther 2016;18(1). https://doi.org/10.1186/s13075-016-1006-1.

150. Cossu M, Andracco R, Santaniello A, et al. Serum levels of vascular dysfunction markers reflect disease severity and stage in systemic sclerosis patients. Rheumatology (Oxford) 2016;55(6):1112–6.

151. Van Bon L, Affandi AJ, Broen J, et al. Proteome-wide Analysis and CXCL4 as a Biomarker in Systemic Sclerosis. New Engl J Med 2014;370(5):433–43.

152. Khadilkar PV, Khopkar US, Nadkar MY, et al. Fibrotic Cytokine Interplay in Evaluation of Disease Activity in Treatment Naive Systemic Sclerosis Patients from Western India. J Assoc Physicians India 2019;67(8):26–30.

153. Abdel-Magied RA, Kamel SR, Said AF, et al. Serum interleukin-6 in systemic sclerosis and its correlation with disease parameters and cardiopulmonary involvement. Sarcoidosis Vasc Diffuse Lung Dis 2016;33(4):321–30.

154. Olewicz-Gawlik A, Danczak-Pazdrowska A, Kuznar-Kaminska B, et al. Interleukin-17 and interleukin-23: importance in the pathogenesis of lung impairment in patients with systemic sclerosis. Int J Rheum Dis 2014;17(6):664–70.

155. Yanaba K, Yoshizaki A, Asano Y, et al. Serum IL-33 levels are raised in patients with systemic sclerosis: association with extent of skin sclerosis and severity of pulmonary fibrosis. Clin Rheumatol 2011;30(6):825–30.

156. Tang J, Lei L, Pan J, et al. Higher levels of serum interleukin-35 are associated with the severity of pulmonary fibrosis and Th2 responses in patients with systemic sclerosis. Rheumatol Int 2018;38(8):1511–9.

157. Moinzadeh P, Krieg T, Hellmich M, et al. Elevated MMP-7 levels in patients with systemic sclerosis: correlation with pulmonary involvement. Exp Dermatol 2011; 20(9):770–3.

158. Matson SM, Lee SJ, Peterson RA, et al. The prognostic role of matrix metalloproteinase-7 in scleroderma-associated interstitial lung disease. Eur Respir J 2021;58(6):2101560.

159. Nakatsuka Y, Handa T, Nakashima R, et al. Serum matrix metalloproteinase levels in polymyositis/dermatomyositis patients with interstitial lung disease. Rheumatology 2019;58(8):1465–73.

160. Manetti M, Guiducci S, Romano E, et al. Increased serum levels and tissue expression of matrix metalloproteinase-12 in patients with systemic sclerosis: correlation with severity of skin and pulmonary fibrosis and vascular damage. Ann Rheum Dis 2012;71(6):1064–72.

161. Kikuchi K, Kubo M, Sato S, et al. Serum tissue inhibitor of metalloproteinases in patients with systemic sclerosis. J Am Acad Dermatol 1995;33(6):973–8.

162. Ren J, Sun L, Sun X, et al. Diagnostic value of serum connective tissue growth factor in rheumatoid arthritis. Clin Rheumatol 2021;40(6):2203–9.

163. Sato S, Nagaoka T, Hasegawa M, et al. Serum levels of connective tissue growth factor are elevated in patients with systemic sclerosis: association with extent of skin sclerosis and severity of pulmonary fibrosis. J Rheumatol 2000;27(1): 149–54.

164. Lambrecht S, Smith V, De Wilde K, et al. Growth differentiation factor 15, a marker of lung involvement in systemic sclerosis, is involved in fibrosis development but is not indispensable for fibrosis development. Arthritis Rheumatol 2014;66(2):418–27.

165. Gamal SM, Elgengehy FT, Kamal A, et al. Growth Differentiation Factor-15 (GDF-15) Level and Relation to Clinical Manifestations in Egyptian Systemic Sclerosis patients: Preliminary Data. Immunol Invest 2017;46(7):703–13.

166. Yanaba K, Asano Y, Tada Y, et al. Clinical significance of serum growth differentiation factor-15 levels in systemic sclerosis: association with disease severity. Mod Rheumatol 2012;22(5):668–75.

167. Nordenbæk C, Johansen JS, Halberg P, et al. High serum levels of YKL-40 in patients with systemic sclerosis are associated with pulmonary involvement. Scand J Rheumatol 2005;34(4):293–7.

168. Alqalyoobi S, Adegunsoye A, Linderholm A, et al. Circulating Plasma Biomarkers of Progressive Interstitial Lung Disease. Am J Respir Crit Care Med 2020;201(2):250–3.

169. Rivière S, Hua-Huy T, Tiev KP, et al. High Baseline Serum Clara Cell 16 kDa Predicts Subsequent Lung Disease Worsening in Systemic Sclerosis. The J Rheumatol 2018;45(2):242–7.

170. Volkmann ER, Tashkin DP, Kuwana M, et al. Progression of Interstitial Lung Disease in Systemic Sclerosis: The Importance of Pneumoproteins Krebs von den Lungen 6 and CCL18. Arthritis Rheumatol 2019;71(12):2059–67.

171. Guiot J, Njock M-S, André B, et al. Serum IGFBP-2 in systemic sclerosis as a prognostic factor of lung dysfunction. Scientific Rep 2021;11(1). https://doi.org/10.1038/s41598-021-90333-0.

172. Kuwana M, Shirai Y, Takeuchi T. Elevated Serum Krebs von den Lungen-6 in Early Disease Predicts Subsequent Deterioration of Pulmonary Function in Patients with Systemic Sclerosis and Interstitial Lung Disease. The J Rheumatol 2016;43(10):1825–31.

173. Kennedy B, Branagan P, Moloney F, et al. Biomarkers to identify ILD and predict lung function decline in scleroderma lung disease or idiopathic pulmonary fibrosis. Sarcoidosis Vasc Diffuse Lung Dis 2015;32(3):228–36.

174. Wu M, Baron M, Pedroza C, et al. CCL2 in the Circulation Predicts Long-Term Progression of Interstitial Lung Disease in Patients With Early Systemic Sclerosis: Data From Two Independent Cohorts. Arthritis Rheumatol 2017;69(9):1871–8.

175. Volkmann ER, Tashkin DP, Roth MD, et al. Changes in plasma CXCL4 levels are associated with improvements in lung function in patients receiving immunosuppressive therapy for systemic sclerosis-related interstitial lung disease. Arthritis Res Ther 2016;18(1). https://doi.org/10.1186/s13075-016-1203-y.

176. De Lauretis A, Sestini P, Pantelidis P, et al. Serum interleukin 6 is predictive of early functional decline and mortality in interstitial lung disease associated with systemic sclerosis. J Rheumatol 2013;40(4):435–46.

177. Nara M, Komatsuda A, Omokawa A, et al. Serum interleukin 6 levels as a useful prognostic predictor of clinically amyopathic dermatomyositis with rapidly progressive interstitial lung disease. Mod Rheumatol 2014;24(4):633–6.

178. Lee JH, Jang JH, Park JH, et al. The role of interleukin-6 as a prognostic biomarker for predicting acute exacerbation in interstitial lung diseases. PLOS ONE 2021;16(7):e0255365.

179. Takada T, Ohashi K, Hayashi M, et al. Role of IL-15 in interstitial lung diseases in amyopathic dermatomyositis with anti-MDA-5 antibody. Respir Med 2018;141:7–13.

180. Shimizu T, Koga T, Furukawa K, et al. IL-15 is a biomarker involved in the development of rapidly progressive interstitial lung disease complicated with polymyositis/dermatomyositis. J Intern Med 2021;289(2):206–20.

181. Peng Q-L, Zhang Y-M, Liang L, et al. A high level of serum neopterin is associated with rapidly progressive interstitial lung disease and reduced survival in dermatomyositis. Clin Exp Immunol 2020;199(3):314–25.

182. Hozumi H, Fujisawa T, Enomoto N, et al. Clinical Utility of YKL-40 in Polymyositis/dermatomyositis-associated Interstitial Lung Disease. The J Rheumatol 2017;44(9):1394–401.

183. Jiang L, Wang Y, Peng Q, et al. Serum YKL-40 level is associated with severity of interstitial lung disease and poor prognosis in dermatomyositis with anti-MDA5 antibody. Clin Rheumatol 2019;38(6):1655–63.

Moving?

Make sure your subscription moves with you!

To notify us of your new address, find your **Clinics Account Number** (located on your mailing label above your name), and contact customer service at:

Email: journalscustomerservice-usa@elsevier.com

800-654-2452 (subscribers in the U.S. & Canada)
314-447-8871 (subscribers outside of the U.S. & Canada)

Fax number: 314-447-8029

Elsevier Health Sciences Division
Subscription Customer Service
3251 Riverport Lane
Maryland Heights, MO 63043

*To ensure uninterrupted delivery of your subscription, please notify us at least 4 weeks in advance of move.

ELSEVIER

Printed and bound by CPI Group (UK) Ltd, Croydon, CR0 4YY

03/10/2024

01040468-0012